ANAESTHESIA AND PHARMACOLOGY

BOERHAAVE SERIES
FOR POSTGRADUATE
MEDICAL EDUCATION
Nr. 12

PROCEEDINGS OF BOERHAAVE COURSES
ORGANIZED BY
THE FACULTY OF MEDICINE, UNIVERSITY OF LEIDEN
THE NETHERLANDS

ANAESTHESIA AND PHARMACOLOGY

WITH A SPECIAL SECTION ON PROFESSIONAL HAZARDS

EDITED BY

JOH. SPIERDIJK, M.D., S.A. FELDMAN, M.D., AND
H. MATTIE, M.D.

1976
LEIDEN UNIVERSITY PRESS

DISTRIBUTED IN THE UNITED STATES BY
THE WILLIAMS & WILKINS COMPANY/BALTIMORE

ISBN-13:978-94-010-1560-8   e-ISBN-13:978-94-010-1558-5
DOI: 10.1007/978-94-010-1558-5

Cover design: E. Wijnans

© 1976 Leiden University Press, P.O,B. 269, the Hague, the Netherlands
Softcover reprint of the hardcover 1st edition 1976

PREFACE

Every specialist, at present, is confronted with the fact that it is continually becoming more difficult to remain 'up to date'. The areas in which he must read are expanding while the individual publications are becoming greater in number, larger in content and appear more frequently.

The choice of the subject was not easy. This time we have selected the pharmacological aspects of anaesthesiology as our main topic, as a continuation of the Boerhaave course in 1971. Although we know that a drug works, the mechanism behind this action is of great importance. The pharmacokinetics and side effects of the drugs we administer affect not only our patients, but also ourselves, our children, and the personnel under our care. In a special section we draw attention to this subject.

We fervently hope that this symposium will further enrich your knowledge of anaesthesia and that through this enrichment you will derive more pleasure from the profession you have chosen and that in the end this will lead to even better care and treatment of the patients entrusted to us.

We wish to express our thanks to Prof. C. M. Conway, Dr. D. T. Popescu, and Prof. D. M. E. Vermeulen-Cranch for their assistance in the editing of some of the chapters in this book.

Joh. Spierdijk
Dept. of Anaesthesiology,
University Hospital Leiden

S. A. Feldman
Dept. of Anaesthetics,
Westminster Hospital London

H. Mattie
Dept. of Clinical Farmacology,
University Hospital Leiden

CONTENTS

CONTRIBUTORS

S. AGOSTON, Institute of Clinical Pharmacology, State University of Groningen, Groningen, The Netherlands.

P. A. BOSSERS, Research Institute for Environmental Hygiene, TNO, Delft, The Netherlands.

T. BURM, Department of Anaesthesiology, University Hospital, Leiden, The Netherlands.

C. M. CONWAY, Magill Department of Anaesthetics, Westminster Medical School, London, United Kingdom.

J. F. CRUL, Institute of Anaesthesiology, University of Nijmegen, Nijmegen, The Netherlands.

S. A. FELDMAN, Department of Anaesthesiology, Westminster Medical School, London, United Kingdom.

F. F. FOLDES, Montefiore Hospital and Medical Center, Bronx, New York, U.S.A.

R. FREY, Institute of Anaesthesiology, Johannes Gutenberg University, Mainz, W.-Germany.

W. K. HAMILTON, Department of Anaesthesiology, University of California, San Francisco, U.S.A.

E. HERRMANN, Institute of Anaesthesiology, Johannes Gutenberg University, Mainz, W.-Germany.

U. W. KERSTEN, Institute of Anaesthesiology, University Hospital, Groningen, The Netherlands.

Z. D. LAZAREVIC, Department of Anaesthesiology, University Hospital, Leiden, The Netherlands.

H. MATTIE, Department of Clinical Pharmacology, University Hospital, Leiden, The Netherlands.

E. L. NOACH, Department of Pharmacology, University Hospital, Leiden, The Netherlands.

D. T. POPESCU, Department of Anaesthesiology, University Hospital, Leiden, The Netherlands.

V. REJGER, Department of Anaesthesiology, University Hospital, Leiden, The Netherlands.

R. S. RENEMAN, Department of Physiology, Faculty of Medicine, Maastricht, The Netherlands.

G. ROLLY, Department of Anaesthesiology, University Hospital, Gent, Belgium.

J. J. SCHWARZ, Bureau of Risk Analysis, TNO, Delft, The Netherlands.

S. E. SMITH, Reader in Pharmacology, St. Thomas Medical School, London, United Kingdom.

W. SOUDIJN, Laboratory of Pharmacological Chemistry, Amsterdam, The Netherlands.

JOH. SPIERDIJK, Department of Anaesthesiology, University Hospital, Leiden, The Netherlands.

L. STAMENKOVIĆ, Department of Anaesthesiology, University Hospital, Leiden, The Netherlands.

E. G. STAR, Department of Anaesthesiology, Johannes Gutenberg University, Mainz, W.-Germany.

L. STRUNIN, Anaesthetic Department, King's College Hospital, London, United Kingdom.

I. R. VERNER, Department of Anaesthesia, The Middlesex Hospital, London, United Kingdom.

CH. WHITCHER, Stanford University Medical Center, Stanford, California, U.S.A.

PART ONE

VOLATILE ANAESTHETICS

1. MECHANISM OF ACTION OF VOLATILE ANAESTHETICS. A REVIEW OF THEORIES OF ANAESTHESIA COMPILED BY A CLINICAL ANAESTHETIST

CHARLES WHITCHER

Much of the material presented in our textbooks on the theories of anaesthesia has been based largely on speculation with very little background in experimental work. At the present time much remains to be learned but extensive experimental work is being done, and much is being learned about anaesthetic action.

A recent text edited by Edmund Eger entitled 'Anesthetic Uptake and Action' (1) includes a chapter called 'Mechanisms of General Anesthesia' written by M. J. Halsey. Many of us would recognize Dr. Halsey as an outstanding researcher in mechanisms of anaesthesia. Halsey begins his chapter:

'An amazing array of inhaled agents produce general anesthesia in all animals. These include potent vapors such as methoxyflurane and halothane and also relatively impotent gases such as nitrogen and hydrogen. Theories of general anesthesia must explain how such diverse compounds can produce the same overall effect.'*

Dr. Halsey proceeds by pointing out that no 'structure-activity' relationship explains the effect of the inhaled agents. In other words, they possess no common structure which is associated with their biological activity. Furthermore, he indicates that anaesthesia alters the function of almost all systems of the body at both a tissue and cellular level, and that these effects may relate to a primary process or may be side effects.

We will first consider where inhalation anaesthetics may act. The site of action can be considered at three different levels including the gross macroscopic level, the cellular level, and the molecular level. At the gross anatomical level, anaesthetics may act at one or more different areas in the central nervous system. The most probable site is the reticular formation of the midbrain with its high concentration of synaptic connections, which are presumably susceptible to altered function due to anaesthesia. A slight

---

* Reprinted with permission from *Anesthetic Uptake and Action*, Edmond I. Eger, II, M.D. Chapter 3, Mechanisms of General Anesthesia, M. J. Halsey, p. 45. The Williams and Wilkins Co., Baltimore, Maryland, 1974. Copyright 1974, Edmond I. Eger, II, M.D.

depression in the function of one neuron, in a series of neurons all slightly depressed, could markedly alter the transmission of impulses over a wide area in the midbrain.

There is no doubt that consciousness depends on excitation in the reticular formation; with inhibition of this area, sleep and anaesthesia result.

Another possible site of anaesthetic action in the brain is the cerebral cortex, where changes in electrical activity due to anaesthesia are readily

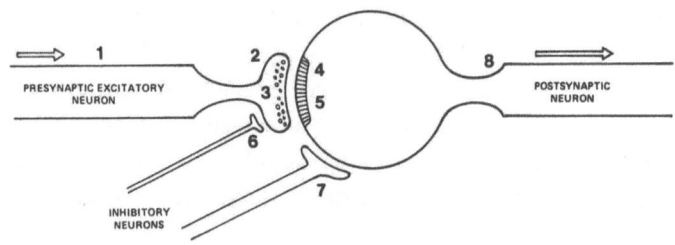

Fig. 1.* Possible sites of anaesthetic action in nerve cells. Arrows indicate the direction of impulse traffic. 1. Conduction of the action potential. All anaesthetic agents block conduction, but at higher concentrations than those at which they block synaptic transmission. 2. Ca^{++}-dependent depolarization-secretion coupling; and 3, subsequent Ca^{++}-independent steps in transmitter release. Several agents (barbiturates and alcohols) decrease the amount of acetylcholine released from presynaptic terminals in sympathetic ganglia. At the neuromuscular junction these agents increase Ca^{++}-independent spontaneous transmitter release. Therefore, 2, Ca^{++}-dependent depolarization-secretion coupling is the probable site of anaesthetic inhibition of transmitter release. 4. Transmitter-receptor interaction. Volatile agents and barbiturates depress the postsynaptic response at the neuromuscular junction and in the central nervous system. The diversity of anaesthetic molecular structures makes a direct action of anaesthetics on the receptor unlikely; however a secondary effect on receptor proteins through derangement of their lipid environment is possible. 5. Electrogenesis in the subsynaptic membrane. There is as yet little evidence about anaesthetic alterations in subsynaptic membrane function. 6 and 7, pre- and post-synaptic inhibition, may be selectively enhanced by barbiturates which may thus indirectly depress excitability. 8. Initiation of the impulse in the postsynaptic neuron. Ether and barbiturates increase the threshold level of depolarization necessary for impulse generation in spinal cord neurons.

seen in the electroencephalogram. Relationship between these changes in electrical activity and anaesthesia and relative importance of reticular formation versus cortex, are not yet clear.

Inhalation anaesthetics may directly inhibit the transmission of impulses in the spinal cord; this is mentioned only for completeness and will not be further explored.

Effects on peripheral nerves are generally thought to be relatively unimportant in inhalation anaesthesia.

A consideration of anaesthetic action at the cellular level will include a brief review of selected aspects of the anatomy of the nerve and the physiology of nerve transmission. A diagram of selected parts of two nerve cells is presented in figure 1. Sensations such as heat, cold, and pain are first sensed or transduced at the peripheral sensory endings. This sensation, whichever it is, is converted into an electrical impulse called an action potential which travels along the axon on its way to a synapse. The propagation of the action potential has been extensively studied. We summarize by saying that with the passage of such a potential there is a transient increase in the permeability of the axon cell membrane to various ions, particularly sodium ions.

The action potential, once initiated, readily passes along the axon but does not directly and immediately traverse the synapse. At this juncture, the release of a chemical transmitter substance occurs, usually acetylcholine or norepinephrine, which subsequently diffuses across the synaptic cleft and acts on the subsynaptic membrane.

Possible levels of anaesthetic action can be considered in this figure. Transduction at the sensory ending could be blocked so that sensations fail to initiate an action potential. As an alternative, anaesthesia could block conduction along the course of the axon. Transmission at the synapse could be affected; or inhibitory neurons could impair transmission by inhibiting either at pre- or postsynaptic sites.

In the event that an action potential courses along an axon to a synapse, a new action potential in the adjacent axon may or may not result depending on the local conditions. For example, inhibitory impulses, acting either at the pre- or postsynaptic membrane, may cause failure of the initiation of a new action potential distal to the synapse. Drugs may reduce the amount of acetylcholine released. Volatile anaesthetics may depress the postsynaptic response. The susceptibility of the postsynaptic neuron to stimulation may be depressed.

In the event that the action potential is finally transmitted to the central nervous system, interpretation and possibly a reaction may take place, such as a muscular contraction or a glandular secretion.

It is thought that blockade along the axon may be a primary site of anaesthetic action. At first glance axon blockade would appear to be an unlikely important site because the concentration required in the peripheral axons, which are generally available for study, is greater than the amount needed for general anaesthesia. The theory of axonal blockade is saved because there is evidence that those axons buried deep in the central nervous system, to which access for study is extremely difficult, may be much more susceptible to blockade with their smaller diameter. At least for local anaesthetics, concentrations which block conduction are inversely related to fiber diameter. It is further suggested that axonal membranes may be specialized; if so, some membranes may be inherently more sensitive to anaesthetics than others. A significant bit of evidence in support of conduction block in the axon is that this blockade can be reversed by pressure (2). Such pressure reversal has not been demonstrated at the synapse.

Pressure reversal is a phenomenon which many clinicians are beginning to be aware of. It has become an important criterion in evaluating theories of anaesthetic action. This phenomenon was first reported by Johnson and Flagler in 1950 (3). These workers showed that with an increase in hydrostatic pressure, anaesthetic requirement is increased. For example, anaesthesia lowers the luminescence of certain bacteria, and luminescence of these

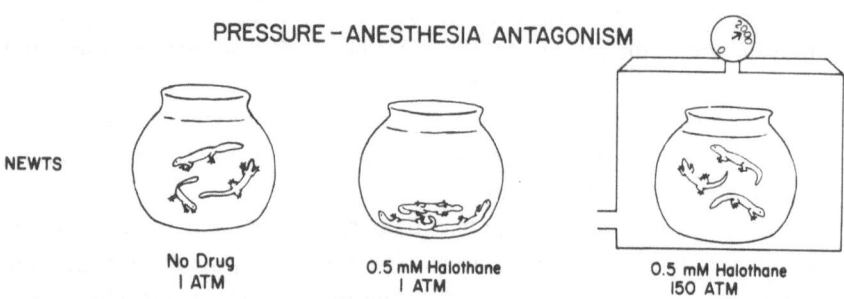

Fig. 2.* Pressure-anaesthesia antagonism. Newts swimming about (left) are anaesthetized with halothane (center). Upon increasing the environmental pressure, activity is restored (right).

* Courtesy of Joan J. Kendig, Ph.D., Assistant Professor of Biology and Anesthesia, Stanford, California.

anaesthetized bacteria is restored at increased pressure. Pressure reversal also occurs in the newt. Figure 2 shows this species immobilized by ethyl alcohol (center panel) and revived and swimming (right panel) when the anaesthetized newt is subjected to increased environmental pressure. Pressure reversal also occurs in higher animals such as mice.

It is widely held that anaesthesia could result from altered synaptic transmission. On the one hand, synaptically-mediated responses in the cord are blocked by low concentrations of anaesthetics in the range of 1 MAC. On the other hand, pressure reversal at the synapse has not been demonstrated, whereas pressure reversal does occur at the axon (4).

To summarize to this point: Each group of researchers in their efforts to pinpoint a primary site of anaesthetic action is apt to find some good reason to champion some particular cellular or gross anatomical site. It is possible that all such sites may be effected by anaesthesia. If indeed one such site should be primary and more important than another, then this distinction is not yet clear.

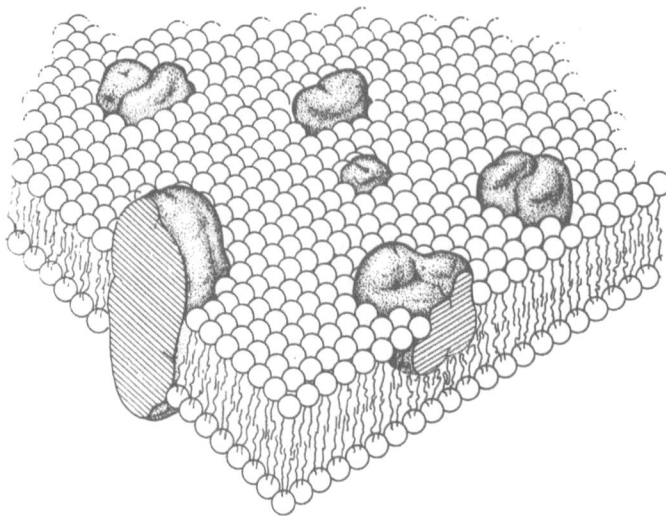

Fig. 3.* Fluid Mosaic model. Shows basic types of protein molecules. Some may partially penetrate the outside of the cell membrane or penetrate all the way through. The latter possibly function as sodium pores.

* Reproduced with permission from Singer, S. J. and Nicholson, G. L., The Fluid Mosaic Model of Structure of Cell Membranes. *Science*, Volume 175, pp. 720-731, Fig., 18 February 1972. Copyright 1972 by the American Association for the Advancement of Science.

We now proceed to consider the molecular basis of anaesthesia which is intimately involved in the structure and function of the nerve cell membrane, diagrammatically represented in figure 3. The inner and outer walls are composed of phospholipids arranged as a bilayer. In the figure it can be assumed that the extracellular fluid bathes the upper layer of the cell membrane and the intracellular fluid is in contact with the lower layer. The membrane itself, which separates these fluid compartments consists of molecular head groups composed of hydrophilic material. These head groups are attached to tails consisting of hydrophobic fatty acids. The hydrophobic inner layers form an efficient barrier to the passage of ions between the extracellular fluid and the intracellular compartments. Inside the nerve cell the concentrations of sodium and chloride are low, and potassium is present in high concentrations. Outside the cell membrane the opposite prevails and the sodium and chloride are high while potassium is low.

This ionic difference is maintained via the sodium pump mechanism which actively extrudes sodium. This active extrusion maintains a difference in potential across the membrane with the intracellular voltage more negative with respect to the extracellular fluid by 70 mv. The action potential causes a momentary reversal of this difference. The pathway through which the sodium ion travels is conceived of as the instantaneous opening of a 'pore' in the membrane. No one has actually seen this pore but its existence is widely accepted.

Anaesthetic action has been explained on the basis of altered properties of this phospholipid bilayer. One group believes that the inhalation anaesthetics alter the phospholipid so that the protein fails to function normally.

The molecular basis of anaesthesia is conveniently studied in model systems. The earliest model system was olive oil, introduced by Meyer (5) and Overton (6) at the turn of the century. It was observed that anaesthetic potency correlated very well with oil/water partition coefficients. Meyer and Overton studied the available anaesthetics, such as ether, chloroform, and nitrous oxide. More recently, Eger and Miller (7) have extended the correlation to include such substances as xenon, nitrogen, and fluorosulphur compounds, relating the oil/gas partition coefficient to MAC. Figure 4 emphasizes this correlation. For the moment attention is called to the right-hand curve in which MAC is expressed as the partial pressure in atmospheres as plotted against the oil/gas partition coefficient. The slope of the curve fits the relation.

MAC × oil/gas partition coefficient equals 2.1

A remarkably linear relationship is shown with close clustering all the way from the most potent anaesthetic, methoxyflurane, through the less potent and less lipid soluble nitrous oxide, and finally to carbon tetrafluoride. A similar effort to relate these agents to the hydrate dissociation pressure (which is another model system) shows a poorer correlation. Despite this phenomenon, Eger has said that the correlation is not bad enough to throw out the hydrate theory of Pauling (8) and Miller (9) on that basis alone.

Recently, models have been prepared which are more like naturally occurring nerves than is olive oil. For example, Seeman (10) has shown that erythrocyte cell membranes are useful in studying anaesthetic action. This preparation is made by haemolizing red cells and washing them, leaving

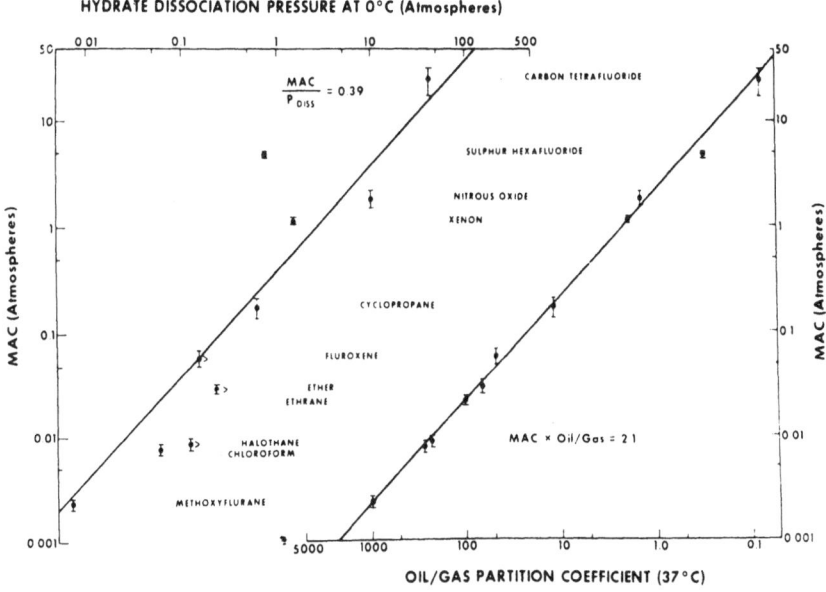

*Fig. 4.** These graphs permit a visual comparison of the correlation of MAC with hydrate dissociation pressure (left graph, upper scale) and lipid solubility (right graph, lower scale). If the data followed the correlation: MAC/hydrate dissociation pressure equals a constant or MAC x oil/gas partition coefficient equals a constant, then the data should lie along the 45°-angle slopes as indicated (Eger, Lundgren, Miller and Stevens, 1969).

* Figure and legend reproduced with permission from *Scientific Foundations of Anaesthesia.* Edited by Cyril Scurr and Stanley Feldman. Chapter 2, Section II, Approaches to a Theory of Anaesthetic Action, J. J. Kendig and J. R. Trudell, p. 281. William Heinemann Medical Books, Ltd., 1974. Copyright 1974, William Heinemann Medical Books, Ltd., 1974.

only the cell membranes. These are called erythrocyte ghosts which consist of a closed sphere of natural protein-containing lipid membrane. With such ghost preparations, as well as intact red cells, the addition of an anaesthetic increases the resistance to cell rupture on exposure to hypotonic solutions. The cell wall thins and increases in area. A corresponding increase in bilayer fluidity in response to anaesthetic exposure has been demonstrated in synthetic membranes as well as other natural membranes.

Another model of the bilayer has been developed to further the study of membranes which can be diagrammatically represented as shown in figure 3. In the context of the present discussion this is called the phospholipid bilayer vesicle preparation (11). Such bilayers are prepared by suspending the desired phospholipid in water and sonicating the solution. The ultrasonic energy allows the phospholipids to reassemble in their normal minimum configuration. Again, this is a double layer sphere with phosphate head groups exposed to water on the inside and the outside of the sphere's shell. The phospholipid hydrocarbon chains meet at the center of the sphere wall, forming a hydrophobic central region. The synthetic phospholipid bilayer preparation offers the researcher control over the physical and chemical characteristics of the bilayer. It is possible to synthesize phospholipids with precisely known hydrocarbon chain lengths and unsaturation. This allows the formation of bilayers of various thicknesses and internal fluidity. By appropriate selection of a head group, the bilayer may be given a surface charge or dipole.

Phospholipid vesicle bilayer preparations are being studied by modern spectroscopic methods. Among these is the electron spin resonance technique (12). A detailed understanding of this technique requires a background in quantum mechanics, not possessed by the writer. It can be said that the electron spin resonance technique provides evidence of the arrangement and motion of the lipid structures. Applying this technique to the study of the phospholipid bilayer preparations, it has been shown that both halothane and methoxyflurane cause an increase in molecular motion. The essence of this phenomenon is an increase in membrane fluidity. This is concentration dependent and occurs at clinically useful concentrations.

Electron spin resonance technique has been applied to further test whether the lipid regions of bilayers are the primary site of anaesthetic action. It has been shown that the disorder induced in the membrane by halothane in spin-labelled phospholipid vesicles is reversed at increased pressures of helium (13). This observation suggests that the phospholipid vesicle is a good model for studying anaesthetic action. Moreover, the close agreement of this phenomenon produced in a pure lipid to that produced in intact animal systems gives weight to the theory that anaesthesia first occurs in the lipid phase. Furthermore, it suggests that pressure reversal occurs in the lipid rather than in the protein regions of the nerve membrane. These results, that inhalation anaesthetics increase the fluidity of the nerve membrane bilayer, is consistent with the anaesthetic-induced increase in membrane surface areas seen in the red cell ghost preparations of Seeman and increased bilayer mobility shown by Metcalfe (14). It is proposed that the application of high pressures decreases the surface area, forcing the chains together, thus decreasing their motion, and providing an explanation of pressure reversal. The small anaesthesia molecule which induces this disorder is not excluded from the membrane. Instead, the hydrocarbon chains are reordered around the anaesthetic molecule.

Electron spin resonance studies of molecular motion in membranes indicate that a three-dimensional view of the motion of the tails of the phospholipid would show a conical motion with the skirt of the cone projecting toward the center of the membrane. The excursion and rate of this motion increases with increasing anaesthetic concentration. This theory can be summarized as the indirect interference with the function of the protein caused by increased motion in adjacent molecular tails.

An alternative theory is the direct interference with the protein. Here the anaesthetic attached to a protein essential to nerve action, directly interfering with its capability to function. It is, of course, possible that both processes are in operation.

Some of the concepts already mentioned are illustrated in figure 5, especially pressure reversal, oil/water solubility, and anaesthesia via inert gases. In this figure, the partial pressure of N_2O necessary to abolish the righting reflex in mice is plotted against increasing partial pressures of the rare gases shown. As the helium pressure increases, so the N_2O requirement increases for abolition of the righting reflex. This indicates antagonism of pressure to the anaesthetic effect of helium. With neon, the effect of pressure is not immediately apparent and a straight line is seen. For hydrogen, the curve is negatively sloped. The explanation is that although these three gases all produce an increasing N_2O requirement under pressure, they also exert an anaesthetic effect. For helium, the least potent and least soluble agent, pressure reversal occurs before its anaesthetic effect is manifested, and so the slope is positive. For neon, which is more soluble and more potent, the two effects cancel, resulting in a straight line. The most soluble of the three

CH. WHITCHER

gases, hydrogen, shows its predominantly anaesthetic effect as a negative slope and its pressure reversal is partially obscured.

A recent theory states that intact nerve function is dependent upon a balance of optimal polarity and viscosity of the membrane bilayer (15).

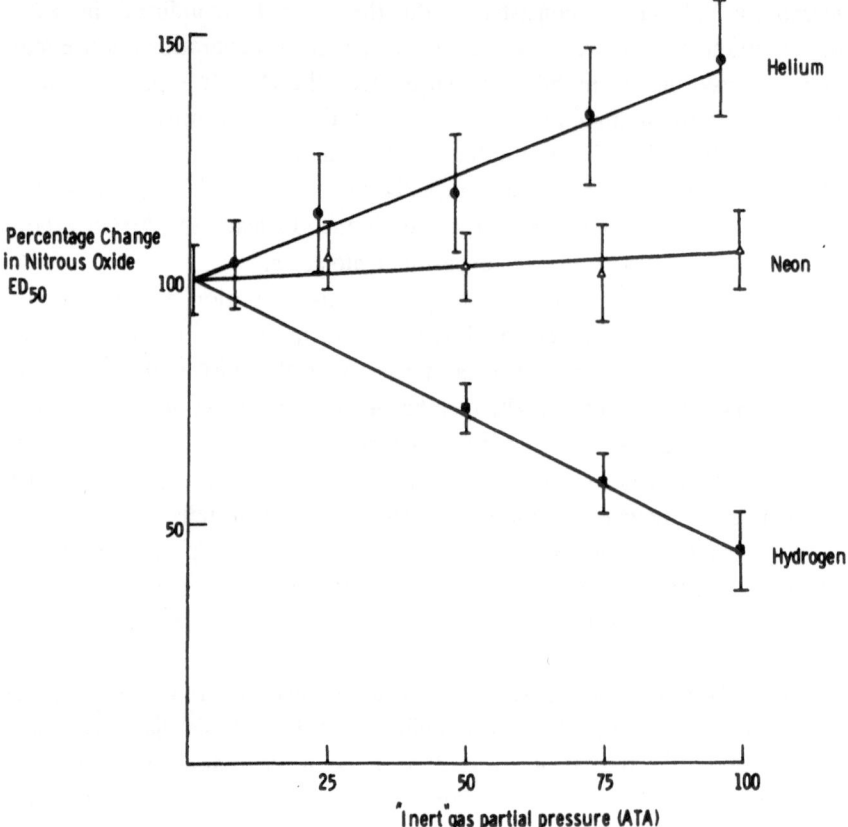

Fig. 5.* The partial pressure of nitrous oxide to produce a loss of righting reflex in mice is plotted against increasing pressures achieved by the addition of helium, neon or hydrogen. Increasing helium pressures increase the nitrous oxide requirement in a linear fashion, indicating that pressure produced with helium antagonizes the effect of anaesthesia. Increase in pressure produced with neon do not alter anaesthetic requirement. Increases in pressure produced with hydrogen reduce anaesthetic requirements as indicated by the decreased partial pressure of nitrous oxide necessary to cause a loss of the righting reflex.

Any perturbation in the protein's environment as by drugs, application of pressure, or change in temperature could inhibit nerve transmission. Once the balance is upset by anaesthesia, any antagonist, such as pressure, tending to restore the optimum conditions would also restore conduction.

In summary, anaesthetic action probably occurs primarily in the reticular activating system of the midbrain and the cerebral cortex. Microscopically, the action most likely occurs along the axon rather than in the synapse, although this is far from settled. From the molecular viewpoint, anaesthetic agents penetrate the inner lipid bilayer of the nerve cell membrane. This disorders the normal function of the protein, including its ability to pass an action potential.

ACKNOWLEDGEMENT

The assistance of Doctors Joan Kendig and James Trudell of the Stanford University Department of Anaesthesia, is gratefully acknowledged in the preparation of this manuscript.

REFERENCES

1. Eger, E. I., II, *Anesthetic Uptake and Action*, Chapter 2, and *Transmission of Messages by the Central Nervous System*, Chapter 3, *IN* Mechanisms of General Anesthesia edited by M. J. Halsey, the Williams and Wilkins Company, Baltimore, 1974.
2. Spyropoulos, C. S., The effects of hydrostatic pressure upon the normal and narcotized nerve. *J. Gen. Physiol.*, 40: 849, 1957.
3. Johnson, F. H. and E. A. Flagler, Hydrostatic pressure reversal of narcosis in tadpoles. *Science*, 112: 91, 1951.
4. Kendig, J. J., J. R. Trudell and E. N. Cohen, Effects of pressure and anesthetics on conduction and synaptic transmission. *J. Pharm. Exptl. Ther.*, 1975. (in press).
5. Meyer, H. H., Zur Theorie der Alkoholnarkose. III. Mitt. Der Einfluss wechselnder Temperatur auf Wirkungsstarke und Teilungskoefficient der Narkotika. *Arch. Exp. Path. Pharmak.*, 46: 338, 1901.
6. Overton, E., *Studien über die Narkose*. Jena: Fisher, 1901.
7. Eger, E. I., C. Lundgren, S. L. Miller and W. C. Stevens, Anesthetic potencies of sulfur hexafluoride. Carbon tetrafluoride, chloroform and Ethrane in dogs: Correlation with the hydrate and lipid theories of anesthetic action. *Anesthesiology*, 30: 129, 1969.
8. Pauling, L., A molecular theory of anesthesia. *Science*, 134: 15, 1961.
9. Miller, S. L., A theory of gaseous anesthetics. *Proc. Natl. Acad. Sci.* (USA), 47: 1515, 1972.
10. Seeman, P., The membrane action of anesthetics and tranquilizers. *Pharmacol. Rev.*, 24: 583, 1972.
11. Hong, K., and W. L. Hubbell, Preparation and properties of phospholipid bilayers containing rhodopsin. *Proc. Nat. Acad. Sci.* (USA), 69: 2617, 1972.

12. Trudell, J. R., W. L. Hubbell and E. N. Cohen, The effect of two inhalation anesthetics on the order of spin-labeled phospholipid vesicles. *Biochim. Biophys. Acta*, 291: 321, 1973.
13. Trudell, J. R., W. L. Hubbell, E. N. Cohen and J. J. Kendig, Pressure reversal of anesthesia: The extent of small-molecule exclusion from spin-labeled phospholipid model membranes. *Anesthesiology*, 38: 207, 1973.
14. Metcalfe, J. C., P. Seeman and A. S. V. Burgen, The proton relaxation of benzyl alcohol in erythrocyte membranes. *Mol. Pharmacol.*, 4: 87, 1968.
15. Trudell, J. R., D. G. Payan, J. H. Chin and E. N. Cohen, The antagonistic effect of an inhalation anesthetic and high pressure on the phase diagram of mixed dipalmitoyl-dimyristoylphosphatidylcholine bilayers. *Proc. Nat. Acad. Sci. USA*, 72: 210, 1975.

GENERAL REFERENCES*

1. Fink, B. and M. D. Raymond, editors; Molecular Mechanisms of Anesthesia. In *Progress in Anesthesiology*, Vol. 1, Raven Press, New York, 1975.
2. Halsey, M. J., R. A. Millar and J. A. Sutton, editors, Molecular Mechanisms. In *General Anesthesia*, Churchill Livingstone, Edinburgh, 1974.
3. Kendig, J. J. and J. R. Trudell, Approaches to a Theory of Anaesthetic Action, Chapter 2. In *Scientific Foundations of Anaesthesia*, Second Edition, edited by C. Scurr and S. Feldman, Year Book Medical Publishers, Inc., Chicago, 1974.

* See also book by Eger (1), cited above.

2. THE UPTAKE AND DISTRIBUTION OF VOLATILE ANAESTHETICS

C. M. CONWAY

The theoretical course of an inhalation anaesthetic can be divided into three phases. There is an initial induction phase during which the anaesthetic agent is transferred from inspired gas into body tissues. This phase concludes when an anaesthetic *tension* equilibrium exists throughout the body and is followed by a maintenance phase during which there is no net exchange of anaesthetic agent. Reduction of inspired anaesthetic concentration to zero leads to a recovery phase when anaesthetic is removed from the body.

In practice anaesthetic equilibrium throughout the body is rarely attained and anaesthetic uptake continues throughout the course of most clinically administered anaesthetics. Depth of anaesthesia can be equated to the tension of anaesthetic in blood supplying the brain. During induction slight and therefore negligible differences exist between alveolar, arterial and cerebral tensions of anaesthetic. Large differences may however exist between inspired and alveolar anaesthetic tensions. The factors governing the ratio of alveolar to inspired anaesthetic tension have a considerable influence upon the clinical course of an inhalation anaesthetic.

Alveolar anaesthetic tension during induction will depend upon the relative masses of anaesthetic agent added to and removed from alveolar gas. The factors controlling the addition of anaesthetic to alveolar gas are the inspired anaesthetic concentration and alveolar ventilation. Anaesthetic is removed from the alveoli by an uptake process which depends upon anaesthetic solubility in blood and on cardiac output. Uptake will also be influenced by the alveolar to mixed venous anaesthetic tension gradient and will thus depend upon venous anaesthetic tension.

INSPIRED ANAESTHETIC CONCENTRATION

At equilibrium the tensions of anaesthetic in inspired gas, alveolar gas, arterial blood, all body tissues and mixed venous blood are equal. Inspired tension is therefore the governing factor in determining eventual depth of anaesthesia. During induction, the greater the inspired concentration the more rapidly will any given brain concentration be attained. This fact is commonly taken advantage of to hasten induction by the use of inspired anaesthetic concentrations considerably greater than those required for maintenance.

Because of the complexities of transfer of anaesthetic or other gases across the alveoli the rate at which alveolar anaesthetic concentration of any given anaesthetic agent approaches that in inspired gas is not necessarily independent of the inspired concentration of that gas. This facet of uptake is discussed below in consideration of the concentration and second gas effects.

ALVEOLAR VENTILATION

The mass of anaesthetic added to alveolar gas will be equal to the product of inspired anaesthetic concentration and alveolar ventilation. Thus at any given inspired concentration increasing alveolar ventilation will tend to hasten uptake. The influence of alterations of alveolar ventilation upon the rate of induction varies for different anaesthetic agents and is greatest in those agents with a high affinity for blood.

BLOOD SOLUBILITY OF ANAESTHETICS

Varying blood solubilities of different anaesthetic agents are the major factors causing differences in the rate of anaesthetic uptake. Blood solubility of an anaesthetic is best expressed as a blood-gas partition coefficient determined at 37°C (fig. 1). It will be seen from table 1 that there are large differences between the blood-gas partition coefficients of the commonly used inhalation anaesthetics. It is convenient to consider separately agents with low blood solubility (cyclopropane and nitrous oxide), the agents which are highly soluble in blood (diethyl ether and methoxyflurane) and those which exhibit an intermediate blood solubility.

If an agent is poorly soluble in blood only small amounts need to be present to exert a high tension. The low affinity of cyclopropane and nitrous oxide for blood means that only small amounts of these agents are removed from alveolar gas during uptake. Alveolar anaesthetic tension will thus rapidly approach that of inspired gas. Conversely because diethyl ether and methoxyflurane have a high blood-gas partition coefficient these agents

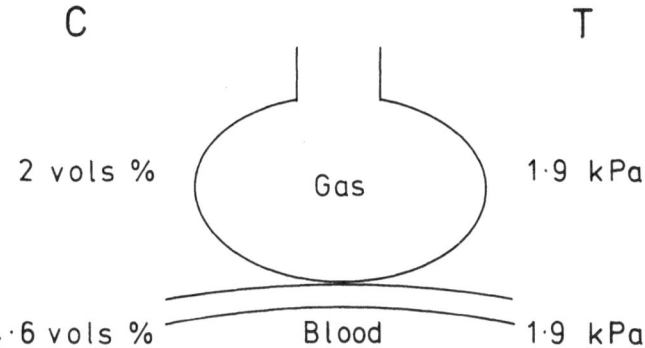

C   T

2 vols %   1·9 kPa
              Gas

4·6 vols %   Blood   1·9 kPa

Fig. 1. The meaning of blood-gas partition coefficient. The figure represents halothane in a gas phase at a concentration (C) of 2 vols %, equivalent to a tension (T) of 1.9 kPa. Blood in equilibrium with this gas at 37°C will contain 4.6 vols % of anaesthetic (blood-gas partition coefficient 2.3). At this equilibrium point there will be no partial pressure difference between gas and blood phases.

Table 1. Blood-gas partition coefficients at 37°C.

Ethylene	0.41
Cyclopropane	0.46
Nitrous oxide	0.47
Fluroxene	1.37
Isoflurane	1.43
Enflurane	1.91
Halothane	2.3
Trichloroethylene	9.15
Diethyl ether	12.1
Methoxyflurane	13

will be removed in large amounts from alveolar gas into pulmonary capillary blood, resulting in large inspired to alveolar anaesthetic tension gradients. As arterial and brain anaesthetic tensions are in virtual equilibrium with alveolar anaesthetic tension it follows that induction will be rapid when anaesthetic agents of low blood solubility are inhaled and slow when highly blood-soluble agents are used.

Not only is induction of anaesthesia rapid when agents of low blood solubility are used, but recovery, the reverse of uptake, is also rapid. During maintenance of anaesthesia with such agents alteration of inspired tension has a rapid effect upon brain anaesthetic tension and therefore on depth of anaesthesia. Alterations in alveolar ventilation have only a slight effect upon the rate at which alveolar approaches inspired anaesthetic tension. Because of the low capacity of blood for insoluble agents, increasing the mass of anaesthetic entering the alveoli by increasing alveolar ventilation only slightly increases the uptake. On the other hand severe imbalance of ventilation-perfusion ratios in the lungs may markedly increase the time taken to reach equilibrium when relatively insoluble anaesthetic agents are used. Slightly increased uptake from relatively well ventilated alveoli will under these circumstances be insufficient to compensate for the reduced uptake from poorly perfused alveoli.

By contrast both induction and recovery are prolonged when anaesthetic agents of high blood solubility are inhaled. Depth of anaesthesia changes slowly in response to alterations in inspired anaesthetic tension. Because during induction with these agents blood leaving the lungs usually has an unsatisfied capacity for anaesthetic, increasing alveolar ventilation and therefore increasing the mass of anaesthetic available for uptake will greatly hasten induction with agents of high blood solubility. For this reason ventilation-perfusion abnormalities have but slight effects on the rate at which arterial tension rises towards inspired tension.

The most useful way of representing the effects of blood solubility upon the duration of the uptake phase is by means of a graph of the ratio of alveolar to inspired anaesthetic tension or fractional concentrations plotted against time. Full equilibrium occurs when the value of the ratio of alveolar to inspired concentrations (F_{AX}/F_{IX}) equals unity. Figure 2 demonstrates the theoretical shapes of these plots under conditions of uniform ventilation and pulmonary blood flow.

CARDIAC OUTPUT

Because an increase in the mass of anaesthetic removed from the alveoli will lower alveolar and therefore arterial anaesthetic tension, any increase in cardiac output will tend to prolong the uptake process. Similarly a reduction in cardiac output will cause alveolar anaesthetic tension to rise more rapidly. However there are differences in the effects of altered alveolar ventilation and altered cardiac output upon the time course of anaesthesia. Whilst increased alveolar ventilation at a constant inspired tension presents an increased mass of anaesthetic to the body, alterations in cardiac output affect the distribution within the body of anaesthetic gas. Although increases in cardiac output will initially slow the rate at which alveolar tension rises

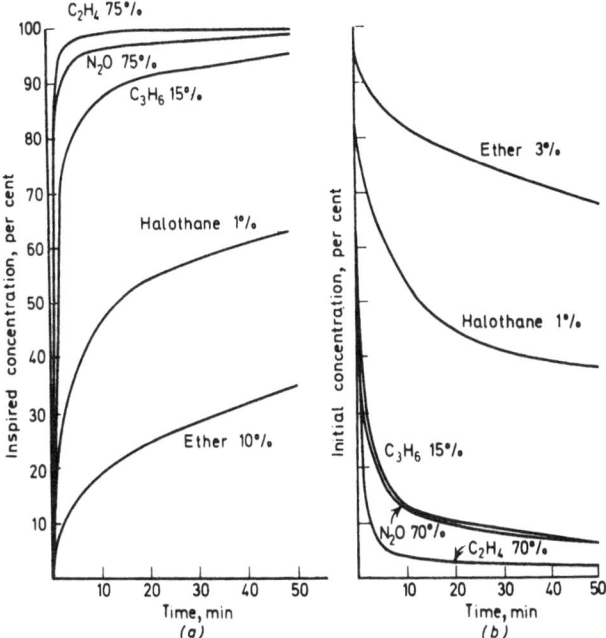

Fig. 2. The rate of change of alveolar anaesthetic tension during induction (a) and recovery (b). The y axis represents alveolar concentration as a percentage of inspired concentration. Note the rapid rise of alveolar tension during induction with agents of low blood solubility (nitrous oxide, cyclopropane, ethylene), the slow rise of alveolar ether concentration, and the intermediate place of halothane. Recovery rates are a near mirror image of induction (From Eger (1)).

towards inspired tension, the greater mass of anaesthetic presented to the tissues will hasten the attainment of an equilibrium state. Alterations in cardiac output are important in the early stages of induction and may account for the ease with which inhalational anaesthesia can be induced in the hypovolaemic patient and the difficulty in sending the fit young hyperdynamic person to sleep. Changes in cardiac output have little effect on the time taken to reach a final equilibrium state.

VENOUS ANAESTHETIC LEVELS

As anaesthetic uptake from the lungs proceeds the concentration of anaesthetics in body tissues increases. In the early stages of uptake circulating blood gives up the majority of its anaesthetic content to the tissues it supplies and mixed venous blood returning to the lungs has a negligible anaesthetic content. As tissue saturation proceeds the anaesthetic tension in blood draining tissues rises. Increasing mixed venous anaesthetic concentration, by lowering the tension gradient across which uptake occurs, limits alveolar anaesthetic uptake. At equilibrium mixed venous and arterial anaesthetic tension levels are equal and uptake ceases.

A less important factor affecting venous anaesthetic levels is metabolism of anaesthetic agent. Whilst metabolic degradation of most anaesthetic agents has now been demonstrated its rate is usually slight and metabolism plays a negligible part in determining venous anaesthetic levels. The only agent with a rate of metabolic transformation great enough to have a significant effect during induction is trichloroethylene.

TISSUE UPTAKE OF ANAESTHETIC

The rate at which the anaesthetic tension in any tissue approaches that of alveolar gas depends upon the tissue solubility of any particular anaesthetic and the blood flow to that tissue. Whilst the solubilities of most anaesthetics vary in different tissues, in general anaesthetic solubility in the principal tissues is close to that in blood. Lipid has a high affinity for all anaesthetics and fatty tissues therefore comprise a large reservoir for inhalational anaesthetics.

Because blood flow varies greatly between different tissues relative perfusion plays a more important role in determining tissue saturation than does tissue solubility. Eger (1) has divided the various body tissues into four groups depending on their blood supply (table 2). The *vessel-rich group*

Table 2.

Tissue group	% body weight	% cardiac output
Vessel-rich	7	70
Muscle	55	25
Fat	20	4
Vessel-poor	18	1

comprises the brain, heart, liver, kidney and endocrine glands, and whilst this group of tissues accounts for only 7% of body mass it receives 70% of the cardiac output. The *muscle group*, in which is included skin, makes up 55% of body weight and receives 25% of cardiac output. The *fat group* of tissues makes up 20% of body weight and receives only 4% of the cardiac output. Finally there is a *vessel-poor* group of tissues made up of cartilage, ligaments and bone, which receives so low a proportion of cardiac output that it can be considered as taking no part in anaesthetic uptake. At the outset of an anaesthetic the bulk of tissue uptake occurs in the vessel rich group and these tissues may reach equilibrium with alveolar anaesthetic tension in 10-15 minutes. For the next few hours the muscle group takes up the largest proportion of anaesthetic. Whilst fat has a high affinity for anaesthetic the low blood supply of most fatty tissues means that equilibrium rarely occurs. Indeed with most inhalational anaesthetics several days would be required for all fatty tissue to become saturated with anaesthetic.

ELIMINATION OF ANAESTHETICS

When inspired anaesthetic concentration is reduced to zero pulmonary excretion of anaesthetic occurs, and is governed by all those factors important during uptake. Thus elimination will be more prolonged in agents which have a high blood-gas partition coefficient and therefore have little tendency to pass from venous blood to alveolar gas. Elimination will be increased if alveolar ventilation or cardiac output are increased. The greater the tissue solubility of an agent the more prolonged will be the process of elimination. The importance of lipid solubility on speed of recovery is well illustrated by considering recovery from nitrous oxide and cyclopropane anaesthesia. The blood solubilities of these two agents are very similar, but cyclopropane is much more soluble in lipids than is nitrous oxide. After a short administration recovery from either agent is rapid. If nitrous oxide is used for several hours recovery is virtually as rapid as after a short administration. Recovery from an equally prolonged cyclopropane anaesthetic is however more prolonged, reflecting the greater uptake of this agent in lipid tissues.

CONCENTRATION EFFECT

During the process of uptake of an anaesthetic gas the composition of alveolar gas will differ from that of inspired gas due to the removal from the alveoli of a mass of anaesthetic agent, resulting in a real or potential reduction in alveolar volume. The final concentration of anaesthetic gas in the

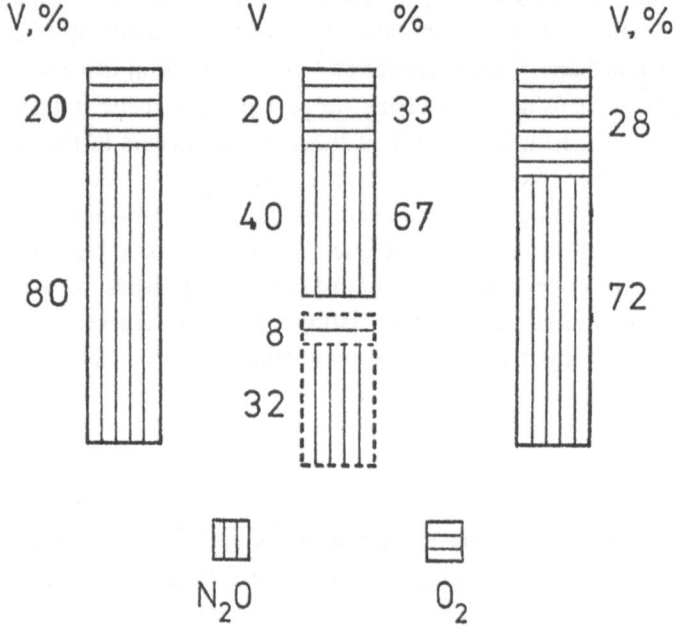

Fig. 3. Concentration and second gas effects during the uptake of 80% nitrous oxide in oxygen. The left hand block represents an initial volume of 100 units of inspired gas. Uptake of half the nitrous oxide causes a volume reduction of 40 units and a large increase in oxygen concentration, shown in the upper portion of the central block. Replacement of this absorbed volume of nitrous oxide by an equal volume of inspired gas (lower part of central block) results in the right hand block in an overall 8% increase in oxygen concentration, and a nitrous oxide concentration which is 90% of the inspired concentration (Modified from Stoetling and Eger (3)).

alveoli will depend on the relative degree of uptake and on the inspired concentration of anaesthetic. The higher the inspired anaesthetic concentration of anaesthetic, the more rapidly will alveolar concentration approach inspired concentration. The reasons for this are illustrated in figures 3 and 4.

Figure 3 shows uptake proceeding in a mythical lung unit of 100 ml volume filled with a mixture of 80% nitrous oxide and 20% oxygen. It is assumed that 50% of nitrous oxide will be absorbed and oxygen uptake has been ignored. Uptake of half the nitrous oxide present results in a volume reduction of 40 ml. The remaining 40 ml of nitrous oxide now represents 67% of the reduced alveolar volume. Thus uptake of 50% of the nitrous oxide has resulted in nitrous oxide concentration falling to 83% of its initial value. This is represented in the upper portion of the middle column of figure 3.

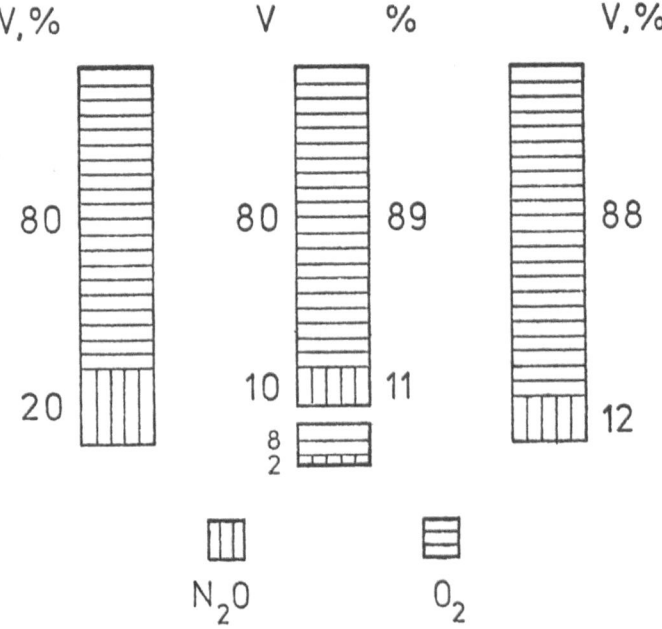

Fig. 4. As for figure 3, but inspired gas is now 20% nitrous oxide in oxygen. Uptake of half the nitrous oxide, because of the smaller changes in volume, results in a final nitrous oxide concentration which is 60% of the inspired concentration.

Under many conditions of induction of anaesthesia there is an excess of inspired gas available as part of the alveolar inspirate. Under these circumstances the potential fall in alveolar volume will be compensated for by an addition aliquot of inspired gas being drawn into the alveoli. The lower portion of the middle column of figure 3 shows an additional 40 ml of inspired gas being added to alveolar gas to restore the alveolar volume to 100 ml. As is shown in the third column of this figure this results in a final nitrous oxide concentration of 72%, which is 90% of the initial inspired concentration.

Figure 4 shows the situation when the inspired mixture contains 20% nitrous oxide and 80% oxygen. Again half the nitrous oxide present is removed by uptake and oxygen uptake is ignored. Nitrous oxide uptake again results in a volume reduction, but this time of a much lesser degree. The residual nitrous oxide represents 11% of the reduced volume and nitrous oxide concentration has fallen to 56% of the initial concentration. Addition of 10 ml of fresh gas to replace nitrous oxide removed by uptake increases nitrous oxide concentration to 12%, that is to 60% of the initial inspired concentration. Thus the greater the initial concentration the greater is the eventual ratio of alveolar to inspired anaesthetic concentration. In theory if the lung is filled with 100% anaesthetic gas the alveolar concentration remains at 100% regardless of the degree of uptake.

The significance of this concentration effect is that the higher the inspired concentration of an anaesthetic, the more rapidly will alveolar concentration approach inspired concentration. In clinical practice the concentration effect is only of importance with those agents which can be used over a wide range of concentrations and whose uptake produces significant alterations in alveolar volume, and is best seen during the uptake of nitrous oxide and diethyl ether.

SECOND GAS EFFECT

The second gas effect is a consequence of the uptake of one component of the alveolar gas mixture upon the concentrations of other components of that mixture. Thus in the example illustrated in figure 3 oxygen has been regarded as an inert gas. Oxygen concentration rises as nitrous oxide is absorbed. Assuming alveolar volume to be maintained by addition of fresh gas the final oxygen concentration is 140% of the initial concentration. In figure 4 the final oxygen concentration is 110% of the initial concentration. If in these two examples the 'inert' fraction contained another anaesthetic, say 1% halothane, nitrous oxide uptake would cause alveolar concentration to rise to 1.4% and 1.1% respectively.

The calculations illustrated above are extreme simplifications of the real case. In practice if a nitrous oxide, oxygen and halothane mixture is inhaled all three components of the mixture would be taken up from the alveoli whilst carbon dioxide and nitrogen would be added to alveolar gas. Because the initial uptake of nitrous oxide would be so much greater than any other changes in the alveoli its effects would predominate at the outset of induction. The concentration and second gas effects due to nitrous oxide uptake would however only prevail for the first few minutes of induction, for as alveolar nitrous oxide concentration approaches that of inspired gas so the mass of nitrous oxide removed from the alveoli falls to low levels.

SUMMARY

Whilst the factors involved in the uptake of anaesthetics from the lungs are many and varied there are no fundamental differences between the factors governing the passage of these gases across the lungs and the pulmonary transport of any other respirable gases. The only difference between the pulmonary exchange of anaesthetics and that of oxygen or carbon dioxide is that anaesthetic uptake or output, unlike that of metabolically active gases, will vary so as to tend to a final equilibrium state of no net anaesthetic exchange.

The factors governing the alveolar concentration of any gas, x, can be expressed in simple mathematical terms as a general alveolar equation:

$$F_{AX} = F_{IX} - \frac{\dot{V}_X}{\dot{V}_A}$$

Where F_{AX} and F_{IX} represent alveolar and inspired fractional concentration of gas x, $\dot{V}_X$ represents uptake of gas x and $\dot{V}_A$ equals alveolar ventilation. If gas x is oxygen this equation leads to one form of the alveolar air equation. Solving the equation for carbon dioxide (assuming no inspired carbon dioxide to be present and carbon dioxide uptake to be negative) gives a form of the Bohr equation. If x is any anaesthetic agent the equation states that the alveolar concentration of anaesthetic will be equal to the inspired concentration minus the ratio of uptake to alveolar ventilation. As anaesthetic uptake will depend on blood solubility, cardiac output and venous blood levels, this equation embraces all the factors discussed in the first part of this chapter.

REFERENCES

1. Eger, E. I., A mathematical model of uptake and distribution. In *Uptake and Distribution of Anaesthetic Agents*, edited by E. M. Papper and R. J. Kitz. Ch. 7. McGraw-Hill, New York, 1963.
2. Kety, S. S., Theory and application of exchange of inert gas at the lungs and tissues. *Pharmacol. Rev.*, 3, 1 (1951).
3. Stoetling, R. K. and E. I. Eger, An additional explanation for the second gas effect. *Anesthesiology*, 25, 273 (1969).

3. ENFLURANE

INTRODUCTION

Anaesthesiologists have always been interested in the development of new
general anaesthetic agents that might replace those in current use and
approach the ideal attributes of an anaesthetic agent (5, 31). Enflurane is
not the ideal anaesthetic agent, but it satisfies most of these criteria and is
being used increasingly all over the world. It was developed in 1963 by
R. C. Terrel (1) in the laboratories of the Ohio Medical Products Company,
and at that time was called Ohio Compound 347. In the same year this new
halogenated ether was used by Krantz (1) in animals and it was later introduced into clinical practise by Virtue (2) in 1966, Dobkin in 1968 (3), and
Botty (4) in 1968. It is now available under the trade name Ethrane (Abbott).

A. PHYSICAL PROPERTIES

Enflurane is a halogenated methylethyl ether with five fluorine atoms and
one chlorine atom in the molecule and has a close chemical resemblance to
methoxyflurane, but in its pharmacological properties it is more closely
related to halothane (1, 3, 30) (fig. 1). It is a clear, colourless liquid with a
pleasant, mild ethereal smell. It is not inflammable or explosive in air or
oxygen or when mixed with oxygen an nitrous oxide in any anaesthetic
concentration at atmospheric pressure and over a temperature range of
21-45°C (9).

Enflurane does not react with soda lime, and its chemical stability is
impressive. It is unaffected by light, has no corrosive action on tin, copper,
brass, aluminium, or iron, and does not need a chemical stabilizer. The
vapour pressure of enflurane is 175 mm of mercury at 20°C, the oil/gas
distribution coefficient is 98.5, the boiling point lies between 56.5° and 57.5°
at atmospheric pressure, and its blood/gas coefficient is 1.91. This means
that enflurane is only moderately soluble in blood and as a result the alveolar

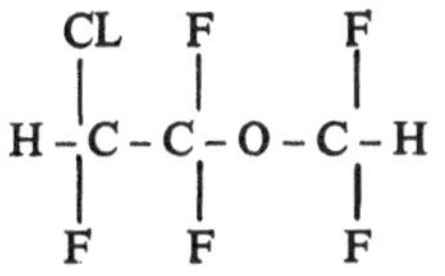

$$
\begin{array}{ccc}
\text{CL} & \text{F} & \text{F} \\
| & | & | \\
\text{H}-\text{C}-\text{C}-\text{O}-\text{C}-\text{H} \\
| & | & | \\
\text{F} & \text{F} & \text{F}
\end{array}
$$

ENFLURANE

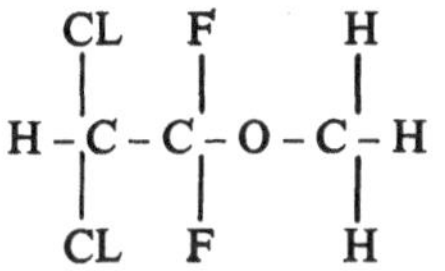

$$
\begin{array}{ccc}
\text{CL} & \text{F} & \text{H} \\
| & | & | \\
\text{H}-\text{C}-\text{C}-\text{O}-\text{C}-\text{H} \\
| & | & | \\
\text{CL} & \text{F} & \text{H}
\end{array}
$$

METHOXYFLURANE

Fig. 1. Structural formulas of enflurane and methoxyflurane.

concentration very rapidly approaches the inspired concentration (6, 7, 8).

The minimal alveolar concentration (MAC) is defined as the alveolar concentration of an anaesthetic agent that abolishes pain reaction to mechanical stimulation in 50% of a group of animals or human subjects. For healthy young men the MAC of enflurane is 1.68% (10, 11). The presence of nitrous oxide in the inspired mixture reduces the MAC of enflurane to 1.17% when 30% N_2O is present and even to 0.57% when 70% N_2O is used. This lowering of the MAC value by N_2O has certain advantages, such as reduction of the enflurane requirement, more rapid recovery, and fewer side effects (13).

B. PHARMACOLOGY

As an anaesthetic agent, enflurane is slightly less potent than halothane. The vapour does not irritate the respiratory tract. The induction of anaesthesia requires 3-5% vapour, and the maintenance level is 1.5-3% for spontaneous respiration and up to 1.5% with controlled respiration.

I. EFFECTS ON THE CARDIOVASCULAR SYSTEM

Depression of myocardial contractility is one of the fundamental effects of inhalation anaesthetic agents. This effect is dose related and reversible, and can be demonstrated both in vitro and in vivo (15). Enflurane has this property too, but to a low degree, than halothane according to some authors

(16, 18, 20, 29). This is attributed by the same authors to heightened sympathetic tone.

The cardiac output and the stroke volume are diminished during the administration of enflurane. In unpremedicated patients the heart rate dropped as induction progressed and became significantly lower than the base value (17, 21, 24). Premedication with atropine counteracts this slowing of the pulse frequency. Since the decreased stroke volume also seems to be the result of a decreased venous return, this must play an important role in the lowering of the blood pressure. After an injection of succinylcholine, the heart rate returns to preinduction values. Atropine given i.v. may accelerate the pulse rate and produce a rise in the blood pressure, but it should be given slowly.

Arterial hypothension under enflurane anaesthesia is the result of diminished cardiac output and, to a lesser degree, of a decrease in the peripheral vascular resistance (7, 8, 14, 30). The fall in blood pressure is moderate and the pressure has a tendency to return spontaneously to initial values. Hypotension occurs mostly when the concentration of enflurane is higher than 3%, and responds well to a pressor drug. The cardiac rhythm, on the other hand, remains very stable under enflurane, which has little effect on the ECG.

The influence of enflurane on the peripheral resistance is uncertain. According to some authors, it has a direct effect on the smooth muscles in the wall of the blood vessels, resulting in a moderate lowering of the systemic resistance. According to other authors, the change in the systemic resistance is slight and has only a small influence on the blood pressure (15).

We investigated cardiac stability during enflurane anaesthesia. During our first 205 enflurane anaesthesias, 7 of the 25 patients in the group with pre-existing ventricular extrasystolies showed a return of the cardiac rhythm to normal during enflurane anaesthesia.

Therefore, the action of enflurane on the cardiovascular system can be summarized as shown in table 2.

Table 2. The effects of enflurane on the cardiovascular system.

1. Decreases the stroke volume and the cardiac output
2. Lowers the peripheral vascular resistance
3. Reduces the systemic arterial blood pressure
4. Has a negative inotropic effect on the myocardium
5. The heart rate remains stable

Enflurane and noradrenalin

One of the characteristics of an ideal anaesthetic agent is the absence of cardiac sensitization to catecholamines. Noradrenalin is frequently used during surgery to achieve local haemostasis, especially during head, neck, and plastic reconstructive surgery. Experience with halothane has shown that serious ventricular arrhythmias or even death can result from the use of noradrenalin (23). Although in man the administration of noradrenalin in the presence of enflurane could also sensitize the myocardium to exogenous catecholamines, the arrhythmygenous dose is much greater than for halothane (22, 25, 26, 28). Furthermore, the types of arrhythmia are different for these two agents, because those induced with enflurane are usually supraventricular in origin.

Enflurane has also been used in a case of pheochromocytoma and apparently did not increase the ventricular sensitivity to endogenous catecholamine challenge, but more experience is required for adequate evaluation here (78).

Under the same precautions, the administration of catecholamines during enflurane anaesthesia can be as safe as during halothane anaesthesia (27). The necessary conditions are: adequate ventilation of the patient; adrenaline dilution 1:100,000 to 1:200,000; adult dose limited to 10 ml in any 10-minute period and to maximally 30 ml per hour. Administration is contraindicated in thyreotoxicosis and in patients with pre-existing heart irregularities and those with diminished cardiac reserve who cannot tolerate tachycardia (Tabel 3).

Table 3. The safety measures for the administrations of catecholamines during enflurane anaesthesia.

1. Adequate ventilation of the patient
2. Epinephrine dilution 1:100000 to 1:200000
3. Adult dose limited to 10 ml in any 10-minute period and no more than 30 ml per hour
4. Contraindications in thyreotoxicosis and in patients with pre-existing cardiac disease, especially those with diminished cardiac reserve who cannot tolerate tachycardia and those in whom pulmonary function will not assure adequate ventilation (avoidance of hypoxia and hypercarbia)

II. EFFECT ON THE RESPIRATORY SYSTEM

Enflurane vapour is well tolerated, does not irritate the respiratory tract, and provides smooth induction of anaesthesia but does not give the rapid depression of the laryngeal and pharyngeal reflexes that permits early insertion of the endotracheal tube. It does not increase tracheobronchial secretion. On the contrary, it inhibits salivary and bronchial secretion and facilitates the maintenance of a patent airway (31).

Generally speaking, the effects of enflurane on respiration do not differ greatly from those of the other inhalation anaesthetic agents. It causes depression but the respiration rate remains relatively stable with a tendency to slow down as anaesthesia becomes deeper. The tachypnoea commonly seen with halothane does not occur. The usual frequency lies in the range of up to 18 per minute (1, 7, 8, 10, 29).

When the plane of anaesthesia is deepened the tidal volume becomes smaller. This volume usually lies in the range of 250-400 ml. An interesting observation is that the 'sigh mechanism' remains relatively intact; the patient retains the ability to take a deep breath spontaneously during surgical planes of anaesthesia. In this respect enflurane resembles diethyl ether (7, 8, 30).

The influence of enflurane anaesthesia on blood gases is reported (83) to lead to a significant CO_2 accumulation as early as after 30 minutes of anaesthesia. In our experience (11) this seldom occurs with lower enflurane concentrations, and if it does happen it is in obese patients or in patients with chronic bronchitis who need higher concentrations (table 4).

There is a reduction in compliance during enflurane anaesthesia, ranging

Table 4. Spontaneous respiration and arterial blood gases under enflurane anaesthesia in 205 patients.

	5 min after induction	30 min after
Minute volume (in litres)	5.2 ± 0.8	4.7 ± 0.7
Respiratory frequency	20 ± 8.7	13.2 ± 4
Capnographic values (in %)	4.7 ± 0.3	5.6 ± 1.0
pH	7.40 ± 0.03	7.36 ± 0.03
pCO_2	42.6 ± 7.3	46.1 ± 7.5
pO_2	88.7 ± 13	92 ± 5
Standard bicarbonate	25 ± 4.0	23.4 ± 3.5
Base excess	0.37 ± 3.6	0.45 ± 4
O_2 saturation	95.2 ± 2.8	95.0 ± 3.2

from 8.3% at 1 vol% to 14% at 2%. This might be due to the effect of the anaesthetic agent on the anti-atelectasis factor (35). The reduced compliance returns to normal rapidly once the administration of enflurane is discontinued (7, 8, 15).

Enflurane has been found to have a slight bronchoconstrictor effect leading to an increase in resistance (84), but Rolly recently reported that enflurane decreases the resistance by as much as 10% (81).

Oxygen consumption is always decreased during general anaesthesia, i.e., below the level observed during normal activity (33). The decrease during enflurane anaesthesia is dose related and amounts to approximately 13-35% (34). This reduction is far below the level observed in the awake basal state. Compared with halothane anaesthesia, oxygen consumption is twice as low with enflurane. This has been attributed to decreased respiratory and cardiac activity and to the muscle relaxation. Factors such as premedication, induction with barbiturates, and spontaneous ventilation can also play a certain role in diminished oxygen consumption.

ANAESTHETIC INDEX

The anaesthetic index, which is the ratio between the alveolar concentration at apnoea and the MAC, is 2:1 for enflurane. This value is lower than that of other inhalation anaesthetic agents, suggesting a wide margin of safety between the levels at which respiratory and cardiac arrest occur. When anaesthesia was carried out experimentally in dogs to the plane of respiratory arrest, artificial pulmonary ventilation with a high concentration of enflurane had to be maintained for approximately 15 minutes before cardiac arrest occurred.

III. EFFECT ON THE CENTRAL NERVOUS SYSTEM

Enflurane is a complete general anaesthetic agent. Induction of anaesthesia is rapid and the recovery of consciousness is equally rapid, but the analgetic effect seems to be weak. This is supported by the fact that the MAC of enflurane is lower when this agent is used in combination with nitrous oxide. In addition, post-operative pain occurs early and an analgetic agent is soon required. Of special interest is the suitability of this agent for neurosurgery. Before an anaesthesia agent can be used in this field, its effects on the physiology of cerebral blood flow and intracranial pressure must be known.

On the one hand, enflurane provides anaesthesia which is light enough for neurosurgery but still deep enough to allow toleration of the endotracheal tube. This is important, because it is well known that any coughing, bucking, breath-holding, or straining can raise the intracranial pressure. On the other hand, enflurane depresses respiration, which results in a rise of the $PaCO_2$ level, which in turn can lead to cerebral vasodilatation, increased blood flow, and elevated intracranial pressure. Investigation with enflurane has shown that although this agent can slightly increase intracranial pressure in patients with normal values, this effect is negligible (38); but in patients with intracranial pathology the elevation can be very marked and cannot be adequately reduced by hyperventilation. This effect is attributed to cerebral vasodilatation, and seems to be directly produced by enflurane. It is thought that shift in the brain circulation might be avoided in patients with intra-cranial hypertension by applying hyperventilation or some other method for reducing the intracranial pressure prior to the use of enflurane, so that an initial rise would start from a lower level. Reinhold, who investigated 5 patients with intracranial pathology (37), found a decrease in the cerebral blood flow varying between 5 and 23%, which could be beneficial for patients undergoing intracranial operations. In our experience, enflurane satisfies a number of the specific requirements for neurosurgical anaesthesia and, with the above-mentioned precautions, can be successfully used in neurosurgery.

CONVULSIONS

Many anaesthetic agents are known to possess both convulsant and ana-esthetic properties. The anaesthetic component takes effect at low concen-trations, whereas excitations predominate at high concentrations. Enflurane produces abnormal muscle movements in some patients. Clinically, these movements are characterized by twitching of certain groups of muscles (in the legs, upper limbs, face and neck, tongue), or tonic-muscular move-ments, or general convulsions resembling the products of paroxysmal epileptiform discharges in the brain. The incidence of this disturbance is probably not as high as was previously thought (3.7%) (1, 3).

Excitations begin at moderate to deep levels of anaesthesia. The implica-tion of these seizures remains undertain. Seizures are generally believed to be associated with an increased utilization of oxygen by the brain, but according to some authors a deficiency of cerebral oxygen can be excluded or is not significant. They also cannot be correlated with a decrease in the cerebral blood flow (44).

Hypocapnia can function as an activating factor. Hyperventilation to a PCO_2 of 22 and a pH of 7.55 increased the frequency, magnitude, and symmetry of spiking electro-encephalographic activity. Hypercapnia, on the contrary, suppressed the spiking activity. It must be kept in mind that hyperventilation significantly decreases the cerebral PO_2 level. The EEG effects ascribed to changes in $PaCO_2$ might be the result of changes in cerebral PaO_2 rather than a direct effect of CO_2 (42, 43).

The effect of enflurane on the EEG is characterized by high voltage and fast activity during light anaesthesia and the appearance of spike and dome complexes and burst suppression for up to 60 seconds at deeper levels. These EEG abnormalities reverted to the normal pattern within a few minutes when the inspired concentration was reduced (36, 39, 40, 41).

IV. EFFECT ON THE MUSCULAR SYSTEM

Enflurane provides good muscular relaxation during mono-anaesthesia, i.e., comparable with that obtained with diethyl ether, cyclopropane, and methoxylflurane. Profound abdominal relaxation can be obtained easily, but generally requires an alveolar concentration higher than 3%.

The effect of non-depolarizing muscle relaxants is potentiated during enflurane anaesthesia (8, 9, 46). Investigation into the effect of enflurane on the neuromuscular twitch response showed a depression of neuromuscular transmission ranging from potentiation of d-tubocurarine at low concentrations of enflurane (1-1.5%) to direct depression of the muscle twitch response at higher concentrations (3%) (45, 47). The potency of the neuromuscular blockade seems to be far greater than has been reported for other volatile anaesthetic agents. Prostigmine is unable to reverse the direct effects of enflurane, which suggests that the neuromuscular block is not of the curare type. It seems more likely that enflurane depresses central nervous system or spinal reflex activity than that it acts on the motor end plate. The clinical importance of these findings lies in the conclusion that the use of non-depolarizing muscle relaxants together with enflurane results in an additive effect, and therefore the dosage of such relaxants should not be higher than one-third of the normal dose. There is no interaction with succinylcholine.

Our material also confirms the reports that enflurane is a potent muscle relaxant at concentrations higher than 2-3%, which makes a cautious use of a non-depolarizing muscle relaxant imperative. The administration of such high concentrations of enflurane also involves the risk of serious hypotension, which could be deleterious for some groups of patients. Therefore, we advise against the use of concentrations higher than 1.5% when enflurane is administered in combination with non-depolarizing muscle relaxants.

MYASTHENIA GRAVIS AND ENFLURANE

The anaesthesiological problems encountered in patients suffering from myasthenia gravis arise mainly from the influence exerted by muscle relaxants, anaesthetic agents and analgetic drugs affecting neuromuscular transmission. Enflurane was used as the only anaesthetic drug throughout surgical procedures in a series of 5 patients with myasthenia gravis (40). The specific oral therapy was interrupted only during the operation and was re-introducted as soon as possible post-operatively. All of the patients recovered very quickly after the administration of the anaesthetic agent was terminated.

It seems justified to conclude that enflurane itself has valuable qualities for use in patients suffering from this rare disease, and that the described method could be adopted as the method of choice in such cases, because it avoids the need for post-operative ventilation.

V. EFFECTS ON THE LIVER AND METABOLISM

The possibility that an anaesthetic agent might damage the liver forms one of the most unpleasant problems confronting the anaesthesiologist. Liver dysfunction associated with anaesthetic agents is, however, very rare. Other factors could be involved, for instance the nutritional status of the patient, hypoxia, hypotension or hypercapnia, blood transfusions, acute or chronic liver diseases, drug addiction, and the use of antibiotics, steroids, phenothiazines, or sedatives (49, 55).

Extensive studies have provided detailed estimations of liver function in patients anaesthetized with enflurane. No changes suggesting a direct toxic effect on the liver have been found up to a month after surgery. Some cases show an increase in serum transaminase values, indicating some degree of liver dysfunction, but these levels have never been as high as would be expected if enflurane were toxic for the lever cell. LDH, SCOT, and SGPT behave similarly. There is a rise in these values, remaining well within normal limits on the first and second post-operative days, but the decrease occurring on the third post-operative day is very distinct. It is interesting that alkaline phosphatase drops below the initial levels (50, 51).

Enflurane is a relatively new anaesthetic agent, and since it is not yet known whether the enflurane molecule or its metabolites are hepatotoxic, cautious and correct evaluation is necessary before any conclusions can be drawn. However, some authors suspect a connection between enflurane and the occurrence of hepatitis (56) and a cross-sensitivity with halothane has not been either excluded or confirmed, but in animals a metabolite (trifluoroacetate) common to halothane, fluorexene, and enflurane has been shown to induce delayed-type hypersensitivity (58).

Biotransformation of enflurane

Clinical studies on enflurane biotransformation in man have shown that it occurs to the extent of 2.4-5%. This biotransformation takes place mainly in the liver via the substrate non-specific NADPH and the oxygen-dependent redox system. The biotransformation products are the sum of inorganic and organic fluoride (52, 63), probably in a ratio of 2:1. Urinary fluoride analysis revealed that most of the recoverable fluoride was in the form of non-volatile organic metabolites. The urinary excretion of inorganic and organic fluoride showed a pattern similar to that seen after the administration of

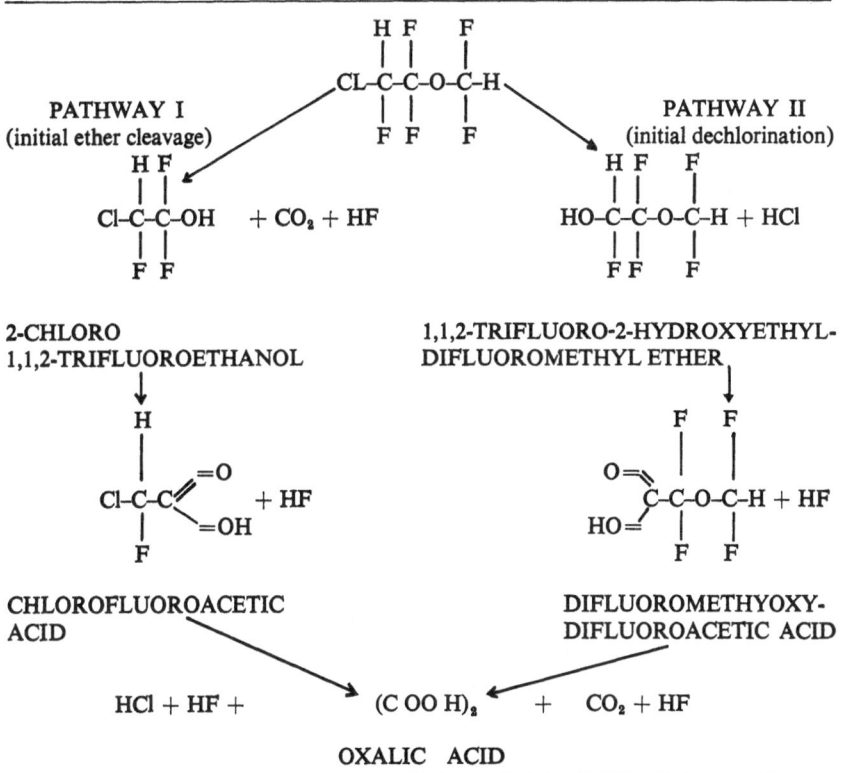

Fig. 2. Proposed metabolic pathways for the biotransformation of enflurane.

methoxyflurane, with a half-life of 1.55 days for inorganic fluoride and 3.69 days for organic fluoride, which suggests tissue and plasma-protein binding of organic fluoride and therefore slower excretion (51, 52, 53).

The metabolic pathway metabolic for enflurane (57) is shown in figure 3. Initial ether cleavage of enflurane (Pathway I) would allow the release of inorganic fluoride. Subsequent dechlorination and oxidation of chloro-fluoroacetic acid would yield oxalic acid as the endproduct of biotrans-formation. Initial dechlorination of enflurane (Pathway II) would result in the formation of oxalic acid.

The very low biotransformation of enflurane is explained by its low fat solubility, a low blood-gas partition coefficient allowing rapid excretion when administration is discontinued, and great chemical stability. The question may eventually arise as to the extent to which these small quantities of metabolites could be toxic.

VI. EFFECT ON RENAL FUNCTION

As for methoxyfluorane, anaesthesiologists are understandably worried about the biotransformation products of enflurane, i.e., fluorides, especially because the configuration of the enflurane molecule resembles that of methoxyflurane and the main products of the biotransformation of the latter are also fluorides. In the case of enflurane, however, the amount of fluorides is very small. Whether this small amount could be sufficient to produce renal dysfunction in some patients is still an open question.

Preliminary studies in animals have shown that prolonged deep enflurane anaesthesia may produce a certain degree of polyuria. The peak levels of the fluoride excretion were, however, reached earlier and returned to con-trol values sooner after enflurane anaesthesia than after methoxyflurane. This too is probably related to the lower tissue solubility of enflurane, which leads to rapid excretion of the agent from the body.

Other experiments have indicated that another factor besides fluoride can play a role in possible renal dysfunction, and this is hypoxia (61). In animals hypoxia in combination with enflurane anaesthesia can lead to severe abnormalities of the cells in the proximal tubuli.

In any case, renal function appears to be completely unaffected by enflu-rane. Numerous observations in man have shown that diuresis neither decreases nor increases and that there is no change in osmolarity or any marked alteration in the electrolyte balance, which could reflect a renal lesion (62). Determination of glomerulal filtration, renal plasma flow, and creatinine and urea clearance, like the other tests, revealed nothing abnormal during and after exposure to enflurane (60). Urinalysis showed that cloudy urine and albuminuria could persist up to 10 days after enflurane anaesthesia in a number of patients, but without any clinical significance.

Nevertheless, in view of the experience with methoxyflurane and the nephrotoxic action of its metabolic fluoride, we do not advise the use of enflurane in cases with severe renal disease or for kidney transplantation, for either donor or recipient. It may be that renal disease interferes with the excretion of fluoride ions, which could lead to accumulation and possibly to damage of renal tubuli (59). Furthermore, a newly transplanted kidney seldom functions normally, especially in the beginning, and it is also possible that the threshold of fluoride nephrotoxicity in a diseased or transplanted kidney is lower than that in a normal kidney.

VII. OTHER EFFECTS

1. Gastro-intestinal tract
Secretory activity in the gastro-intestinal tract is depressed by enflurane, even when atropine is not given as premedication. The motility of the gastro-intestinal tract itself is slightly inhibited. Enflurane may depress intestinal contractions by an action on both nerves and muscles (64).

The incidence of post-operative nausea, vomiting, and hiccups after enflurane anaesthesia has been very low in our material, which is contrary to the high incidence reported in the first clinical studies on this anaesthetic agent.

2. Body temperature
A mild reduction of the body temperature occurs under enflurane anaesthesia, but usually not amounting to more than 1°C below the initial value. The incidence of shivering is quite low if there is no further drop in temperature.

One important question concerns the connection between enflurane and the syndrome of malignant hyperthermia (66). This syndrome is associated with most general anaesthetic agents, and the findings in a very recently published case suggest that enflurane too may be an inductor of malignant hyperthermia (65). The pathogenesis of this syndrome is still unclear. A patient subject to malignant hyperthermia does not necessarily develop rigidity after the administration of succinylcholine. An abnormal production of heat in the soda-lime canister, together with tachycardia, rapid elevation of the body temperature, and hypertonicity of skeletal muscles during anaesthesia, are warning signs and constitute indications for immediate treatment of this syndrome.

3. Uterus

The effect of enflurane on the pregnant uterus is controversial. Devoghel found a dose-related and reversible reduction of spontaneous or oxytocin-induced contractions at any stage of labour, leading to possible uterus atony or post-partum haemorrhage (69), but earlier reports by some Latin American authors did not indicate any significant effects of enflurane on uterine or foetal dynamics (67, 68, 70).

4. Blood

There is an increase in the numbers of leucocytes and polymorphonuclear cells during enflurane anaesthesia. This increase is without importance, however, because it has been seen for all potent anaesthetic agents (1, 3, 7, 8). The haemoglobin level, haemotocrit value, and red cell count drop slightly on the first post-operative day, to below pre-operative levels. The prothrombin time, the thrombin test, and the activity of coagulation factors I, II, and V show slight but non-significant changes (71). Serum sodium and chloride levels do not change. A slight to moderate reduction of the serum potassium level has been reported. This occurs with other inhalation and i.v. anaesthetic agents as well, and has been attributed to the effect of respiratory alkalosis, but it is also seen in the absence of respiratory disturbances and during mild hypercapnia (71).

5. Glucose metabolism

Investigations on human growth hormone (HGH) in plasma have shown that during anaesthesia enflurane does not increase the level of this hormone significantly over a 45-minute period before the operation, but the slight rise continued and reached a peak two hours after the start of the operation (72, 73). It is known that the anterior pituitary growth hormone (which is anabolic and increases the uptake and synthesis of amino acids) also has diabetogenic and anti-insulin effects, thus reducing the peripheral utilization and uptake of glucose, decreasing the glucose tolerance, and increasing the retention of glycogen. This hormone also stimulates the mobilization of free fatty acids (FFA), which promotes glycolysis and gluconeogenesis.

Plasma insulin levels did not increase very markedly during anaesthesia with enflurane alone, but tended to rise at the end of the operation period. Blood glucose levels did not change significantly during such anaesthesia, but rose markedly during the operation; plasma FFA levels fell significantly, but tended to rise during the recovery period. In patients suffering from diabetes mellitus, HGH exerts a diabetogenic effect. Because enflurane does not give an increase of the plasma HGH or blood glucose and does not decrease plasma insulin, it may be preferred for diabetic patients.

Camu, who studied the influence of enflurane anaesthesia in dogs, found that enflurane significantly increased plasma glucose levels and reduced the level of circulating immuno-reactive insulin. Glucose tolerance was also impaired. He concluded that carbohydrate intolerance during enflurane anaesthesia results from an inhibitory effect of the anaesthetic agent on insulin secretion, partially mediated by an alpha-adrenergic activity (74).

6. Intra-ocular pressure

Most of the general anaesthetic agents cause a decrease in the intra-ocular pressure and very few of them increase it (ketamine, N_2O, chloralhydrate). A study done in young patients has shown that enflurane effectuates only a mild to moderate reduction of the intra-ocular pressure (75). It also permits central positioning of the eyes early in the period of administration, which together with the rapid emergence from anaesthesia, makes it suitable for eye operations.

USE OF VAPORIZER

Like all the volatile general anaesthetic agents, enflurane must be converted into vapour before use. A special vaporizer has been designed for the controlled administration of enflurane, the maximal limit being fixed at 5%, which is sufficient to allow the broadest use (76). The performance of the Enfluratec vaporizer (Cyprane Ltd.) was assessed in our laboratory with a gas chromatograph (Hewlett-Packard 5750). For high flows (9 1/min) the concentrations were much lower than indicated by the control knob, but at a lower concentration range (round 1%) the results were acceptable (fig. 3).

A halothane vaporizer can also be used for enflurane, but it should of course be emptied and cleaned before re-filling (77). To determine the delivered concentration, the number on the dial should be multiplied by 0.72 (example: 1.5 vol % halothane $\times$ 0.72 = 1.08 vol % enflurane).

Fig. 3. Test of the vaporizer (Enfluratec – Cyprane Ltd.).

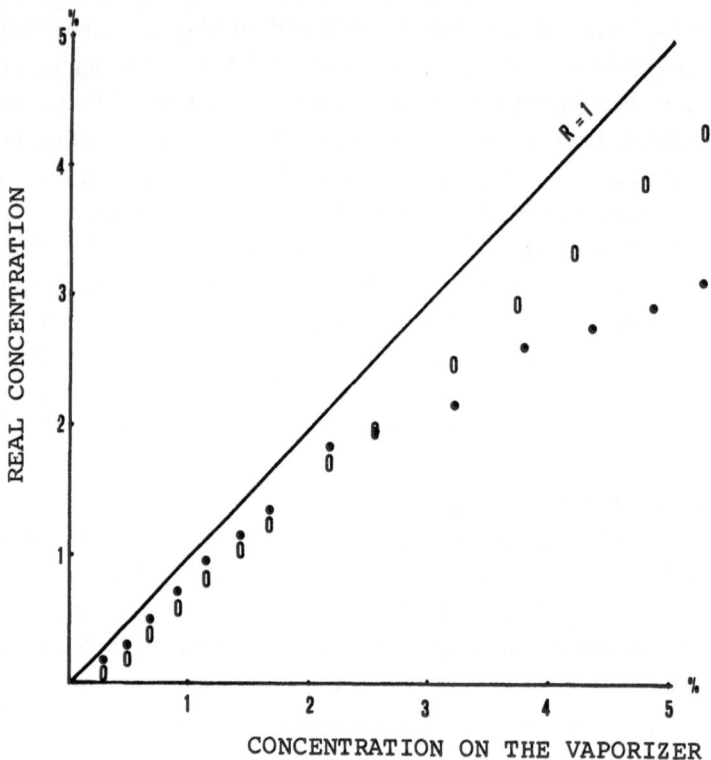

CONCENTRATION ON THE VAPORIZER

0 = 6 l/min.
• = 9 l/min.
R = 1 IDEAL VALUE

PREMEDICATION AND INDUCTION

Many kinds of premedication have been used prior to enflurane anaesthesia, according to the accepted practice in medical centres and the popularity of drugs. At our hospital, a combination of fentanyl and droperidol or of droperidol and atropine is usually applied. When a sedative is also given, particulary one with a potent hypnotic activity, delayed recovery from anaesthesia must of course be expected (78).

Enflurane can also be given without premedication. It should be kept in mind that premedication with atropine counteracts the effects by which enflurane shows the pulse frequency.

Induction of anaesthesia is obtained easily with one of the intravenous induction agents. For this purpose we usually use Penthotal® 4 mg/kg, Althesin® 50 microl/kg, or etomidate (Hypnomidate®) 0.20 mg/kg. Induction of anaesthesia by the inhalation method is easily achieved with enflurane combined with either oxygen alone or with an oxygen-nitrous oxide mixture. We recommend starting with an enflurane concentration of 0.5% and raising it after every few inspirations by 0.5% until surgical anaesthesia is produced. In general, an inspired concentration of between 3.5 and 4.5% enflurane produces surgical anaesthesia in 7 to 10 minutes.

MAINTENANCE DOSAGE

Surgical levels of anaesthesia can be attained with 1.5-3% concentrations. Higher levels are not desirable and must be avoided. If relaxation is also required, a supplemental dose of a muscle relaxant may be used in a lower dosage than usual. Ventilation to keep the arterial-blood CO_2 tension in the 35-45 mmHg range is to be preferred to hyper- or hypoventilation to minimize possible CNS excitation.

The blood-pressure level during maintenance of anaesthesia is an inverse function of the enflurane concentration in the absence of other complications, and any hypotension can be easily corrected by lightening the level of anaesthesia.

CONCLUSIONS

Enflurane is an inhalation anaesthetic that satisfies the anaesthetic requirements for both long and short procedures very well (80). Induction of and recovery from enflurane anaesthesia are rapid, and the level of anaesthesia can be changed rapidly. Enflurane reduces ventilation as the depth of anaesthesia increases. There is a dose-related hypotension, but the cardiac rhythm remains remarkably stable. The safety of catecholamines used topically or parenterally during enflurane anaesthesia has not yet been established in man; in animals it is safer than halothane. Muscle relaxation is adequate, and the action of non-depolarizing relaxants is augmented by enflurane. Damage to parenchymatous organs such as the liver and kidneys seems unlikely, but warnings are found in the literature.

Enflurane is a very stable anaesthetic agent; metabolization amounts to about 2.4-5%. Increasing depth of anaesthesia produces a change in the EEG but, unlike the other inhalation anaesthetic agents, enflurane decreases the cerebral blood flow. The side-ffects of enflurane are few and relatively unimportant.

Enflurane is a relatively new anaesthetic agent and is already widely used in anaesthetic practice, but additional large-scale studies are required to determine its real place in anaesthesiology.

REFERENCES

1. Dobkin, B., K. Nishioka, D. Gengaje, D. Sook, W. Evers and J. Israel, Ethrane (Compound 347) Anaesthesia: A clinical and laboratory review of 700 cases. *Analg. and Anaesth.*, vol. 43: 3, 477 (1969).
2. Virtue, W., O. Lund, M. Phelps, K. Vogel, H. Beckwit and M. Heron, Difluoromethyl 1,1,2-trifluoro-2-chlorethyl ether as an anaesthetic agent: Results in dogs and a preliminary note on observation in man. *Canad. Anaesth. Soc. J.* 12: 233 (1966).
3. Dobkin, A., G. R. Heinrich, S. J. Israel, A. Levy, J. F. Neville and K. Ounkasem, Clinical and laboratory evaluation of a new inhalation agent: Compound 347. *Anaesthesiology*, vol. 20: 2: 275 (1968).
4. Botty, C., B. Brown, V. Stanley and C. R. Stephen, Clinical experiences with Compound 347, a halogeneted anaesthetic agent. *Anaesth. and Analgesia*, 47: 499 (1968).
5. Temmeran, de P., Introduction on the pharmacology of Compound 347 or Enflurane. *Acta Anaesth. Belg.*, vol. 25: 2: 170 (1974).
6. Drug Commentary, Evaluation of a general anaesthetic, Ethrane. *JAMA*, vol. 225: 8 (1973).
7. Hanquet, M., F. Bortem and Vidouqe, General properties of Ethrane. *Anaesth. and Resuscitation*, vol. 84 (Ethrane): 6, Springer Verlag, New York.
8. Lawin P., General Aspects of Enflurane. *Acta Anaesth. Belgica* 2: 175 (1974).
9. Leonard, P., The lower limits of flammability of Halothane, Ethrane and Isoflurane. *Anaesth. and Analg.*, vol. 54: 2: 238 (1975).
10. Torri, G., Uptake and elimination of Enflurane at constant inspired and alveolar concentration. *Acta Anaesth. Belgica* 2: 190 (1974).
11. Popescu, D. T., J. Nauta and J. Spierdijk, Spontaneous ventilation during Ethrane and Halothane/Nitrous oxyde anaesthesia. *Anaesthesia and Resuscitation*, vol. 84: 203 (1974).
12. Gion, H., C. Saidman, The minimal alveolar concentration of Enflurane in man. *Anaesthesiology*, vol. 35: 4 (1971).
13. Torri, G., G. Damia and M. L. Fabiani, Effect of Nitrousoxide on the Anaesthetic requirement of Enflurane. *Brit. J. Anaesth.*, 46: 468, (1974).
14. Brown, B., R. Crout, A comparative study of the effects of five general anaesthetics on the myocardial contractility: Isometric conditions. *Anaesthesiology*, vol. 34: 3 (1971).
15. Marchal, B., P. Cohen, H. Klingenmair, J. Neigh and J. Pender, Some pulmonary and cardiovascular effects of Enflurane anaesthesia with varying pCO_2 in man. *Brit. J. Anaesth.* 43: 996 (1971).
16. Iwatsuki, N., S. Shimasato and B. Etstein, The effects of changes in time interval of stimulation on mechanics of isolated heart muscle and its response to Ethrane. *Anaesthesiology*, 32: 1: 11 (1971).

17. Ribeiro, C., M. De Luz, M. Labrunie, J. Cukier, N. Treiger and P. de Andrande, Inhalation agent: Ethrane – Compound 347. *Rev. Bras. Anaesthesiologica*, 21: 376 (1971).
18. Shimosato, S., N. Sugai, N. Iwatsuki and B. Etstein, The effect of Ethrane on cardiac muscle mechanics. *Anaesthesiology*, vol. 30: 5: 513 (1969).
19. Scovteid, P., H. Price, The effects of Ethrane on the arterial pressure, Preganglion sympathetic activity and barostatic reflexes. *Anaesthesiology*, vol. 36: 3: 257 (1972).
20. Millar, R., J. Worden, C. Couperman, H. Price, Further studies of sympathetic actions of anaesthetics in intact and spinal animals. *Brit. J. Anaesth.*, vol. 42: 366 (1970).
21. Levesque, P., V. Nanages, C. Shanks, S. Shimosato, Circulatory effects of Enflurane in normocarbic human volunteers. *Canad. Anaesth. Soc. J.*, vol. 21: 6: 580 (1974).
22. Konchigeri, H., M. Shaker, A. Winnie, Effect of Epinephrine during Enflurane Anaesthesia. *Anaesth. and Analgesia*, vol. 53: 6: 894 (1974).
23. Forbes, A. M., Halothane, Adrenalin and cardiac arrest. *Anaesthesia* 21: 22 (1966).
24. Graves, C., N. Downs, Cardiovascular and renal effects of Enflurane in surgical patients. *Anaesthesia and Analgesia*, vol. 53: 6: 898 (1974).
25. Lipman, M., L. Reisner, Epinephrine injection with Enflurane anaesthesia: Incidence of cardiac arrhytmias. *Anaesth. and Analg.*, vol. 53: 6: 886 (1974).
26. Matorras, A., Comparative study of myocardial sensinitization to norepinephrine under Halothane and Enflurane anaesthesia. *Brit. J. Anaesth.* 38: 712 (1966).
27. Katz, R. C. and G. J. Katz, Surgical infiltration of pressor drugs and their interaction with volatile anaesthetics. *Brit. J. Anaesth.*, 38: 712 (1966).
28. Van de Wall, J. and H. Delooz, Enflurane and the heart. *Acta Anaesth. Belg.*, vol. 25: 2: 266 (1974).
29. McDowell, S. A., K. D. Hall and C. R. Stephen, Difluoromethyl 1,1,2-trifluoro-2-chloroethyl ether: Experiments in dogs with a new inhalation anaesthetic agent. *Brit. J. Anaesth.* 40: 511 (1968).
30. Helrich, M., H. Cascorbi, Crossover study of Ethrane and Halothane in volunteers. *Anaesthesiology*, vol. 31: 4: 370 (1969).
31. Lebowitz, M., C. Blitt, J. Dillon, Clinical investigation of Compound 347 (Ethrane). *Anaesth. and Analg.*, vol. 49: 1: 1 (1970).
32. Lind, H. W., V. E. Lamb, The search for better anaesthetic agents: Clinical investigation of Ethrane. *Anaesthesiology*, vol. 32: 6: 555 (1970).
33. Waltemath, C., The effect of nitrous oxyde, halothane and ethrane on haemoglobin function. *Anaesth. and Analg.*, vol. 50: 3: 426 (1971).
34. Rolly, C., L. Renders-Verscichelen and P. Van der Aa, Oxygen consumption during Ethrane anaesthesia. *Acta Anaesth. Belg.*, vol. 25: 2: 246 (1974).
35. Gasparetto, A., G. Barusco, Effect of Ethrane, Halothane and Penthrane on alveolar surfactants. *Anaesth. and Resuscitation*, vol. 84: 212, 1974, Springer-Verlag, New York.
36. Bostem, F., M. Hanquet, J. P. Gollez, Ethrane and EEG. *Acta Anaesth. Belg.*, vol. 25: 2: 233 (1974).
37. Reinhold, A., M. de Rood, A. Capon, E. Mouwade, J. Fruhling and A. Verbist, The action of Ethrane on cerebral blood flow. *Acta Anaesth. Belg.*, vol. 25: 2: 257 (1974).
38. Zattoni, J., C. Siani, C. Rivano, The effects of Ethrane on intracranial pressure. *Anaesthesiology and Resuscitation*, vol. 48: 272, 1974, Springer-Verlag, New York.
39. Clark, D., E. Hosick, B. Rosmer, Neurophysiological effects of different anaesthetics in unconscious man. *Journ. Appl. Physiol.*, vol. 31: 6: 884 (1971).
40. Hosick, E., D. Clark, N. Adam and B. Rosmer, Neurophysiological effects of different anaesthetics in conscious man. *Journ. Appl. Physiol.*, vol. 31: 6: 892 (1971).

41. Joas, T. A., W. C. Stevens, E. I. Eger, EEG seizure activity in dogs during anaesthesia. *Brit. J. Anaesth.*, 43, 739 (1971).
42. Lebowitz, M., Blitt., Dillon., Enflurane induced CNS excitation and its relation to carbon dioxide tension. *Anaesth. and Analg.*, vol. 51: 3: 355 (1972).
43. Neigh, J., J. K. Garman, J. R. Harp, The electroencephalographic pattern during anaesthesia with Ethrane/Effects on depth of anaesthesia, pCO_2 and N_2O. *Anaesthesiology*, vol. 35: 5: 482 (1971).
44. Smith, A., H. Woelman, Cerebral blood flow and metabolism. *Anaesthesiology*, vol. 36: 4: 378 (1972).
45. Cohen, P. J., D. V. Heisterkamp, P. Skovsted, The effect of general anaesthetics on the response to tetanic stimulus in man. *Brit. J. Anaesth.*, 42: 543 (1970).
46. Egilmez, A., A. Dobkin, Ethrane (Compound 347) in man. *Anaesthesia*, vol. 27: 2: 171 (1972).
47. Lebowitz, M., C. Blitt, L. Walts, Depression in twitch of response to stimulation of the ulnar nerve during Ethrane Anaesthesia in man. *Anaesthesiology*, vol. 33: 1: 52 (1970).
48. Wahlin, A., K. G. Häkermank, Ethrane anaesthesia in patients with myasthenia gravis. *Acta Anaesth. Belg.*, vol. 25: 2: 215 (1974).
49. *Summary* of the National Halothane study, *JAMA* 197: 775 (1966).
50. Heyner, L., S. Johansson, A. Wahlin, The effect of Ethrane on liver function. *Anaesthesiology and Resuscitation*, vol. 84: 150, 1974. Springer-Verlag New York.
51. Soares, R. E., M. Dessai, Variations in serum enzyme (SGPT, SGOT, LDH and GT) levels during Ethrane anaesthesia in man. *Anaesth. and Resuscitation*, vol. 84: 150, 1974. Springer-Verlag New York.
52. Chase, R. E., D. Holaday, V. Viserova-Bergerova, L. Saidman, F. Mack, The biotransformation of Ethrane in man. *Anaesthesiology*, vol. 35: 3: 262 (1971).
53. Halsey, M., D. Sawyer, I. Eger, S. Behlman, D. Impelman, Depatic metabolism of Halothane, Methoxyflurane, Cyclopropane, Ethrane and Forane in miniature Swine. *Anaesthesiology*, vol. 35: 1: 43 (1971).
54. Cohen, E., Metabolism of the volatile anaesthetics. *Anaesthesiology*, vol. 35: 2: 193 (1971).
55. Linde, H., L. Berman, Non-specific stimulation of drug metabolizing enzymes by inhalation anaesthetic agents. *Anaesthesia and Analgesia*, vol. 50: 4: 656 (1971).
56. Sadove, M., S. Kim, Hepatitis after use of the two different fluorinated anaesthetic agents. *Anaesthesia and Analgesia*, vol. 53: 2: 336 (1974).
57. Cousins, M., R. Mazze, Biotransformation of Ethrane and Isoflurane (Forane). *International Anaesthesiology Clinics*, vol. 12: 2: 111 (1974).
58. Mathie, A., D. di Padua, B. D. Kahan and J. Mills, Humoral immunity to a metabolite of halothane, fluoroxene and enflurane. *Anaesthesiology*, 45: 5: 612 (1975).
59. Loehning, R., R. Mazze, Possible nephrotoxicity from Ethrane in a patient with severe renal disease. *Anaesthesiology*, vol. 40: 2: 203 (1974).
60. Barr, G. A., M. J. Cousing, R. I. Mazze, A comparision of the renal effects and metabolism of Ethrane and methoxyflurane in fischer 344 rats. *Jour. Pharmac. Exp.* 188: 257 (1974).
61. Dvoracek, B., R. Ducardus, U. J. M. van Haelst, K. Kubat, H. Lip, W. van de Pluijn, The effects of Ethrane on renal function, an experimental comparasion with Penthrane in pigs. *Anaesthesiology and Resuscitation*, vol. 84: 158, 1974, Springer-Verlag, New York.
62. Granberg, P. O., A. Wahlin, The effects of Ethrane on renal function with special reference to tubular rejection of sodium. *Anaesthesiology and Resuscitation*, vol. 84: 172 (1974).

63. Dobkin, A., D. Kim, J. Choi, A. Levy, Blood serum fluoride levels with Enflurane and Isoflurane anaesthesia during and following major abdominal surgery. *Can. Anaesth. Soc.* Journal, vol. 20: 4494, 1973.
64. Schwartz, M., T. M. Mackrell, Potency of Compound 347 (Ethrane) in inhibition of frog gastric secretion. *Proc. Soc. Exp. Biol. Med.* 136: 9294 (1971).
65. Pan-Tai-Hsiung, A. Wallacl, J. Demarco, Malignant hyperthermia associated with Enflurane anaesthesia: A case report. *Anaesthesia and Analgesia*, vol. 54: 1 (1975).
66. Relton, J. E. S., B. A. Britt, D. J. Steward, Malignant hyperthermia. *Brit. J. Anaesth.* 45: 269 (1973).
67. Xavier, L., Halogenados en obstetrica. *Revis. Brasil. de Anaesth.*, 20: 4: 525 (1970).
68. Figuerola, M., P. Tamay, C. Ortix, Evaluation of Compound 347 (Ethrane) in cesaerean section. *Rev. Mexic. de Anaesth.*, 19: 332 (1970).
69. Devoghel, J. C., Ethrane in obstetrics. *Acta Anaesth. Belgica*, vol. 25: 2 (1974).
70. Fortuna, A., Ethrane for obstetric anaesthesia. *Excerpta Medica*, Int. Congress Series, Nr. 261, Vth World Congress of Anaesthesiologistst, Kyoto, 1972, p. 172.
71. Von Hahn, H. Foirtrik, Wirkung von Ethrane auf die Blutgezinnung. *Anaesthesiology and Resuscitation*, vol. 84: 173 (1974).
72. Oyama, T., A. Matsuki, M. Kuod, Effects of Enflurane anaesthesia and surgery on carbohydrate and fat metabolism in man. *Anaesthesia*, vol. 27: 2179 (1972).
73. Kimura, K., A. Maeda, T. Oyama, Effects of Ethrane anaesthesia on endocrine, hepatic and renal function in man. *Exc. Medica*, Vth World Congress of Anaesthesiologists, Kyoto, 1972, p. 126.
74. Camu, F., Influence of Enflurane anaesthesia on carbohydrate metabolism in dogs. Nordisk Anaesthesiologisk Forening, Abstracts of the XIIth Congress of the Scandinavian Society of Anaesthesiologists, Oulu, 1975, p. 29.
75. Radtke, N., J. Waldman, The influence of Enflurane anaesthesia on intraocular pressure in youths. *Anaesthesia and Analgesia*, vol. 54: 2: 212 (1975).
76. Dobkin, A. B., D. Kim, A. A. Levy, P. A. Byles, Studies on the calibretion of Enflurane vaporizers. *Anaesthesia and Analgesia*, vol. 52: 3: 317 (1973).
77. Oehmig, H., Technische Fragen der Ethrane Anwendung, *Anaesthesiology and Resuscitation*, vol. 84: 228, 1974. Springer-Verlag, New York.
78. Kim, D., A. Dobkin, Effects of premedication on duration of anaesthesia with halogenated vapors: Chloroform, Trichcloroethylene, Halothane, Methoxyflurane, Enflurane and Isoflurane. *Can. A. Soc. Journ.*, vol. 20: 4: 389 (1973).
79. Kopriva, C. I., R. Eltringham, The use of Enflurane during resection of a Pheochromocytoma. *Anaesthesiology* vol. 41: 4: 399 (1974).
80. Dobkin, A., How to use Enflurane (Ethrane) – Experience with 5000 cases. *Anaesthesiology* 4: 108 (1974).
81. Rolly, G., B. Malcolm-Thomas and J. P. Meert, Ervaring met de continue monitoring van long compliance en luchtwegenweerstand. Congress of the Belgium Society of Anaesthesiologists, 11-13 September 1975, Brussel (Bruxelles).
82. Popescu, D. T., Symposium over Enflurane, Den Haag, juni 1975.
83. Erhorn, E., Wirkung von Ethrane auf die Blutgase bei Spontanatmung in Ethrane *Anaesthesiology and Resuscitation*. vol. 84, page 195 – Springer Berlin 1974.
84. Rugheimer, E., J. Himmler, K. Greiner, Einfluss von Ethrane auf die Atmung in Ethrane. *Anaesthesiology and Resuscitation*, vol. 84, page 186. Springer Berlin 1974.

4. CRITICAL COMPARATIVE REVIEW ABOUT ANAESTHETIC AGENTS, INCLUDING HALOTHANE

LEO STRUNIN

This review concerns serious unwanted effects. All the agents discussed will, in combination with an intravenous induction agent, produce good general anaesthetic conditions such that one is not distinguishable from another. Minor side effects, for example those on the cardio-respiratory system, are easily recognised and serious consequences are usually avoidable. Therefore one may ask why are the current halogenated hydrocarbons not entirely acceptable and why have the early agents, for example chloroform, fallen into disuse? The answer rests with the effects of these drugs on specific organs of the body, for example the kidney and liver. Damage to these organs is not necessarily apparent at the time of anaesthesia and surgery but may manifest itself in the immediate post-operative period. Clearly an agent which is always associated with organ damage would not remain in clinical use. The difficulty is that organ damage is intermittent, the mechanism is often not clear and other factors relating to disease or surgical procedures may be involved.

MECHANISMS OF ORGAN DAMAGE

A direct toxic effect is the most easily understood and liver damage associated with chloroform anaesthesia was initially thus described. However this now seems unlikely and metabolic and/or hypersensitivity reactions are the more recent explanations. Metabolism of volatile anaesthetics has been extensively studied and indeed toxic metabolites have been found in some instances. Animal models show effects of drug metabolising enzyme induction and inhibition related to increased or decreased toxicity. It has, however, always seemed to the author that such animal models, particularly relating to enzyme induction have little bearing on the situation in man. The environment is seething with enzyme inducing substances and it must be a rare patient whose liver has not undergone some enzyme induction.

It therefore seems unlikely that this alone is a significant factor in organ toxicity.

Anaesthesia and the immune response is currently a fashionable topic. That the immune response is altered by anaesthesia and surgery is beyond question. Whether this alteration is relevant in post-operative organ damage is unresolved as is a relationship to hypersensitivity. It is suggested that repeated exposure to halothane at short intervals is potentially harmful (1), and a hypersensitivity response has been implicated. So far it is not known whether this is true for all agents, but it may be that if a valuable agent is preferred this may alter the timing of surgical procedures.

CHLOROFORM

It is of interest that chloroform began to replace diethyl ether as early as 1847 (2). The reason was that deaths (cause unknown) were occurring frequently in association with ether. It was not long before similar problems arose with chloroform. These were not, however, hepatic or renal problems – they were cardiac (3). Liver and kidney damage is rare after chloroform anaesthesia but the mechanism is metabolic (4). There is free radical formation with covalent binding to tissue macromolecules and subsequent damage. Usually this is reversible. Thus we have a situation where the cardiac effects of chloroform in sensitising the myocardium to circulating catechol amines may readily cause death and renal and liver damage may occur under some circumstances. However, if care is taken it is possible to anaesthetise a small number of patients with chloroform and avoid such ill-effects (5). Nevertheless, even a cursory glance at the literature will show why chloroform is not really acceptable.

METHOXYFLURANE

This agent was first used around 1960. After some initial popularity its use has declined and indeed some have felt that it ought to be withdrawn from clinical use (6). The reason for this criticism relates to postoperative renal damage. Methoxyflurane is extensively metabolised in the body and among the metabolites are fluoride and oxalic acid. These are both nephrotoxic substances and fluoride toxicity, in particular, has been extensively studied in relation to various industrial processes. It is now clear that renal damage after methoxyflurane is dose related (in excess of 2 MAC hours will result in renal damage) (7, 8, 9, 10). Pre-existing renal damage is obviously relevant as is interaction with other nephrotoxic drugs.

Hepatitis after methoxyflurane anaesthesia has occurred. Joshie and Conn (11) have recently reviewed 24 cases. Two-thirds were obese women, half had been exposed previously to either methoxyflurane or halothane, eosinophilia was present in 20%, the liver histology was similar to viral hepatitis and there was a 58% mortality. The similarity of this hepatitis to unexplained hepatitis following halothane (UHFH) is obvious. One might ask is such hepatitis specific to the anaesthetic agents involved or an indication that in certain 'obese women' repeated anaesthesia is more than their liver can tolerate?

ENFLURANE (ETHRANE) AND ISOFORANE (FORANE)

These two compounds, isomers of each other, are the newest halogenated hydrocarbons (12, 13). Experience with isoforane is limited, but enflurane has been widely used in the USA and Europe. If one takes halothane as a reference drug then enflurane and isoforane have similar properties, cardio-respiratory depression is, however, more marked and enflurane produces EEG changes when given in high dosage with a reduced arterial carbon dioxide tension (14). The crucial point of difference relates to metabolism. Enflurane and isoforane are chemically very stable substances but nevertheless do undergo some biotransformation in man (15). Fluoride is one of the main metabolites. The actual amount metabolised is very small and it was suggested that this would result in a low incidence of toxic effects. Clinical experience has not borne this out and already cases of renal and liver damage have been reported (16, 17, 18, 19). The similarity of these case reports to those concerning methoxyflurane and halothane is obvious. If renal damage is ascribed to fluoride, could the hepatic damage be further evidence of a specific 'liver response' to anaesthesia in some individuals?

HALOTHANE

This agent has been widely available for nearly 20 years. Clinical usage and investigation has been on an unprecedented scale as compared with any other anaesthetic drug. The limitations of halothane are easily identified, with the exception of liver damage, and one does not need to be in anaesthetic practice long to realise why it is widely used. Nevertheless, the spectre of unexplained hepatitis following halothane (UHFH) has lead to restrictions on halothane usage, particularly with respect to repeated exposure. Are such precautions necessary, what is the present position with regard to UHFH?

Four papers in 1971 (20, 21, 22, 23) and the recent (1974) analysis of reports to the Committee on Safety of Medicines (1) provide the background to the problem. In summary, retrospective studies seem to show that unexplained hepatitis may occur in rare instances when halothane anaesthesia is repeated within a short period. However, there is no evidence available to show that a second anaesthetic involving halothane carries a greater overall risk to a patient than one involving other anaesthetic agents. Similarly no data is available concerning repeated non-halothane anaesthetics. Although the findings of Joshie and Conn (11) on methoxyflurane associated hepatitis may be significant the mechanism of UHFH is unknown.

Metabolism of halothane in man has not been studied extensively. As yet no hepatotoxic metabolite has been demonstrated (24). Immunological studies of patients with UHFH have failed to demonstrate a hypersensitivity response (25). Nevertheless these mechanisms cannot be ruled out and further work is required.

Prospective studies, although desirable, raise considerable technical and ethical problems if halothane and non-halothane anaesthesias are to be compared. Regrettably two such studies (26, 27) have not been very contributory. All patients received halothane at least once and most were suffering from neoplasia. Therefore, when the need for repeated anaesthesia within a short time arises, it remains a matter for the clinical judgement of the anaesthetist concerned to decide whether a further halothane or non-halothane anaesthetic is in the best overall interests of the patient. Clearly this judgement will relate to all the clinical circumstances.

CONCLUSION

All currently used volatile agents in the course of producing general anaesthesia may have unwanted effects. It is probably pharmacologically and physiologically naive to suppose that an 'ideal agent' can be developed. Therefore the imperfections of existing drugs should be carefully investigated, so that a reasoned judgement on choice may be made in a given situation to cause the least harm.

REFERENCES

1. Inman, W. H. W. and W. W. Mushin, Jaundice after repeated exposure to halothane: An analysis of reports to Committee of Safety of Medicines. *Brit. Med. J.* 1, 5 (1974).
2. Rook, A., The first experiences with ether anaesthesia in Cambridgeshire and West Suffolk 1847. *Anaesthesia* 30, 677.
3. Matsuki, A. and E. K. Zsigmond, The first fatal case of chloroform anaesthesia in the United States. *Anaesth. and Analges.* 53, 152 (1974).
4. Inhett, K. F., W. D. Reid, I. G. Sipes and G. Krishna, Chloroform toxicity in mice: Correlation of renal and hepatic necrosis with covalent binding of metabolites to tissue macromolecules. *Exp. Molec. Path.* 19, 215 (1973).
5. Smith, A., P. P. Volpitto, Z. W. Gramling et al., Chloroform, halothane and regional anaesthesia: A complete study. *Anaesth. and Analges.* 52, 1 (1973).
6. Desmond, J. W., Methoxyflurane nephrotoxicity. *Canad. Anaesth. Soc. J.* 21, 294 (1974).
7. Mazze, R. I., G. L. Shut and S. H. Jackson, Renal dysfunction associated with methoxyflurane anaesthesia: A randomised, prospective clinical evaluation. *J.A.M.A.* 216, 278 (1971).
8. Mazze, R. I. and M. J. Cousins, Renal toxicity of anaesthetics: with specific reference to the nephrotoxicity of methoxyflurane. *Canad. Anaesth. Soc. J.* 20, 64 (1973).
9. Robertson, G. S. and W. F. D. Hamilton, Methoxyflurane and renal function. *Brit. J. Anaesth.* 45, 55 (1973).
10. Cousins, M. J. and R. I. Mazze, Methoxyflurane nephrotoxicity: a study of dose response in man. *J.A.M.A.* 225, 1611 (1973).
11. Joshie, P. H. and H. O. Conn, The syndrome of methoxyflurane associated hepatitis. *Ann. Intern. Med.* 80, 395 (1974).
12. Dobkin, A. B., R. Nishioka, D. B. Gengaje and D. S. Rim, Ethrane (Compound 347) Anaesthesia: A clinical and laboratory review of 700 cases. *Anaesth. and Analges.* 48, 477 (1969).
13. Dobkin, A. B., P. H. Byles, S. Chanvoni and D. A. Valubuena, Clinical and laboratory evaluation of a new inhalation anaesthetic: Forane (Compound 469). *Canad. Anaesth. Soc. J.* 18 264, (1971).
14. Joas, T. A., W. C. Stevens and E. I. Eger, Electroencephalographic seizure activity in dogs during anaesthesia. *Brit. J. Anaesth.* 43, 739 (1971).
15. Chase, R. E., D. A. Holaday and V. Fiserora-Bergerova, The biotransformation of Ethrane in man. *Anaesthsiology* 35, 262 (1971).
16. Loehning, R. W. and R. I. Malle, Possible nephrotoxicity from enflurane in a patient with severe renal disease. *Anaesthesiology* 40, 203 (1974).
17. Mazze, R. E. and R. W. Loehning, Enflurane toxicity. *Anaesthesiology* 41, 102 (1974).
18. Van Der Reis, L., S. J. Askin, G. N. Freckar and W. J. Fitzgerald, Hepatic necrosis after enflurane anaesthesia. *J.A.M.A.* 227, 76 (1974).
19. Sadove, M. S. and S. I. Kin, Hepatitis after use of two difference fluorinated anaesthetic agents. *Anaesth. and Analges.* 53, 336 (1974).
20. Mushin, W. W., M. Rosen and E. V. Jones, Post-halothane jaundice in relation to previous administration of halothane. *Brit. Med. J.* 3, 18 (1971).
21. Sharpstone, P., D. R. R. Medley and R. Williams, Halothane hepatitis: A preventable disease? *Brit. Med. J.* 1, 448 (1971).
22. Sherlock, S. Progress report: Halothane hepatitis. *Gut* 12, 324 (1971).
23. Simpson, B. R., L. Strunin and B. Walton, The halothane dilemma: A case for the defence. *Brit. Med. J.* 4, 96 (1971).
24. Strunin, L. and B. R. Simpson, Halothane in Britain today. *Brit. J. Anaesth.* 44, 919 (1972).

25. Walton, B., D. C. Dumonde, C. Williams, D. Jones and J. M. Strunin, Lymphocyte transformation: Absence of increased response in alleged halothane jaundice. *J.A.M.A.* 225, 494 (1973).
26. Wright, P., O. E. Eade, M. Chisholm, M. Hawksley, M. Lloyd, T. M. Mole, J. C. Edwards, M. J. Gardner, Controlled prospective study of the effect on liver function of multiple exposure to halothane. *Lancet* 1, 817 (1975).
27. Trowell, J., R. Peto and A. Crampton Smith, Controlled trial of repeated halothane anaesthetics in patients with carcinoma of the uterine cervix treated with radium. *Lancet* 1, 821 (1975).

PART TWO

DRUGS USED IN LOCAL ANAESTHESIA

5. PHARMACOLOGY, TOXICITY, CLINICAL USE

D. T. POPESCU

Medicine started as an empirical science, based on observation and determined by the therapeutic possibilities at any given time.

For many years, after its discovery in 1884, cocaine was the only chemical local anaesthetic (fig. 1). Progress came 20 years later when Einhorn synthe-

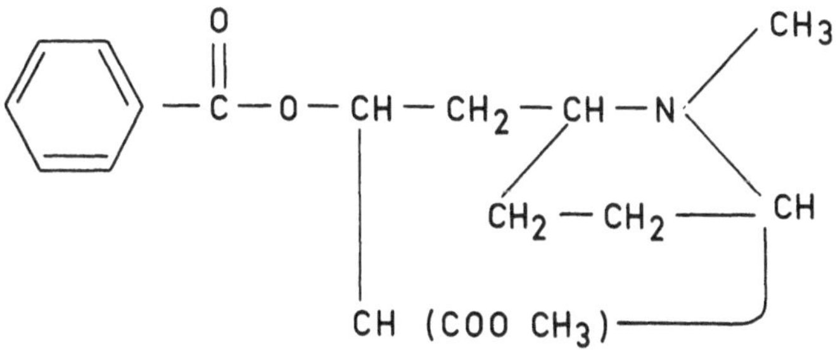

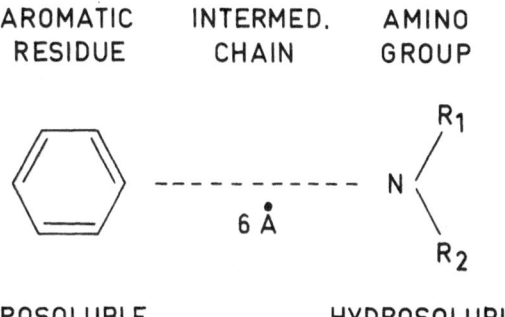

Fig. 1. Cocaine.

sized procaine. It was later recognised that there are three important characteristics of the bulky cocaine molecule (also found in procaine) (fig. 2): the aromatic residue (liposoluble pole of the molecule), the amino group (hydrosoluble pole) and the intermediate chain, which is an ester linkage (later Lofgren discovered that its length is 6 Å (1)).

AROMATIC   INTERMED.   AMINO
RESIDUE   CHAIN   GROUP

LIPOSOLUBLE   HYDROSOLUBLE

Fig. 2. Early structural formula of local anaesthetics.

When it was established that the intermediate chain can also be an amido linkage (fig. 3), dibucaine (nupercaine) was produced (1928) but it was another 20 years before a safe and widely accepted drug was synthesized: lidocaine (1946). Since then industry has produced a large number of local anaesthetics and today, it seems to be difficult for the anaesthetist to choose between them. Some authors (2, 3) look for an 'ideal local anaesthetic'. We

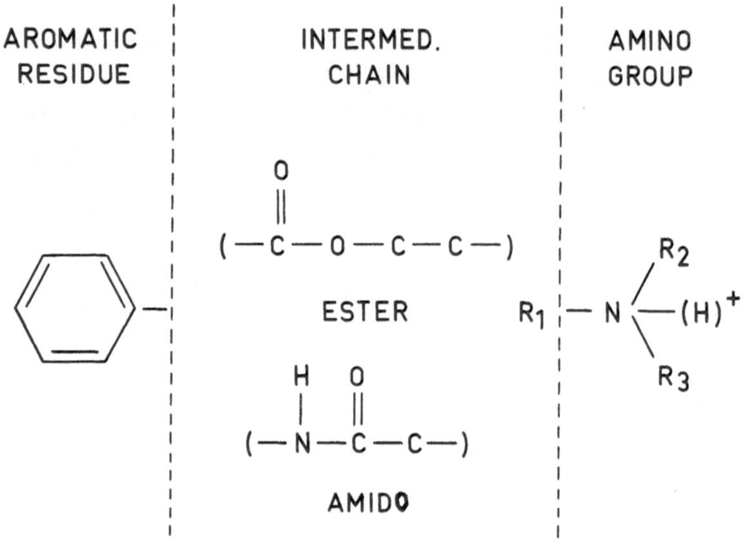

| AROMATIC | INTERMED. | AMINO |
| RESIDUE | CHAIN | GROUP |

Fig. 3. Complete structural scheme. H⁺ = ionised form.

believe that in 1975 we may not make the mistake of earlier medical specialists who years ago called every tumour 'cancer' and thus looked for an universal therapy. Different operations demand different types of analgesia and/or muscle relaxation. Various local anaesthetic techniques require different qualities of the drug in use. Our knowledge of the molecular mechanism of action of anaesthetics is incomplete. It is wiser under these conditions to understand the pharmacology and the different qualities of various local anaesthetics as thoroughly as possible and to make good use of them.

The definition of local anaesthetics is: drugs that reversibly block nerve conduction when applied locally to nerve tissue in the appropriate concentration (3). Due to the fact that this action is bound to the chemical bipolar structure shown above (fig. 3), a large number of drugs demonstrate local anaesthetic activity: phenothiazines, alpha and beta blockers, parasympatholytics, spasmolytics, analgesics, tranquilizers, antiseptics, antibiotics, etc.

Since the main action of many of these lies elsewhere, the number of drugs listed as local anaesthetics is smaller and yet some feel that there are still too many on the market (3).

PHARMACOLOGICAL ACTION

We can distinguish here between the local anaesthetic (or blocking) action and the general effects, regarded mostly as side-effects.

Local action
It is easy to say that nerve impulse generation and conduction are both prevented by these drugs but this does not explain their mechanism of action.

It is better to say that local anaesthetics interfere with the transient but marked increase in the permeability of membranes for sodium and potassium ions which is produced by nerve action (depolarisation).

That other ions can be important (calcium) has also been demonstrated (3). Not only the action potential is reduced or blocked but the resting

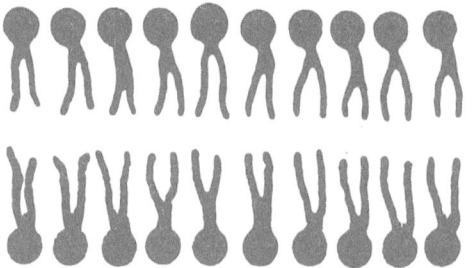

Fig. 4. The lipid bilayer.

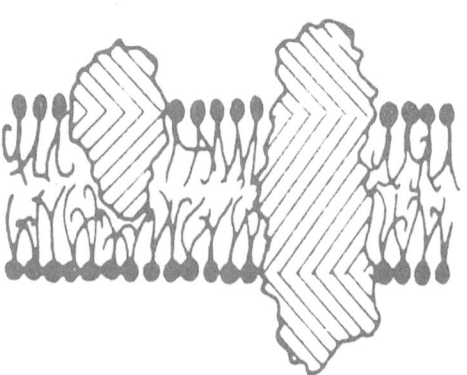

Fig. 5. The lipid bilayer with dynamic sodium channels. After Meymaris (4) with kind permission of the author and editor.

potential is also influenced. The effect depends on the physiological state of the nerve before the block. Straub (cit. 3) demonstrated that procaine produces a slight rise in potential in a normal nerve, a slight drop in a nerve in a catelectrotonic state and no change in a nerve in an anelectrotonic state. This can also be explained by the reduction of the permeability of the resting membrane for sodium, potassium and other ions.

The precise mechanism whereby a local anaesthetic influences the permeability of the membrane is not yet fully understood. It is however quite useful to enumerate the successive steps, as our understanding of the molecular structure of the membrane progressed from the simple lipid bilayer theory of Gorten-Grendel (4) (fig. 4) to the dynamic fluid mosaic model of Singer and Nicholson with sodium channels (fig. 5). In the days when membranes were thought to be simple bilayers of lipids the *surface charge theory* was accepted. This stated that the local anaesthetic agent is bound to the membrane presumably by the lipophilic end of the molecule, its cationic head remaining outside the cell. The resting potential of the cell remains constant but the transmembrane potential increases considerably, thus blocking the possibility of depolarisation (5). With our present-day knowledge of the molecular structure of the membranes it is less probable that this explains the blocking mechanism.

Recently Takman (6) used new concepts to establish an exhaustive classification of all local blocking agents (fig. 6).

I. POOR PENETRATING THROUGH MEMBRANES.

    A. ACTING AT THE EXTERNAL OPENING OF Na CHANNEL,

                Tetrodotoxin, Saxitoxin.

    B. ACTING AT THE INTERNAL OPENING OF Na CHANNEL,

        (RECEPTOR), Quaternary ammonium ions (Permanent + charge).

II. PENETRATING WITH RELATIVE EASE.

    C. ACTING THROUGH PHYSICO - CHEMICAL PROP.

        (RECEPTOR INDEPENDENT) (NO ELECTRICAL CHARGE),

                Benzocaine.

   B.C. ACTING BOTH AT RECEPTOR AT INSIDE Na CHANNEL

       AND THROUGH PHYSICO - CHEMICAL MECHANISM,

              Local anaesthetics.

Fig. 6. After Takman (6) with kind permission of the author and editor.

The amino (basic) group of the local anaesthetics is secondary or tertiary (bound to two or three radicals) and exists in aqueous solutions as a mixture of the two forms, uncharged base (fig. 7) and the charged ionic or acid form, according to an equilibrium characterised for every drug by its dissociation constant (pKa). In other words in a solution of lidocaine (for example) we will find both forms, ionised and non-ionised (fig. 8), which

$$(BH^+) + H_2O \rightleftharpoons B + H_2OH^+$$

$$\text{tot Conc} = (BH^+) + (B)$$

$$\text{Log} \frac{(BH^+)}{(B)} = pKa - pH$$

Fig. 7. Local anaesthetic drug in solution.

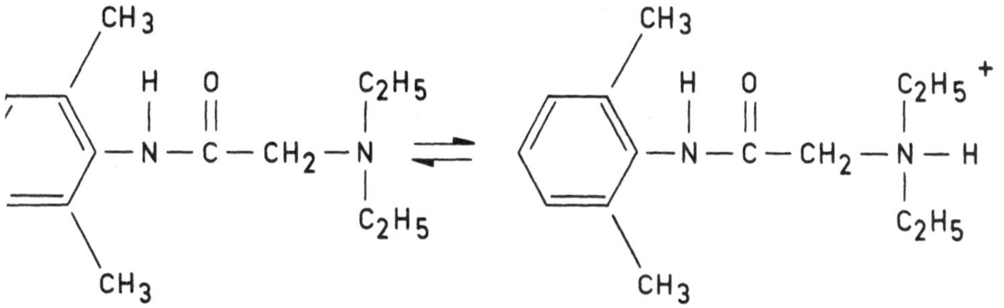

UNIONISED   IONISED

Fig. 8. Lidocaine in solution.

explains its pharmacological quality (blocking properties outside and inside the sodium channels) and its classification in group BC.

It is easier for us, as nonchemists, to understand this phenomenon if we remember that in the form of a free base local anaesthetics are poorly soluble and unstable: they are therefore prepared as water soluble salts, usually hydrochlorides. These salts are acid and easily dissociable.

There is abundant evidence that the acid salts must first be neutralised in the tissues to liberate the free base, before the drug can penetrate nerves and produce its blocking action. Whether the local active form is the true base or the ionised form is still debatable.

The necessary break-down of the acid form explains the known fact that local anaesthetics are less active (or inactive) when injected into an inflammed area (local tissular acidosis) or in patients with renal insufficiency (general acidosis but also neuritis).

This also explains why some laboratories have tried to introduce carbonated salts in the place of hydrochloric salts. A shorter latency and more intense sensory and motor blocks were attributed by some to these salts (7, 8, 9).

A second theory to explain the precise mechanism of action is *the membrane expansion theory*, which was proposed by Shanes (1958) (5). The penetration of the lipophilic pole of the local anaesthetic into the membrane causes a mechanical expansion which constricts the sodium channels. Johnson and Miller (cit. 5) postulate that the anaesthetic agent increases the freedom of movement (disorder) within the lipid molecules leading to expansion of the lipids which produces corresponding changes in the proteinic pores (constriction of sodium channels). The fact that pressure reverses local anaesthesia – as well as general anaesthesia – and our search for an unique explanation of the mechanism of action make this theory very attractive.

Specific receptor theory

A specific receptor for local anaesthetics was suggested by Ehrlich and Einhorn as early as 1894 (cit. 6). Recent experiences with various substances with local anaesthetic action, which have very dissimilar molecules but a similar ammonium pole, suggest the existance of a specific receptor existing in the nerve membrane.

That the receptor must be on the inner surface of the membrane is demonstrated by the local anaesthetic action of quaternary ammonium compounds which are unable to penetrate the membrane and are active only when applied from inside (10). That this receptor is at, or near, the sodium channel was demonstrated by Strichartz (cit. 5).

We have tried to summarize the last two theories on the following slide (fig. 9), a modification of Ritchie. The two forms, pure base (B) and ionised base (BH$^+$), are present in the extraneural space (e). Only the pure base penetrates the nerve sheath where it dissociates (Bp $\rightleftarrows$ BH$^+$P). The pure base penetrates the membrane (Bm) producing expansion (disorder) of the lipid layers with narrowing of the sodium channel. The pure base further penetrates the axoplasm (Bi) where it dissociates (BH$^+$ i); the dissociated

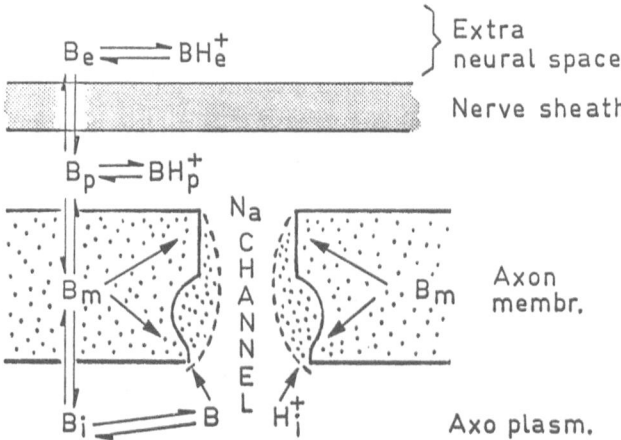

Fig. 9. Working mechanism of local anaesthetics modified after Ritchie (5) with kind permission from author and editor.

form reacts with the receptors and blocks (from inside) the sodium channel.

In connection with subcellular mechanisms, I would like to mention the experiments of Haschke and Fink (11) who demonstrated a dose-dependent reversible uncoupling of the oxidative phosphorylation by lidocaine (5-10 mM) in the porcine brain mitochondria and an inhibition of the electron transport rate (50% at 8mM) at the NADH-dehydrogenase level. Their conclusion is that the depression by lidocaine of the rapid axonal transport is due to the depression of oxidative metabolism.

PHARMACOKINETICS

Fate of local anaesthetics
Chemical structure is extremely important for the metabolic pathway of inactivation. With the exception of cocaine man rapidly inactivates *ester compounds* (procaine, chloroprocaine) in blood by hydrolysis with plasma cholinesterase. We can do it 4 to 20 times faster than other animals (12).

This explains their reputed low toxicity, their short duration of action and the difficulties encountered in the measurement of the concentration of these compounds in blood (13).

Amido bound anaesthetics (anilide type; lidocaine, mepivacaine, bupivacaine, etidocaine) are mainly inactivated in the liver by microsomal enzymes after a somewhat longer period.

This explains their reputation of higher toxicity, their longer duration of action, the possibility of a precise determination of blood levels and the possibility of correlating these concentrations with the toxic effects. Enzyme induction by phenobarbital has been demonstrated in dogs: 50% of a lidocaine dose was metabolised in induced dogs in comparison to 25% in normal living animals (14).

The symptoms the anaesthetist does not want to see are the side-effects of local anaesthetics. As there is generally a direct relationship between plasma concentration and adverse reactions (15), we shall concentrate a little longer on various factors affecting this parameter. The actual plasma concentration is the result of (fig. 10) the dynamic equilibrium between absorption, distribution, metabolism and excretion.

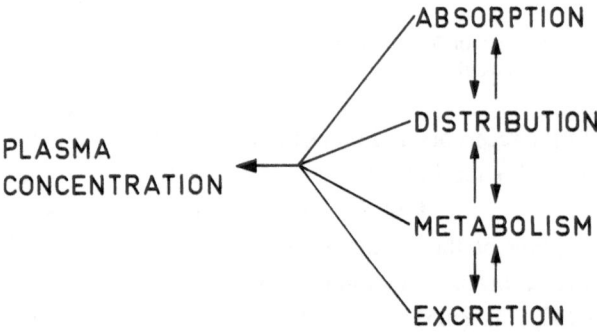

Fig. 10. Actual plasma concentration.

Even for anilide-type anaesthetics, which are characterized by a slow excretion, this factor plays only a negligible role in the equilibrium during the initial hours after administration.

Absorption, distribution – redistribution and metabolism are important and of course the rate at which they occur is the most significant point.

For the ester linkage types metabolism is very rapid, and therefore the rate of absorption is the most important factor. Since it is also important for the amido linkage types, let us concentrate on this factor.

Absorption can be influenced by the patient, the anaesthetist and the drug (fig. 11). Patients who are dehydrated, have a high cardiac output (high temperature (16)) or are alkalotic will have high absorption rates; they will be even higher if the drugs are administered in highly vascularized areas.

The anaesthetist can produce high absorption rates by giving the drug directly intravenously or intramuscularly, giving repeated injections, using plain solutions or adding hyaluronidase (17).

ABSORPTION

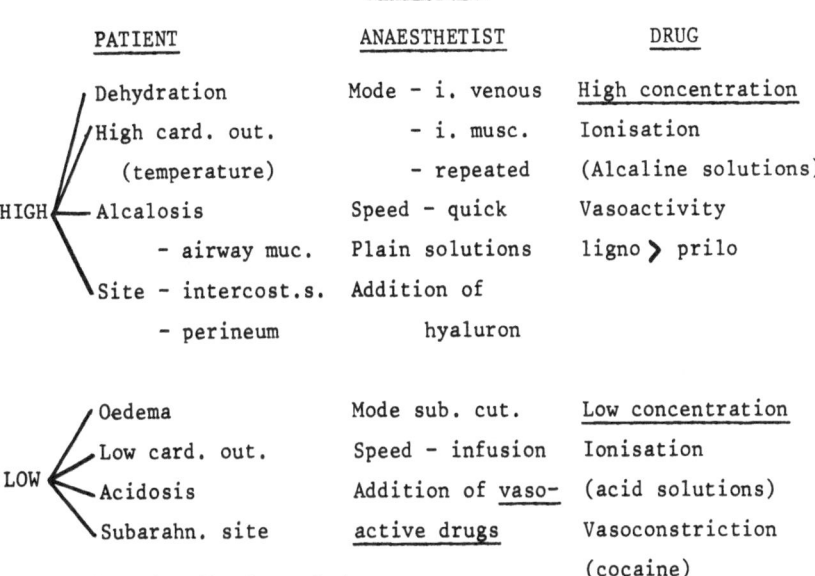

PATIENT	ANAESTHETIST	DRUG

Dehydration   Mode - i. venous   High concentration

High card. out.   - i. musc.   Ionisation

(temperature)   - repeated   (Alcaline solutions)

HIGH — Alcalosis   Speed - quick   Vasoactivity

    - airway muc.   Plain solutions   ligno ⟩ prilo

Site - intercost.s. Addition of

    - perineum   hyaluron

Oedema   Mode sub. cut.   Low concentration

Low card. out.   Speed - infusion   Ionisation

LOW — Acidosis   Addition of vaso- (acid solutions)

Subarahn. site   active drugs   Vasoconstriction

                                              (cocaine)

Fig. 11. Absorption of local anaesthetics.

As far as the drug is concerned: high concentrations, alkaline solutions and vasoactive anaesthetics (lidocaine) are absorbed more quickly.

One apparently paradoxical effect should be mentioned here: acidotic patients have slow absorption rates, thus lower plasma levels, but higher toxicity. This is due to the fact that absorption is slower (only in the unionised form) but once it has penetrated into the cells, intracellular acidosis causes marked ionisation of the anaesthetic and thus the effect is pronounced. The toxic effect is due to the ionised active form which is 'trapped' (18) in the acidotic cells of vital organs.

Distribution of local anaesthetics is not yet fully understood but some data are pertinent. It is probably influenced by the drug through its plasma protein binding coefficient (fig. 12).

We have to remember that there is always an equilibrium in plasma between the bound and the unbound part of the molecule. This equilibrium is specific for each drug: 92.2% for bupivacaine, 82,3% for mepivacaine, 70.6% for lidocaine (19) and 94% for etidocaine. Only the unbound fraction of the drug will pass through membranes. This means a low tissue blood coefficient for drugs with high protein binding. These drugs (bupivacaine, etidocaine) will have a slower onset of action, a longer duration and a slow metabolism.

Placental passage is also correlated to protein binding because again only

64   D. T. POPESCU

DISTRIBUTION

DRUG	PATIENT	ANAESTHETIST
PROTEIN BINDING	ACIDOSIS	CHOICE OF DRUG
influences	more hydrophilic fr.	ON
- ONSET	more anaesth. in	PHARMACOLOGY
- DURATION	lungs, erythroc.	
- METABOLISM	HEPATIC PERFUSION	
- PLACENTAL	- CARDIAC OUTPUT	
TRANSFER	- SPLANCHNIC FLOW	
High: bupivac.	HEPATIC INSUFFIC.	
etidoc.		

Fig. 12. Distribution of local anaesthetics.

the unbound fraction will pass freely into the foetal circulation. The maternal foetal coefficient is high for lidocaine and mepivacaine (about 1%) and low for bupivacaine (0.25-0.30%) (15, 20).

Comparing blood levels after peridural anaesthesia for delivery, Brown et al., (21) recently demonstrated that when equal doses are administered to the mother 23% more mepivacaine than lidocaine is found in the newborn.

Distribution of local anaesthetics can also be influenced by the patient's condition. It was demonstrated that during acidosis the ratio of the hydrophilic to the lipophilic component is elevated. This can interfere with capillary diffusion which explains the higher concentration of bupivacaine found in the lungs of acidotic patients (15). The higher concentration of these drugs in erythrocytes in acidotic patients may also reflect a pH-dependent change in the membrane transport. Since amido derivatives are metabolised mainly in the liver, their distribution will also depend on hepatic circulation; low cardiac output syndromes, low splanchnic circulation and hepatic insufficiency will diminish the clearance of these drugs giving rise to high plasma concentrations and toxic effects even when low doses are administered. The anaesthetist can use these pharmacological data and choose his anaesthetic judiciously on the basis of the clinical condition of the patient. We must remember that the newborn child has a lower capacity for metabolising local anaesthetic agents than the mother.

SIDE-EFFECTS

We anaesthetists consider as side-effects all pharmacological actions of these drugs other than the local anaesthetic activity.

CARDIOVASCULAR EFFECTS

We used to regard local anaesthetics as myocardial depressants and with the exception of cocaine as vasodilators. Recent investigations involving plasma concentration contradict this theory in many respects. Studies on isolated atrial and ventricular muscle reveal that local anaesthetics resemble chinidine in their cardiac actions: they increase the effective refractory period, raise the threshold for stimulation and prolong conduction time. This led to the use of lidocaine in cardiology.

But the cardiac effect in a healthy man (or animal) is more complex. Jorfeld et al. (22) demonstrated that subconvulsive doses of lidocaine in man and dogs (4-6 micro g/ml) produce an increase in heart rate and occasionally an increased systemic vascular resistance.

With higher doses (5-7 micro g/ml) Klein et al. (23) demonstrated an increased mean arterial pressure and systemic vascular resistance without any indication of altered myocardial function. These effects can be explained by the stimulating effect (or depression of the inhibitory activity) of the drugs on the central nervous system, evoked through the sympathetic system (24). Higher doses of local anaesthetics will cause cardiac depression.

The increase in the peripheral resistance can be explained by the increase in the tone of the capacitance vessels (also of the resistance vessels if administered intra-arterially). It is important to remember that local anaesthetics will produce vasoconstriction in a vascular bed whose tone has been experimentally decreased. These vasoactive effects seem to be due to alteration of the cytoplasmic concentration of free calcium ions (24). Special anaesthetic techniques (peridural, spinal) may have important cardiovascular effects due either to the quantity of the anaesthetic (higher in the peridural technique) the extent of the sympathetic block or the addition of adrenalin to the anaesthetic solution (25).

Effects on ventilation
The effect on the rate and depth of respiration parallels the other effects on the central nervous system (26).

The bronchodilatation effect has been described for some local anaesthetics (procaine) but has no clinical significance in the treatment of asthmatic patients (3).

This effect is stronger when the anaesthetic is applied locally and most probably is due to a stablizing effect on the membrane of smooth muscles in the trachea and bronchi.

Effect on liver function
When administered correctly local anaesthesia has no adverse effects on liver function. The effect of hypotension (collapse, shock) during local anaesthesia can be as deleterious as it is during other anaesthetic techniques.

Effects on kidney function
Local anaesthetics influence kidney function only in special techniques (peridural, spinal) when high levels are reached (above T 5) through the sympathetic block. Addition or omission of the vasopressive agent to the anaesthetic solution can also modify this action.

Effects on the inflammatory response
Recent studies have demonstrated that local anaesthetics in clinical doses can interfere with the inflammatory response, inhibiting nucleic acid synthesis (27), phagocytosis and metabolism (28) of human leukocytes in vitro. The importance of these findings for the clinician is not clear; it is unlikely that systemic resistance to infection will be modified, but local effects could be important.

Effect on neuromuscular junction, and ganglionic synapse
Past investigations (Harvey 1939, cit. 3) demonstrated that procaine reduced the response to nerve stimulation but did not affect direct muscular stimulation. Jaco in 1974 (cit. 3) suggested that procaine diminishes the production of acetylcholine in the motor nerves. Similarly procaine blocks ganglionic transmission and reduces the production of acetylcholine by preganglionic stimulation (3).

Effect on smooth muscle
Local anaesthetics depress contraction of the smooth muscles in vitro and in vivo. Depression of tracheobronchial muscle has already been mentioned. It is not clear whether this depression in vivo is due solely to the direct effect on the membrane of the muscle cells, or is a combined effect of this with the local blocking of the nervous reflexes.

Effects on the central nervous system

Classically local anaesthetics have a biphasic action on the central nervous system: initial stimulation, followed by depression and death, usually due to respiratory failure (3).

Clinical experience and more recent studies (79) have demonstrated that we should also consider an initial depression period characterised by: sleepiness, sensation of cold, feeling of pressure on the forehead, numbness of the lips and tongue as well as difficulties in talking.

This period is followed by an excitation period with: restlessness, tremor, convulsions which can lead to opisthotonus. Death can occur in this phase due to the failure of ventilation movements. This period is explained by Frank and Sanders (cit. 3) and de Jong (30) by the depression in the first instance of inhibitory neurons in the central nervous system. Wikinsky (31) claims that a subcortical depressant effect causes the convulsions. The last phase is the depression of central activity: sleep or coma, respiratory failure (of central origin) and if everything goes well amnesia follows.

Recent electro-encephalographic studies (37) confirmed this clinical evolution and showed only small differences between the four anaesthetics tested. Sakabe (33) demonstrated that low doses depress while high (convulsant doses increase cerebral oxygen consumption.

INTERACTION WITH OTHER DRUGS

Combinations of local anaesthetics

Some authors recommend this approach in order to combine the short onset of one (choroprocaine) with the longer duration of another (bupivacaine) (34) or to lessen the doses and thus the probability of toxic reactions (35), or to combine an ester type with an amido type (chloroprocaine, bupivacaine) (36).

In our opinion combinations are to be avoided because we still do not know everything about these drugs and the reactions may be additive (37) and unpredictable (38).

CARDIOVASCULAR DRUGS

Interactions with chinidine can lead to severe bradycardia, since local anaesthetics have the same effect on the myocardium.

68 D. T. POPESCU

VASOCONSTRICTORS

Local anaesthetics are often combined with vasoconstrictors in order to reduce their rate of absorption (39) and thus to minimize toxic reactions. Addition of vasopressors prolongs the duration of anaesthesia (40, 41) and produces a better block in peridural techniques (42). Addition of vasoconstrictors to short lasting anaesthetics (lidocaine, mepivacaine) seems to be indicated. For the newer, long lasting compounds opinions differ: Kier (43) found no advantages for bupivacaine, but Bromage (44) did, while Bridenbaugh sees (39) no use for etidocaine in peridural techniques.

When combining vasoconstrictors and local anaesthetics we should always remember that vasoconstrictors:
- have contra-indications: hypertension, tachycardia, extrasystoles.
- are not always necessary: bupivacaine, plexus blocks (45).
- do not diminish the frequency of toxic reactions (46).
- have their own side-effects: local (ischaemia, oedema, gangrene) as well as general (hypertension, tachycardia) (47).
- concentrations above 1:100,000 produce more side-effects (47) whereas concentrations above 1:200,000 have no stronger vasoactive effect (46).

Claims have appeared in the past few years that ornithinvasopressin (POR 80) is superior to adrenalin since it has fewer side-effects (48, 49, 50).

GENERAL ANAESTHETICS

The technique of intravenous infusions of local anaesthetics during general anaesthesia was introduced for cardiac stabilisation (procaine) (N. de Bouchet) and/or better intraoperative (lidocaine) (51, 52) or postoperative analgesia (53). It was found that the combination diethylether – procaine can be deleterious, just as any combination of ether with adrenergic blockers. With thiopentone, nitrous-oxide or halothane techniques no adverse effects are mentioned by some (54). Others (55) stress that barbiturates administered together with halothane result in cardiovascular depression.

Neither the duration of sleep nor the requirements of postoperative analgesics were influenced (52) by intravenous infusion of lidocaine.

MUSCLE RELAXANTS

A reduction in the required dose of relaxant was reported for both succinyl-choline 13-17% (52, 56) and d-tubocurarine (3). Both types of local ana-esthetic (esters and amidos) have the same effect (3, 52, 56).

The explanation may be that they have the same metabolizing enzyme (esters and succinylcholine) or that they diminish the acetylcholine produc-tion at the motor end-plate (3); it is also possible that they both interfere with the cellular mechanisms of calcium ions (24).

PHENOTHIAZINES

Association with chlorpromazine should increase the toxicity of local anaesthetics (57).

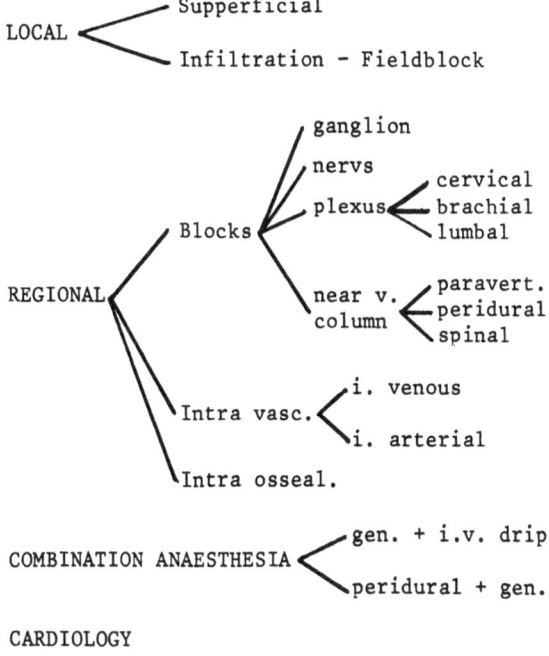

Fig. 13. Clinical use.

CLINICAL USE

Before starting to use local anaesthetics, it is wise to remember that however minor it may seem, the decision to use anaesthesia for diagnostic, surgical or therapeutic purposes is a truly medical one. It is also necessary to be able to answer positively the following seven questions:
– do I know the patient and the operation to be performed?
– do I know the regional anatomy?
– do I know the pharmacology of the drug?
– do I master the technique?
– do I have the necessary instruments?
– do I know the possible complications?
– am I ready to treat the side-effects and complications?
Figure 13 summarizes the use of local anaesthetics.

Pure local anaesthesia: as superficial (drips, spray, instillations, pommade) or as infiltration anaesthesia.

Regional anaesthesia: blocks can be achieved in some ganglions (superior cervical, gasserian), in many nerves (radial, median, ulnar, femoral, etc.), in some plexus (cervical, brachial, lumbar), and near the vertebral column (paravertebral, peridural, spinal). Intravascular techniques (intravenous or intra-arterial) and intra-osseal techniques (calcaneus) also give good results.

Local anaesthetics can be used in combination anaesthesia (intravenous drip adjuvant for general anaesthesia) or as regional blocks complemented with light general anaesthesia.

As clinical anaesthetists we should be aware of the possible *toxicity* of local anaesthetics, but also remember that there is no general agreement about the notion 'toxicity'.

For us, bradycardia is a symptom of toxicity while the cardiologist administers lidocaine in order to produce bradycardia. There are important differences between species (and many toxicological studies are performed in various species), differences in the techniques of administration (subcutaneous, peridural, intravenous, etc.) and differences in the interpretation of the gravity of the symptoms. We have to consider acute symptoms of toxicity and delayed toxic effects (neuropathy (59)). We must remember that for the local effects, it is impossible to define the boundary between functional changes and permanent toxic effects. Fink, Aasheim and Ngai (60, 61, 62) describe the local inhibition of the microtubular transport of various enzymes as the possible mechanism of anaesthesia but warn that if experimental 'anaesthesia' of the rabbit vagus nerves with 0.6% lidocaine is prolonged for more then 90 minutes (60) permanent damage of the axonal transport occurs. This can be in their opinion the mechanism of postanaesthetic neuropathy. Adams et al. (63) demonstrated that local degenerative lesions in the spinal cord are produced only by highly concentrated solutions.

From the practical point of view, we anaesthetists are most interested in the general symptoms of acute toxicity. Any adverse functional (or structural) change in an organ or functional system due to the direct effect of the local anaesthetic or its metabolites (64) should be considered a toxic effect.

We must be able to recognise the symptoms quickly to understand the pathophysiological changes and to treat them immediately.

Prevention is better than treatment and therefore it is desirable to start prevention with premedication. Prevention of convulsions (the most dangerous toxic effect) is not provided by barbiturates, gamma OH, Thalamonal or ketamine – in rats (65). Prevention cannot be achieved by prior administration of oxygen (66) although it is efficient once convulsions begin (33). Nitrous oxyde and diazepam raise the seizure threshold for lidocaine more than twofold in various species (65, 67, 68), thus offering real prevention against convulsions although not protecting against cardiovascular effects (69). It seems from the preceding that the best premedication should be diazepam. In practice however the patient becomes too sleepy with diazepam which hampers assessment of the analgetic level; therefore we prefer the combination Thalamonal-atropine which offers the advantage of preventing reactive vasoconstriction in the non-anaesthetised regions during spinal and peridural techniques. After regional anaesthesia is established and the desired level of analgesia is reached, we use diazepam for hypnosis and protection against eventual toxic reactions.

It is generally agreed that for anilide derivatives, toxic reactions correlate with the plasma level of the free fraction of the anaesthetic (not bound to proteins (Scott disagrees – 70)). With lidocaine convulsions appear when the plasma level is higher than 10 microg/ml (71). Although it was generally agreed that procaine is less toxic than lidocaine, Cahill et al. (72) demonstrated that when expressed in mg/kg/min lidocaine is the less toxic drug.

We have to distinguish between the specific toxic effects of the individual drugs. Prilocaine (propitoxaine, Citanest) which was introduced 11 years ago (under the name of L. 67) was reputed to be of lower toxicity than lidocaine and mepivacaine (73). When larger doses were given however it appeared that this drug produces methemoglobinaemia (74, 75) and cyanosis. Chlorprocaine has a low toxicity (ester compound) but is not suited for regional intravenous anaesthesia because it causes thrombophlebitis (76).

The symptoms of acute toxicity can be classified as slight and severe. Slight symptoms can be subjective: circumoral and tongue numbness, lightheadedness, disorientation and objective: muscle twitching, slurred speech, nystagmus. Severe symptoms are:

– apnoea
– bradycardia or cardiac arrest
– convulsions.

The treatment of toxic reactions must be rapid and efficient. It must start with the prevention of toxic effects by means of an adequate premedication (diazepam – atropine) and the prevention of high plasma concentrations by using a faultless technique, vasopressors when not contraindicated and the lowest active concentration of the drug for every technique (77). Tucker and Boas (78) observed that when the same quantity of lidocaine was administered, plasma concentrations were 40% higher when intravenous regional anaesthesia was performed with a 1% solution instead of a 0.5%. Activive treatment should begin, when possible, with interruption of the administration or with isolation of the extremity. An intravenous route must be started or the existing one checked for patency. Moreover the patient must be observed and various manifestations treated adequately, thus allergic reactions by infusions, anti-allergic drugs or hydrocortisone and cardiovascular troubles by vasopressors (preferably drugs with combined alpha and beta effects) or atropine and plasma expanders.

Cardiac compression is the only treatment for asystole. Ventilation should be supported, if necessary after the intubation of the trachea (respiratory analeptics are not indicated since apnoea is a symptom of central nervous exhaustion); convulsions are to be treated by oxygen administration, intravenous diazepam (less depression of the ventilation than barbiturates) and sometimes even muscle relaxants and controlled ventilation.

Because the metabolism of local anaesthetics is not under our control we can only try to promote renal excretion by generous fluid administration.

SPECIAL INDICATIONS FOR VARIOUS ANAESTHETICS

For contact anaesthesia we have to use drugs with good penetrating qualities: lidocaine 4-6% gives the best results.

For infiltration anaesthesia drugs with low resorption, in a weak dilution and, if not contra-indicated, in combination with vasopressors: lidocaine 0.24% $\pm$ 1/200,000 adrenalin.

For blocks, good penetrating drugs: lidocaine 1-1.5%, mepivacaine 1%. For peridural anaesthesia, depending on the duration of the operation: mepivacaine 2%, etidocaine 1%. If a good motor block is desired a combination of mepivacaine and adrenalin is mandatory or the spinal technique should be used (lidocaine 5% or mepivacaine 4%).

For obstetrical analgesia, when motor blocks should be avoided, bupivacaine 0.125 to 0.25% is the drug of choice.

For intravascular techniques a drug with a high protein binding coefficient is the best: etidocaine 0.5%.

CHOICE OF THE CONCENTRATION

When choosing the concentration of the drug for local anaesthesia we must navigate between Scilla and Charibda. Higher concentrations improve the quality of the block (79) while giving rise to higher plasma concentrations and thus increasing the risk of toxic effects (77, 78).

MAXIMAL DOSE

There is no unique answer to this question and this explains the large discrepancies found in the literature (for procaine: between 2 g and 15 g). (57). We saw in the discussion of pharmacokinetics that many factors influence absorption (plasma concentration) and we need only remember the tremendous individual variations in the duration of anaesthesia (540-1680 minutes, More 1970) to understand the large variation in the individual sensibility. The pharmaceutical companies provide tables, based on the considerable experience of various authors, which offer some orientation in this field.

We should not forget that these are mean values and that biological material presents an exceedingly wide range of reactions.

We are medical doctors and we must try to treat individual patients with the lowest efficient dose of any drug. This can only be achieved by careful clinical observation of the patient's reaction to the administered dose and not by administering standard (maximal) doses. I would like to end with words of Covino (80): improved training of physicians in the use of local anaesthetics may be the most important factor in their clinical safety.

REFERENCES

1. Geddes, I. C., Chemical structure of local anaesthetics. *Brit. Journ. Anaesth.* 34: 4: 229 (1962).
2. Bonica, J. J., *The management of pain.* Philadelphia. Lea & Febiger. 1954.
3. Goodman, L. S., A. Gilman, *The pharmacological basis of therapeutics.* London – Toronto. Macmillan 1970.
4. Meymaris, E., Chemistry and physiology of local anaesthesia. Chemical anatomy the nerve membrane. *Brit. J. Anaesth.* Suppl. 47, p. 164 (1975).
5. Ritchie, J. M., Mechanism of action of local anaesthetic agents and biotoxins. *Brit. Journ. Anaesth.* Suppl. 47, 191 (1975).
6. Takman, B. H., The chemistry of local anaesthetic agents: classification of blocking agents. *Brit. Journ. Anaesth.* Suppl. 47, p. 183 (1975).
7. Schulte-Steinberg, O., J. Hartmuth, L. Schütt, Carbon dioxide salt of lignocaine in brachial plexus block. *Anaesthesia*: 25: 2: 191 (1970).
8. Bromage, P. R., A comparison of the hydrochloride and carbon dioxide salts of lignocaine and prilocaine in epidural anaesthesia. *Acta Anaesth. Scand.* Suppl. 16: 55 (1965).
9. Bromage. P. R., M. F. Burfoot, D. E. Crowell, A. P. Truant, Quality of epidural blockade III. Carbonated local anaesthetic solutions. *Brit. Journ. Anaesth.* 39: 197 (1967).
10. Frazier, D. T., T. Narahashi, M. Jamada,,ᶦThe site of action and active form of local anaesthetics. *J. Pharmacol. Ewp. Ther.* 171:45 (1970).
11. Haschke, R. H., B. R. Fink. Lidodaine effects on brain mitochondrial metabolism in vitro. *Anesthesiology* 42: 6 : 737 (1975).
12. Foldes, F. F., D. L. David. O. J. Plekss. Influence of halogeen substitution on enzymatic hydrolysis. *Anesthesiology* 17 : 187 (1956).
13. Tucker, G. T., L. E. Mather, Pharmacology of local anaesthetic agents. *Brit. Journ. Anaesth. Suppl.* 47, 213 (1975).
14. Cosmo, A., Di Fazio, R. E. Brown, Lidocaine metabolism in normal and phenobarbital pretreated dogs. *Anesthesiology* 36: 3: 238 (1972).
15. Widman B., Plasma concentration of local anaesthetic agents in regard to absorbtion, distribution and elimination, with special reference to bupivacaine. *Brit. Journ. Anaesth. Suppl.* 47: 231 (1975).
16. Adriani, J., R. Zepernick, E. Hyde, Influence of the status of the patient in systemic effects of local anesthetic agents. *Anesth. and Analg.* 45: 1: 87 (1966).
17. Goldman, J. A., A rare toxic effect of local anaesthesia with lignocaine. *Brit. Journ. Anaesth.* 30: 377 (1958).
18. Catchlove. R. F. H., The influence of CO_2 and pH on local anaesthetic action. *Journ. Pharmacol. Exp. Ther.* 181: 298 (1972).
19. Tucker, G. T., R. N. Boyes, Ph. O. Bridenbaugh, D. C. Moore, Binding of anilide-type local anesthetics in human plasma. *Anesthesiology* 33: 3: 287 (1970).
20. Bromage, P. R., S. Datta, L. A. Dunford, Etidocaine: an evaluation in epidural analgesia for obstetrics. *Canad. Anaesth. Soc. J.* 21: 535 (1974).
21. Brown, W. U. Jr., G. C. Bell, A. O. Lurie, J. B. Weiss, J. W. Scanlon, M. H. Alper, Newborn blood levels of lidocaine and mepivacaine in the first postnatal day following maternal epidural anesthesia. *Anesthesiology* 42: 6: 698 (1975).
22. Jordfeld, L., B. Löfström, B. Pernow, B. Persson, J. Wahren, B. Widman, The effect of local anaesthetics on the central circulation and respiration in man and dog. *Acta Anaesth. Scand.* 12: 153 (1968).
23. Klein, S., R. I. L. Sutherland, J. Morch, Haemodynamic effects of intravenous lignocaine in man. *Canad. Med. Assoc. J.* 99: 14 (1968).

24. Blair, M. R., Cardio-vascular pharmacology of local anaesthetics. *Brit. Journ. Anaesth. Suppl.* 47: 247 (1975).
25. Bonica, J. J., P. U. Berges, K. Morikawa, Circulatory effects of peridural block. *Anesthesiology* 33: 6: 619 (1970).
26. Lee, A. J., R. S. Atkinson, *A synopsis of anaesthesia.* Bristol. Joh. Wright & Sons. p. 313 (1968).
27. Cullen, B. F., P. B. Chretien, B. G. Leventhal, The effect of lignocaine on P. H. A. stimulated human leukocyte transformation. *Brit. Journ. Anaesth.* 44: 1247 (1972).
28. Cullen, B. F., R. H. Haschke, Local anaesthetic inhibition of phagocytosis and metabolism of human leukocytes. *Anesthesiology* 40: 2: 142 (1974).
29. Eriksson, E., S. Englesson, S. Wahlqvist, B. Örtengren, Study on the intravenous toxicity in man. Some in vitro studies on the distribution and adsorbability. *Acta Chir. Scand.* Suppl. 358: 25 (1966).
30. de Jong, R. H., R. Robles, R. W. Corbin, Central actions of lidocaine. Synaptic transmission. *Anesthesiology* 30: 1: 19 (1969).
31. Wikinsky, J., J. E. Usubiaga, R. L. Morales, A. Torrieri, L. E. Usubiaga, Mechanism of convulsions elicited by local anaesthetic agents. *Anesth. and Analg.* 49: 3: 504 (1970).
32. Englesson, S., M. Matousek, Central nervous effects of local anaesthetic agents. *Brit. Journ. Anaesth.* Suppl. 47. 241 (1975).
33. Sakabe, T., T. Mackaw, T. Ishikawa, H. Takeshita, The effects of lidocaine on canine cerebral metabolism and circulation related to the electroencephalogram. *Anaesthesiology* 40: 5: 433 (1974).
34. Cunningham, N. L., J. A. Kaplan, A rapid onset, longacting regional anesthetic technique. *Anesthesiology* 41: 5: 509 (1974).
35. Moore, D. C., L. D. Bridenbaugh, Ph. O. Bridenbaugh, G. E. Thompson, G. T. Tucker, Does compounding of local anesthetic agents increase their toxicity in humans? *Anaesth. and Analg.* 51: 4: 579 (1972).
36. Villa, E. N., G. T. Marx, Chloroprocaine – bupivacaine sequence for obstetric extradural analgesia. *Canad. Anaesth. Soc. Journ.* 22: 1: 76 (1975).
37. Akamatsu, T. J., K. H. Siebold, The synergistic toxicity of local anaesthetics. *Anaesthesiology* 28: 1: 238 (1967).
38. Brecher, M. J., R. A. Greenberg, N. M. Greene, Drug interactions (toxicity) associated with drug combination. *Acta Anaesth. Scand.* 16: 1: 22 (1972).
39. Bridenbaugh, Ph. O., G. T. Tucker, D. C. Moore, L. D. Bridenbaugh, G. E. Thompson, R. J. Balfour, Role of epinephrine in regional block anaesthesia with etidocaine. *Anesth. and Analg.* 53: 3: 430 (1974).
40. Egbert, L. D., Th. C. Deas, Effect of epinephrine upon the duration of spinal anaesthesia. *Anesthesiology* 21: 4: 345 (1960).
41. Moore, D. C., L. D. Bridenbaugh, Ph. A. Bagdi, Ph. O. Bridenbaugh, H. Stander, Prolongation of spinal blocks with vasoconstrictor drugs. *Surg. Gynaec. Obst.* 124: 983 (1966).
42. Bromage, P. R., Spread of analgetic solutions in the epidural space and their site of action. *Brit. Journ. Anaesth.* 34: 3: 161 (1962).
43. Kier, L., Continuous epidural anaesthesia in prostatectomy. Comparison of bupivacaine with and without adrenaline. *Acata Anaesth. Scand.* 18: 1: 1 (1974).
44. Bromage, P. R., P. O'Beirn, L. A. Dunford, Etidocaine a clinical evaluation for regional analgesia in surgery. *Canad. Anaesth. Soc.* Journ. 21: 523 (1974).
45. Dhuner, K. G., J. G. L. Harthon, B. G. Herbing, T. Lie, Blood levels of mepivacaine after regional anaesthesia. *Brit. Journ. Anaesth.* 37: 10: 746 (1965).
46. Dhuner, K. G., Mepivacaine and vasocontrictors in regional anaesthesia. *Acta Anaesth. Scand.* Suppl. 48: 1-52 (1972).

76 D. T. POPESCU

47. Stevenson, A., J. Adriani, E. Hyde, The efficacy and adverse effects of vasoconstrictors used as adjuncts in regional anaesthesia. *Anaesth. and Analg.* 43: 5: 495 (1964).
48. Nolte, H., J. Dudeck, Th. Dudeck, B. Hüthwohl, Ornithin - 8 - Vasopressin als Vasoconstringens in der regionalen Anaesthesie. I. Teil. *Der Anaesth.* 21: 9: 398 (1972).
49. Nolte, H., J. Dudeck, Th. Dudeck, B. Hüthwohl, Ornithin -8 - Vasopressin als Vasoconstringens in der regionalen Anaesthesie. II. Teil. *Der Anaesth.* 21: 9: 402 (1972).
50. Coleman, A. J., L. W. Baker, Some cardiovascular effects of ornithine - 8 - vasopresin, a new surgical vasoconstrictor agent. *Brit. Journ. Anaesth.* 45: 511 (1973).
51. Gilbert, C. R. A., I. R. Hanson, A. B. Brown, R. A. Hingson, Intravenous use of Xylocaine. *Anaesth. and Analg.* 30: 6: 301 (1951).
52. Phillips, O. C., A. T. Nelson, W. B. Lyons, Intravenous lidocaine as an adjunct to general anaesthesia. *Anesth. and Analg.* 39: 4: 317 (1960).
53. Bartlett, E. E., O. Hutaserani, Xilocaine for the relief of postoperative pain. *Anesth and Analg.* 40: 3: 296 (1961).
54. Howat, D. D. C., *Complications associated with high extradural block for upper abdominal surgery.* 3e Int. Symp. Wepion-Namur, p. 207 feb. 1974.
55. Scott, D. B., Drug interactions with local anesthetics; in *Anesthésiques locaux en anesthésie et réanimation* 2nd Ed. p. 145. Paris. Libr. Arnette (1974).
56. de Clive-Lowe, S. G., J. Desmond, J. North, Intravenous lignocaine in anesthesia. *Anesthesiology* 13: 138 (1958).
57. Killian, H., Die Komplikationen der Lokalanaesthesie. *Der Anaesth.* 10: 10: 294 (1961).
58. Nolte, H., H. Oehmig, *Die Lokalanaesthesie in Lehrbuch der Anaesthesiologie.* Editors Frey-Hügin-Mayrhofer. Ed. Springer-Berlin-Heidelberg-New York. III ed. p. 291-297 (1972).
59. Fink, B. R., Acute and chronic toxicity of local anaesthetics. *Canad. Anaesth. Soc. Journ.* 20: 1: 5 (1973).
60. Fink, B. R., R. D. Kennedy, A. E. Hendrikson, M. E. Middaugh, Lidocaine inhibition of rapid axonal transport. *Anesthesiology* 36: 5: 422 (1972).
61. Aasheim, G., B. R. Fink, M. Middaugh, Inhibition of rapid axoplasmic transport by procaine hydrochloride. *Anesthesiology* 41: 6: 549 (1974).
62. Ngai, S. H., W. Dairman, M. Marchelle, Effects of lidocaine and etidocaine on the axoplasmic transport of catecholamine-synthetising enzymes. *Anesthesiology* 41: 6: 542 (1974).
63. Adams, H. J., A. R. Mastri, A. W. Eicholzer, G. Kilpatrik, Morphologic effects of intrathecal etidocaine and tetracaine on the rabbit spinal cord. *Anesth. and Analg.* 53: 6: 904 (1974).
64. Jenkins, L. C., Toxicity of anaesthetics. Introduction to symposium. *Canad. Anaesth. Soc. Journ.* 20: 1: 2 (1973).
65. Aldrete, J. A., W. Daniel, Evaluation of premedicants as protective agents against convulsive doses of local anesthetic agents in rats. *Anesth. and Analg.* 50: 1: 127 (1971).
66. Munson, E. S., P. A. Pugno, J. H. Wagman, Does oxygen protect against local anaesthetic toxicity? *Anesth. and Analg.* 51: 3: 422 (1972).
67. de Jong, R. H., J. E. Heavner, L. F. de Oliviera, Effects of nitrous-oxide on the lidocaine seizure threshold and diazepam protection. *Anesthesiology* 37: 3: 299 (1972).
68. Maekawa, T., T. Sakabe, H. Takeshita, Diazepam blocks cerebral metabolic and circulatory responses to local anesthetic induced seizures. *Anesthesiology* 41: 4: 389 (1974).
69. de Jong, R. H., J. E. Heavner, Diazepam and lidocaine - induced cardiovascular changes. *Anesthesiology* 39: 6: 633 (1973).

70. Scott, D. B., Evaluation of toxicity of local anaesthetic agents in man. *Brit. Journ. Anaesth.* 47: 1: 56 (1975).
71. Bromage, P. R., J. G. Robson, Taux sanguin de le lignocaine au cours de l'anesthésie régionale et locale. *Anesthésie, Analgésie, Réanimation* 17: 3: 371 (1960).
72. Cahill, J. F., J. G. Aldos, A. S. Wenning, Relation between acute toxicity and critical rate of disposal of several local anesthetics. *Canad. Journ. Physiol.* 43: 343 (1965).
73. Crawford, O. B., Comparative evaluation in peridural anaesthesia of lidocaine, mepivacaine and L. 67. *Anesthesiology* 25: 3: 321 (1964).
74. Lund, P. C., J. C. Cwik, Citanest, a clinical and laboratory study. *Anesth. and Analg.* 44: 6: 712 (1965).
75. Bromage, P. R., A comparison of the hydrochloride salts of lignocaine and prilocaine for epidural analgesia. *Brit. Journ. Anaesth.* 37: 10: 753 (1965).
76. A.S.T.R.A., *Symposium on intravenous regional anesthesia.* Worchester. Mass. (1966).
77. Adriani, J., *The pharmacology of anesthetic drugs.* Ch. C. Thomas, Springfield Ill. 3th. ed. p. 86 (1952).
78. Tucker, G. T., R. A. Boas, Pharmacokinetic aspects of intravenous regional anesthesia. *Anesthesiology* 34: 6: 538 (1971).
79. Fink, B. R., G. Aasheim, S. J. Kish, T. S. Croley, Neurokinetics of lidocaine in the infraorbital nerve of the rat in vivo. *Anesthesiology* 42: 6: 731 (1975).
80. Covino, B. G., Comparative clinical pharmacology of local anesthetic agents. *Anesthesiology* 35: 2: 158 (1971).

6. CEREBROSPINAL FLUID AND PLASMA LEVELS OF ETIDOCAINE AFTER PERIDURAL ADMINISTRATION

F. F. FOLDES AND P. PORGES

Etidocaine hydrochloride (Duranest) is a new, amide-type local anaesthetic agent of long duration of action. Its use for peridural block was investigated by Lund et al. (1). They found that 1% etidocaine had a rapid (about 4 min) onset and relatively long (4-6 hours) duration of action.

The purpose of the present study was the determination of the cerebrospinal fluid (CSF) and plasma concentrations of etidocaine in patients operated upon under peridural block. Observations were also made on the plasma levels and systemic toxicity of intravenously injected etidocaine.

MATERIALS AND METHODS

Peridural anaesthesia with etidocaine was administered to 21 male patients undergoing surgery on the lower half of the body. Their mean age was 53 (23 to 85) years and their mean weight 72 (49 to 90) kg. Another 10 unpremedicated patients to be operated on under general anaesthesia received intravenous etidocaine. Five of these were males and 5 females. Their mean age was 57 (20 to 86) years and their mean weight 59 (48 to 70) kg.

Patients who received peridural block were premedicated with 75 to 100 mg pentobarbital sodium, 25 to 75 mg meperidine hydrochloride and 0.3 to 0.6 mg atropine sulfate. On arrival to the operating room an intravenous infusion was started and heart rate and systolic and diastolic blood pressure was recorded. After this, with the patient in the lateral position, polyvinylite catheters were introduced through No. 18 thin wall needles into the subarachnoid and peridural spaces at the second and third lumbar interspace respectively. The patient was then turned into the supine horizontal position and CSF and heparinized venous blood samples were obtained before and at 5, 10, 20, 50 and 90 minutes and subsequently at 60 minute intervals after the peridural injection of 0.5 ml/kg 1.0 percent etidocaine containing 1:200,000 adrenaline. The sampling was continued in the recovery room until the termination of analgesia to pin prick at the 12th thoracic (T_{12}) dermatome. Heart rate and blood pressure were also recorded at these times. The time of onset of sensory anaesthesia at T_{12}, the time of development of the highest level of sensory anaesthesia, the time of onset and termination of motor anaesthesia and the time when the patient started to complain of wound pain were also recorded.

After the level of sensory anaesthesia regressed to T_{12} the catheter was very slowly withdrawn from the subarachnoid space. When the drop forming on the hub of the needle inserted into the proximal end of the catheter ceased to increase in size, indicating that the distal end of the catheter was just outside the dura, 5 ml of the patient's freshly drawn venous blood was injected through the catheter to 'seal' the opening of the dura (2).

The 10 unpremedicated patients in whom the plasma level and systemic toxicity of etidocaine was studied after slow intravenous administration received 1.25 mg/kg etidocaine, diluted to 20 ml with 0.9 percent sodium chloride, at the rate of 4 ml (0.25 mg/kg)/min. Heart rate systolic and diastolic blood pressure were observed before and at 0.5, 1, 2, 3, 4, 5, 7, 10, 15 and 60 minutes and heparinized blood samples were obtained for etidocaine determinations before and at 5, 10, 20 and 60 minutes after the start of the etidocaine injection.

The blood samples obtained from both groups of subjects were centrifuged, the plasma and CSF specimens were stored at $-30°C$ until airmailed from Vienna to the Astra Research Laboratories in Sweden where their etidocaine concentrations were determined by a gas chromatographic method similar to the one developed for the determination of lidocaine (3).

Subjects of both groups were carefully observed for signs and symptoms attributable to systemic toxicity to local anesthetic agents.

RESULTS

The first 13 patients of the first group were operated on under peridural block without supplementation. The time course of the peridural block, which extended from the 5th sacral to the 4th to 2nd thoracic dermatome, summarized in Table 1 indicates that etidocaine in the volume and concentration administered rapidly produced sensory and motor block of relatively long duration of action. The mean duration of the sensory block was 320 ± 23 (SEM) and that of the motor block 282 ± 29 minutes. Despite the fact that the sensory block included almost all dermatomes from which the sympathetic outflow originates, the incidence and severity of circulatory

Table 1. The course of sensory and motor block after the peridural administration of etidocaine.[1]

	Sensory block			Motor block		Duration of surgery	Start of wound pain
	Time of onset[2]	Time to highest level	Duration	Time of onset	Duration		
Mean[3]	6.31	12.92	320.38	9.15	281.76	89.53	322.15
S.E.M.	0.69	1.14	22.65	1.36	29.01	18.62	38.64

1. 5 mg (0.5 ml of a 1% solution) per kg body weight.
2. Times in min from the start of peridural injection.
3. Of observations on 13 patients in whom peridural block was not supplemented.

changes was very low. Only 4 of the 13 patients required a single moderate
dose of vasopressor (10 to 20 mg methoxamine or 25 to 50 mg ephedrine
intramuscularly). No signs or symptoms of central nervous system toxicity
were observed in any of the 21 patients who received peridural block. There
were no postanaesthetic complications (e.g., headache, backache, prolonged
urinary retention) attributable to the peridural block.

CSF samples were obtained from 10 of the 13 patients. In 3 others sampling
was not possible because of technical reasons. From the point of view of the
time courses of the CSF concentrations the 10 samples could be divided into
two distinct groups. In 7 the highest mean concentration, 95.4 μg/ml was
reached 10 minutes after the end of injection. In the remaining 3 the highest
mean CSF concentration, 895.9 μg/ml was reached at 5 minutes. It was
assumed that in the second group etidocaine penetrated into the subarachnoid place through a tear in the dura caused by the needle through which the
subarachnoid catheter used for sampling was inserted. The CSF concentrations measured in the first group of 7 subjects are presented in figure 1.

Plasma samples were obtained from 20 of the 21 subjects who received
peridural etidocaine. The plasma concentration of etidocaine after its peridural administration reached a maximum of 1.4 ± 0.16 μg/ml at 20 minutes

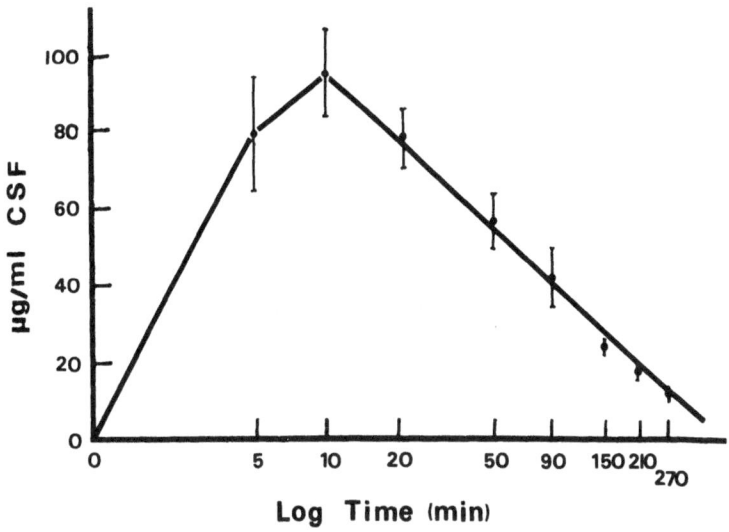

Fig. 1. The cerebrospinal fluid (CSF) concentration of etidocaine after the peridural
administration of 0.5 ml/kg 1% etidocaine. Each point represents the mean and vertical
bars 2 SEM of concentrations measured in 7 subjects.

Table 2. Circulatory changes after the intravenous administration of etidocaine.[1]

	Control	Minutes after the start of intravenous injection								
		0.5	1	2	3	4	5	7	10	20
Pulse rate	82.4[2] ± 7.0	76.8 ± 6.8	78.0 ± 6.6	81.4 ± 5.8	82.8 ± 6.6	82.8 ± 6.5	82.4 ± 6.6	79.9 ± 5.8	80.4 ± 6.1	79.6 ± 5.9
Systolic blood pressure	139.5 ± 8.5	140.5 ± 9.5	134.5 ± 8.6	133.0 ± 7.3	139.0 ± 8.0	140.0 ± 7.2	137.0 ± 6.1	139.0 ± 6.8	141.5 ± 6.8	137.5 ± 10.7
Diastolic blood pressure	80.0 ± 2.6	76.5 ± 3.2	78.5 ± 3.6	80.5 ± 3.6	81.5 ± 3.6	81.5 ± 4.0	80.5 ± 4.2	82.0 ± 3.6	80.0 ± 3.4	78.5 ± 4.3

1. 0.125 mg/kg dissolved in 20 ml 0.9% NaCl injected over 5 min.
2. Mean ± SEM of 10 subjects.

after the start of its peridural administration and gradually decreased to 0.44 ± 0.03 μg/ml by 270 minutes.

In none of the 10 subjects who received etidocaine intravenously were there any signs or symptoms of significant systemic toxicity. Heart rate, systolic and diastolic blood pressure remained stable (table 2). The only CNS effects were slight tremor beginning at 7 minutes after the start of intravenous injection of etidocaine and lasting 2 minutes in two and 1 minute in one patient, and sleepiness of short duration in one 86 year old patient. The plasma etidocaine concentrations, because of some mishap during transit could only be determined in 8 of the 10 subjects. The results shown in figure 2 indicate that the maximal plasma level of etidocaine was 3.96 ± 0.54 μg/ml at the end of injection. By 60 minutes the plasma concentration decreased to 0.8 ± 0.11 μg/ml. The anaesthetic and postanaesthetic course was uneventful in all 10 patients.

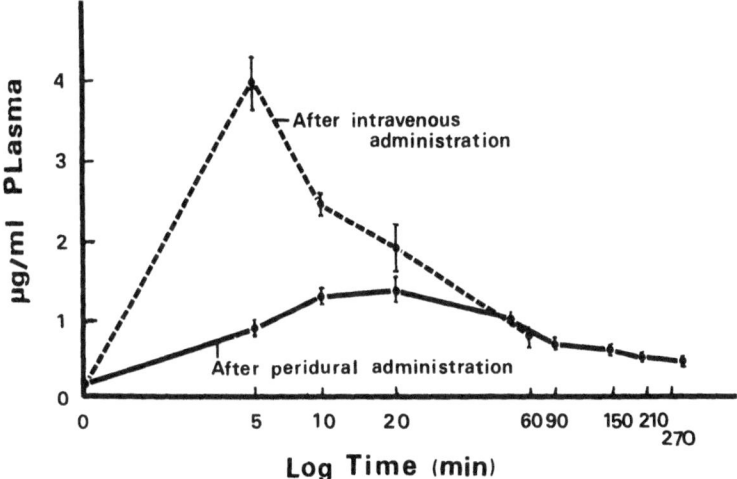

Fig. 2. The plasma levels of etidocaine after the peridural administration (20 subjects) of 5 mg/kg or the intravenous injection (8 subjects) over a 5 min period of 1.25 mg/kg etidocaine.

DISCUSSION

One percent etidocaine produced satisfactory peridural block of rapid onset and satisfactory duration of action. Etidocaine induced peridural block was not accompanied by the degree of hypotension encountered during peridural anaesthesias of comparable extent with other local anaesthetic agents.

Others (Dr. H. Nolte, Personal Communication) also observed that the intensity and duration of the sympathetic blocking action of etidocaine is relatively low. It occurred to us that the peripheral sympatholytic effect of etidocaine may be antagonized by central sympathomimetic effects. This possibility, however, could be excluded since after its intravenous infusion plasma levels of etidocaine which were almost three times higher than those reached after epidural administration had no significant circulatory effects (table 2). At the present time we have no explanation for the lack of significant sympathetic blocking activity of etidocaine. It is conceivable that the membrane structure of sympathetic fibers is different from those of the sensory and motor fibers. Such differences may explain the preferential absorption of various local anaesthetic agents of different chemical structure into one or the other type of nerve fiber.

Although, by choice, 40 to 60 percent larger volumes of etidocaine were used in this study than those commonly employed for epidural block, no signs or symptoms of CNS toxicity were encountered. The absence of systemic toxicity is in agreement with the finding that the highest plasma levels of etidocaine observed after epidural administration were 2 to 3 times lower then the plasma levels which produced mild, transient signs of CNS toxicity in 4 out of 10 subjects after intravenous administration. These observations indicate that, except for inadvertent intravenous administration of large doses of etidocaine, significant systemic toxicity is unlikely to occur when peridural block is induced with etidocaine.

SUMMARY

One percent etidocaine produces peridural block of rapid onset and long duration of action. Circulation remains unexpectedly stable under etidocaine induced peridural block. The highest plasma level of etidocaine after peridual administration of 40 to 60 percent larger volumes than those usually employed in clinical anaesthesia was two to three times lower than the marginally toxic concentration produced by its slow intravenous infusion. In agreement with this no signs or symptoms of systemic toxicity had been observed in 21 patients after the peridural injection of 0.5 ml/kg 1 percent etidocaine.

REFERENCES

1. Gormley, J. B., Treatment of postspinal headache. *Anesthesiology* 21, 565 (1960).
2. Lund, P. C., J. C. Cwik and R. T. Pagdanganan, Etidocaine – A new long-acting local anesthetic agent: A clinical evaluation. *Anest. Analg.* 52, 482 (1973).
3. Keenaghan, J., The determination of lidocaine and prilocaine in whole blood by gas chromatography. *Anesthesiology* 29, 110 (1968).

PART THREE

DRUGS USED IN GENERAL ANAESTHESIA

7. PHARMACOKINETICS: GENERAL ASPECTS

H. MATTIE

To understand the action of drugs, it is necessary to know something about the relationship between the concentration of the drug at the receptor site and the magnitude of the effects of drug-receptor interaction. This knowledge is readily obtained from in vitro experiments, but in the clinical situation the concentration of a drug at the receptor site usually cannot be determined directly. Here we are limited to the determination of such quantities as the dose, the concentration in blood or serum, time, and certain known effects. Besides, in clinical medicine there are very often several steps between the direct effect caused by receptor activation and a measurable effect. Quantitative relationships between these variables can be visualized as highly simplified models, mechanical models as it were, which can be expressed as mathematical equations; some of which seem very complicated, but all of them are a gross simplification of biological reality. It is one thing, for instance, to describe the time course of serum concentrations mathematically, but it is another thing to arrive at a specific model from this mathematical expression. This can be illustrated by an example. When a drug has been completely absorbed after administration, the concentration declines in a non-linear way. In other words, the decline of the concentration differs during different successive intervals. Many concentration time curves take the form of an exponential decline, best described by the general equation:

$$C_t = C_0 \times e^{-kt} \tag{1}$$

The reason why this is called an exponential decline is that the variable time is in the exponent. The same formula can be written as:

$$\ln C_t = \ln C_0 - kt \tag{1a}$$

in which:
C_t = the concentration at any time t after time zero,
C_0 = the concentration at time zero,
e = the base of the natural logarithms, and
k = a rate constant.

From this equation it can be seen why semi-logarithmic paper is so often used to make graphs of drug concentrations in blood: on this graph paper the time course is linear. The reason why e is used as a base is that although any number would work, with e it can be derived directly from equation 1 that:

$$dC/dt = - k \times C \tag{2}$$

which means that the rate of decline of the concentration is directly proportional to the concentration itself.

This is a good mathematical expression for what can actually be seen; the reason why can best be shown by an example. A drug of small molecular size is filtered by the renal glomeruli in the same way as creatinin, so that its renal clearance will be about 100 to 120 ml/min. When this clearance is fairly constant, the amount of drug in the filtrate is proportional to the concentration in the filtrate and – the concentration in the filtrate being equal to the concentration in plasma – the amount of drug in the filtrate will be proportional to the concentration in plasma. So it is quite easy to understand that when a drug is cleared by the kidneys and the glomerular filtration rate is constant, the elimination rate of the drug is indeed proportional to the concentration. The same principle evidently holds for liver metabolism, because drugs that are cleared mainly by the liver usually show the same kind of decline in plasma concentration. At least at relatively low concentrations, the blood flow through the liver is the rate-limiting factor for the metabolic clearance. But at much higher concentrations it is quite possible that the amount of enzyme is rate-limiting, and at very high concentrations in the blood the metabolizing enzymes of the liver can be saturated. Elimination then becomes linear, because there is a maximal amount of drug to be eliminated by the liver. One important drug that is eliminated in this way, at least at pharmacologically active concentrations, is ethyl alcohol. Pharmacokinetic terminology may seem rather misleading in this respect: a concentration-time course is usually non-linear, but because semi-logarithmic plots giving straight lines are always used, the term non-linear elimination has been generally adopted in this field for elimination that is non-linear on semi-logarithmic plots, and as a result alcohol elimination, which is described here as linear, is called non-linear in pharmacokinetic terminology.

In the example just given the drug is cleared by the kidney at the same rate as creatinin, but this is often not the case. There are two possible explanations for this: the first is that the filtration rate of the drug is different from that of creatinin, and the second is that total elimination is not equal to filtration. But why should filtration of the drug be not the same as that of creatinin? Most drugs have a small molecular size, so that could not be the cause. Many drugs are, however, bound more or less strongly to serum proteins. Although this binding is usually completely reversible during the filtration process, part of the drug is free and part of it is bound to the plasma protein molecules and therefore will not be filtered. In quantitive terms: when 50% of the drug is bound to plasma protein, the glomerular filtration of the total amount of the drug will be only 50% of creatinin filtration. In many cases, however, this explanation is still insufficient to explain why renal clearance of some drugs is so small. The reason for this is that when the primary filtrate is concentrated in the renal tubuli, water reabsorption leads to a rise in the concentration of the drug, and since the primary filtrate is concentrated about 100 times, this implies that the concentration of the drug would become 100 times higher in the urine than in the plasma. This results in a steep *concentration gradient* of the drug between the urine in the collecting tubuli and the blood surrounding the tubuli, which can lead to diffusion of the drug back into the blood. Whether this happens or not depends on a very definite property of the drug, namely its socalled lipid solubility. For the kinds of drug discussed in this book, this is a very important property. The more lipophilic the drug, the more readily it passes through cell walls and cells. Thus, where the lipid solubility of a drug is very high, there will be considerable back diffusion. The same lipid solubility often leads, moreover, to a high degree of protein binding, so that there are two ways in which lipid solubility influences the renal clearance of a drug. But for the kinetics of a drug there is a third consequence of lipid solubility, i.e., the binding of the drug to all kinds of tissue, for instance fat and muscles, is also dependent on its lipid solubility. Binding to tissues means disappearance from the blood, which in turn leads to low blood concentrations. Since for this kind of drug low concentrations are found in the plasma, glomerular filtration, which is proportional to plasma concentration, must be low. Moreover, protein binding may occur, which leaves a still smaller fraction to be filtrated, and in the end back diffusion occurs. When a high proportion of the drug is bound to tissue, the volume of distribution or, preferably, the apparent volume of distribution is said to be large. This term can be misleading, however, because it suggests that there is a certain space in the body that contains a drug at a certain concentration, and that this concentration is the same as the concentration in the serum; and it also suggests that the rest of the body is devoid of the drug. In many

instances nothing is further from reality. Actually, the volume of distribution is only calculated as though the drug was distributed in this way, i.e.:

$$\text{AVD} = \frac{\text{dose}}{\text{concentration}} \tag{3}$$

Of course, the volume of distribution is indeed dependent on physical
factors, but the value of the calculated volume of distribution (given in
litres or percentage of body weight) usually has no physical reality.

The mathematical relationship between the parameters discussed so
far is rather simple:

$$k = \frac{\text{clearance}}{\text{AVD}} \tag{4}$$

i.e., the elimination rate constant is dependent on the elimination mechanisms and the distribution in the body. The parameter k is expressed as
time^{-1}, which is difficult to visualize. Therefore, another parameter is often
substituted, which is the half-life time. The half-life time ($T\frac{1}{2}$) is defined
as the time required to eliminate half of the amount of the drug present
in the body. The value of $T\frac{1}{2}$ can be derived directly from k by dividing the
natural logarithm of 2 by k. The advantage of the use of $T\frac{1}{2}$ as parameter is
that it is concrete and has some practical value. For instance, the dose
interval for a maintenance dose of 50% of the starting dose of a certain
drug is equal to the half-life time. When a drug has a $T\frac{1}{2}$ of 24 hours and
the starting dose is 200 mg, for example, the maintenance dose should be
100 mg every 24 hours.

The serum concentration-time course of a drug often shows an extra
peak in the initial part of the semi-longarithmic plot. This too can be expressed
as a – still rather simple – mathematical expression, i.e., a so-called bi-
exponential curve:

$$C_t = Ae^{-\alpha t} + Be^{-\beta t} \tag{5}$$

This equation has no direct biological meaning. It suggests that elimination
is initially faster, but since elimination from the body is not faster the drug
must be eliminated from the plasma, where the drug is sampled, but not
from the body. A mechanical model in which the drug can diffuse from the
central plasma compartment to a peripheral compartment, can be derived
from the constants in this equation. If this model is valid, it would mean that
up to a certain time the concentration of active drug is lower in the peripheral

compartment than in the central compartment, and that after that moment the reverse is the case. In this context it is important to know whether the concentration at the receptor site behaves like the concentration in the central compartment or like that in the peripheral compartment. This is especially important because central-compartment concentrations tend to be much higher after i.v. administration than after i.m. or s.c. injection. It can be shown, at least for this model, that the difference between i.v. and i.m. injection is smaller in the peripheral than in the central compartment, and that fluctuations caused by intermittent administration are as it were dampened in the peripheral compartment.

The very first phase of the concentration time course, preceding the so-called distribution phase, is the absorption phase. The shape of any concentration time curve is strongly influenced by the mode of absorption, which again is often exponential: absorption slows down when the concentration at the site of injection (or in the gastro-intestinal tract after oral administration) diminishes, but can of course take any shape, e.g. it may be linear during continuous infusion. The rate of absorption is also dependent on physical qualities of the drug, especially when it is administered orally, and again lipid-soluble drugs are absorbed more easily than drugs that have less lipid solubility. As already mentioned, lipophilic drugs that are easily absorbed are excreted very slowly by the kidneys, and this explains why the liver plays an important part in the elimination of drugs. It is often stated that the liver detoxifies, but it would be very remarkable if the liver could change a large number of relatively newly developed toxic substances into an equally large number of non-toxic substances, which is certainly not the case. The liver changes all such substances into other, also potentially toxic, substances even though many such substances are devoid of the desired pharmacological activity. However, the most important change brought about by the liver makes the drugs less lipophilic, which means that they can be handled more easily by the kidneys.

The renal excretion of lipophilic drugs can also be enhanced by two modes of treatment. The first of these is called forced diuresis; when 12 litres of fluid are administered to a patient over a 24-hour period, the concentration of the drug in the urine will be kept much lower than normal, which greatly reduces back diffusion, and, in addition, the urine flow becomes more rapid, which shortens the time in which the drug can be reabsorbed. The second method is to change the pH of the urine by administering an alkalizing or acidifying substance. This influences the degree of ionization of the drug, and when a lipophilic drug becomes partially ionized, reabsorption is greatly reduced because the ionized part is much less lipophilic than the non-ionized fraction. Moreover, it is now clear when haemodialysis can be effective, namely, when a drug filtered effectively by the glomeruli is reabsorbed rapidly. Under these conditions haemodialysis can have a strong effect on the total elimination, because the concentration of the drug in the dialysate fluid is much lower than that in the urine. However, when a drug has a large distribution volume and is therefore not very accessible to the artificial kidney, haemodialysis should have a long duration, although this is often impractible. Haemodialysis is also not very effective when protein binding is extensive.

8. PHARMACOKINETICS AND METABOLISM OF HYPNOTIC AND PSYCHOTROPIC DRUGS

S. E. SMITH

Drugs with actions on the central nervous system, whether anaesthetic, hypnotic, tranquilliser or antidepressant, are characterised by high degrees of lipid solubility. This makes them largely insusceptible of renal elimination because they are realsorbed in the renal tubules down the concentration gradient which is established there by removal of water. The vast majority are consequently metabolised in the liver by the addition of polar groups which render them more water soluble and more readily excretable.

To a certain extent the addition of polar groups to psychotropic drugs reduces their pharmacological activity. The reduction achieved by any one step, however, is often slight and there are many instances in which the opposite effect results; the drug actually becomes more potent. Over several steps, however, activity is usually largely abolished and the overall rate of metabolism therefore has a decisive effect on both the intensity and duration of the drugs action.

General pharmacokinetic considerations indicate that once absorption and distribution have occurred the plasma drug concentration (C) which follows administration of a single dose can be derived from the formula:

$$C = C_0 \cdot e^{-kt}$$

where C_0 is the equilibrium concentration at time (t) zero and k the elimination constant. In the present context k is a function of hepatic enzyme activity. Furthermore:

$$C_0 = \frac{F. \text{Dose}}{V_D}$$

where F is the fractional absorption of the drug (taking into account both bioavailability of the drug and its first pass metabolism) and V_D the equilibrium distribution volume. Rearrangement gives:

$$C = \frac{F. \text{Dose}}{V_D \cdot e^{kt}}$$

Following repeated drug administration accumulation occurs until the drug reaches a mean steady-state concentration (C_{ss}) at which the overall rate of absorption is balanced by the rate of elimination. Then:

$$C_{ss} = \frac{F.\ Dose}{V_D \cdot k \cdot T}$$

where T is the dosage time interval.

It is apparent that, whether drugs are given in single or in multiple doses, the concentration achieved is inversely related to the distribution volume and to the elimination constant or its logarithmic function. To the extent that drug effects must be related to drug concentrations at tissue sites and therefore indirectly to plasma concentrations, volumes of distribution and elimination constants assume paramount importance. Each is here considered in turn.

Distribution volumes of different drugs range widely according to their physical properties. On the one hand, drugs such as neuromuscular blocking agents which are fully ionised at physiological pH remain within the extracellular water and have distribution volumes of the order of 14-22% of body weight. On the other hand, drugs with lipid solubility are distributed more widely, crossing freely into the intracellular fluid and being concentrated in lipid membranes and fat depots. Such compounds have distribution volumes which are much larger, often greater than that of the whole body. Tricyclic antidepressants, being amines, are concentrated in intracellular water because of the pH differential and are highly bound to intracellular organelles; their distribution volumes are very large indeed. Plasma protein binding tends to hold drug within the circulation and thus to reduce the distribution volume. Some values are shown below.

drug	V_D (L/Kg)	$t_{\frac{1}{2}}$ (hr)
nortriptyline	21.1	34.2
pentobarbitone	2.0*	42.0
buthalitone	1.8	21.7
thiopentone	1.2*	4.0
tubocurarine	0.14	0.8

*approximate values

The enormous distribution volume of nortriptyline is of interest and of considerable importance in one respect. It implies that at equilibrium less than 1% of the drug is in the circulation; the remainder is all in the tissues. This explains why in antidepressant poisoning forced diuresis or haemodialysis is of no use in removing the drug; such a small proportion of the whole is available for ready removal.

Routes of drug metabolism are complex but conveniently divisible into two categories, Phase I and Phase II, as shown here:

Phase I – oxidation
reduction
dealkylation
hydroxylation

Phase II – conjugation

Phase I processes are predominantly oxidative, adding or exposing functionally reactive groups that are then available for the synthetic (conjugating) mechanisms of Phase II. These metabolic stages are clearly seen in the metabolism of phenacetin, which is first dealkylated to form paracetamol (with its reactive hydroxyl group) and subsequently conjugated with glucuronic acid. By contrast the metabolism of psychotropic agents is much more complex. The molecule of diazepam, for example, is readily attacked in at least three places. As a result several different metabolites are formed, some of them with sedative potencies comparable with the parent drug. One of them, N-demethyldiazepam, is eliminated from the body with a half-life of 100 hours whereas diazepam itself has a half-life of 24 hours. Following repeated administration of the parent drug, therefore, much of the pharmacological effect is due to this metabolite, for it accumulates to reach steady-state concentrations which are at least 50% higher than those of diazepam itself. The same may also be true of imipramine, the deaminated metabolite of which, desipramine, is probably responsible for much of the drugs therapeutic activity. Recent research indicates that even the 2-hydroxy-metabolite possesses much pharmacological potency, though in the body it is unlikely to exert much effect because of rapid elimination by conjugation. In the case of chlorpromazine at least 50 different metabolites have already been identified and others may yet exist. Investigations reveal that steady-state concentrations of this drug decline as time goes by because of hepatic enzyme induction. In such a situation it is difficult to find out which of the many metabolites contributes to, or is responsible for, the pharmacological action.

In practical medicine the rates at which these metabolic processes proceed is subject to wide interindividual variability, and the complexity of the metabolic patterns involved makes analysis very difficult. Both inherited and acquired influences, some brought about by interactions with other drugs and chemicals, are responsible for wide differences in distribution volume and hepatic enzyme activity. Thus 10-fold or greater differences in steady-state concentrations are found with many of these drugs and it is commonly believed that such differences account for the variability of drug response so readily observed. Direct correlations between plasma drug concentrations and their effects are, however, difficult to find except in a few instances. They are well documented with cardiovascular drugs like procainamide and digoxin, with anticonvulsants and with some central depressant agents such as ethanol. Close correlations between nortriptyline concentrations, atropine-like side-effects and inhibition of tyramine pressor responses have been described and relationships proposed with therapeutic effects. Such observations need confirmation and the proposition that the routine measurement of plasma concentrations would assist drug therapy substantially is unproven. Evidence with other centrally active drugs is scanty and perhaps likely to remain so considering the problems involved.

Though this lack of interindividual correlation at present limits the usefulness of monitoring plasma concentrations in clinical practice, pharmacokinetic studies are slowly contributing to our understanding of the fundamentals of drug action in man. As a tool this methodology is of clear importance.

9. PSYCHOTROPIC AND RELATED DRUGS IN ANAESTHESIOLOGICAL PRACTICE

E. L. NOACH

In this review, interactions between psychotropic and related drugs and general anaesthetics will be discussed from two points of view. The first and principal part will be about 'useful' interactions, so the use of psychotropic drugs within the framework of general anaesthesia and related tasks of the anaesthesiologist. In the second and much shorter part, possible harmful interactions will be discussed of psychotropic drugs, which for psychiatric reasons are given to patients who have to undergo anaesthesia for an intercurrent surgical procedure. As a non-clinician, I wish to call your attention to pharmacological *principles* which may lead to favourable or unfavourable *possibilities* which you, in the clinic, may encounter.

With a view to possible future developments, some drugs or categories of drugs will be mentioned which are still in the experimental phase but may before long be available for clinical use.

BENEFICIAL USES OF PSYCHOTROPICS IN ANAESTHESIOLOGY: NEUROLEPTICS, MINOR TRANQUILLIZERS AND NOOTROPICS

In the pre-anaesthetic phase, psychotropic drugs are used for sedative purposes and, in combination with analgesics, to obtund pain. During this phase, drugs may already be administered for purposes needed in later stages of the anaesthesiological procedure.

During surgical anaesthesia, in addition to the general anaesthetic, administration of other drugs may be desirable for the following reasons:

- potentiation of the anaesthetic
- analgesia (especially neuroleptanalgesia)
- muscular relaxation
- hypotension or hypothermia
- prevention or therapy of harmful effects of the anaesthetic on respiration and circulation.

In the post-anaesthetic phase, psychotropic and/or analgesic drugs may be used for the treatment of pain, restlessness, nausea and insomnia.

In this enumeration of possible uses of psychotropic drugs, I would like to go into the so-called 'potentiation of anaesthesia'. It is a matter of dispute whether potentiation of any drug is an advantage, if it only means the enhancement of desired as well as undesired effects. If less of an anaesthetic is needed to obtain full surgical anaesthesia, but also to get into trouble with respiration or circulation, such 'potentiation' by another drug would only be a matter of finance: is the combined price of two drugs in a smaller dosage less than the cost of the anaesthetic alone? In most cases, the general anaesthetic is the cheaper of the two, so not much is gained in a *medical* sense, if no other advantages can be made evident. Potentiation in anaesthesiology is only of value when a *desired* effect, for instance on consciousness or pain, is potentiated selectively and harmful or otherwise undesired effects are left unpotentiated, in other words, when the *margin of safety* of the anaesthetic drug is enhanced. In this context, some thoughts could also be given to drug-specific side effects such as liver toxicity. I am not aware of data proving a *clear* dose-dependency of hepatotoxic effects of any anaesthetic. This means that it is questionable whether the dose of such a hypothetical anaesthetic may be lowered so much by the use of a concomitant depressant drug that we land in the non-toxic range.

It should also be remembered that in diminishing the toxicity of one drug, new toxic potentialities of the other may be introduced. In this connection, I may remind you of the hepatotoxicity of phenothiazines such as chlorpromazine. Summarizing, simple potentiation of the effect of an anaesthetic may be advertised as a benefit, a blessing or a financial advantage, but given the class of anaesthetics as a whole no real profit is gained by such an interaction.

After these general comments, it is necessary to give a survey of the classes of drugs which will be discussed. These are: 1. the psychotropic drugs in the generally accepted classification plus a new addition, the 'nootropic drugs'; the latter have made a promising start in animal experiments, but clinical experience is not yet wide enough to make a definite evaluation possible; 2. the analgesic drugs, but only as far as new developments are concerned. *Hypnotics* will at most be mentioned briefly, since their use, abuse and interference with anaesthetic drugs are sufficiently familiar to anaesthesiologists. Likewise, *lithium*, in use for maniacal psychoses, will be left out because its interactions with anaesthetic medication have not been sufficiently investigated.

Fig. 1. Classification of Neuroleptics (major tranquillizers) (with some examples).

Group	Example (Generic name)	Trade names ® (only preparations obtainable in The Netherlands)
Phenothiazines	Chlorpromazine	Largactil
Thioxanthenes	Chlorprotixene	Taractan, Truxal
Butyrophenones	Haloperidol	Serenase
Fluspiridoles	Pimozide	Orap
Rauwolfia alkaloids	Reserpine	Serpasil

Neuroleptics (see fig. 1). Not much can be said about this class which is not yet common medical knowledge. The group of neuroleptics may be subdivided into various sub-groups without too many qualitative differences. Common to all of them is their strong sedative and anti-psychotic effect, anti-emesis, disregulation of body temperature, in many cases also their sympatholytic action causing a slight or moderate lowering of blood pressure. The toxic effects, parkinsonism, mostly reversible liver damage etc., are also generally known, so further discussion is not necessary.

Fig. 2. Classification of Ataractics (minor tranquillizers) (with some examples).

Group	Example (generic name)	Trade names ® (only preparations obtainable in The Netherlands)
Benzodiazepines	Chlordiazepoxide	Librium
	Diazepam	Valium, Levium
	Nitrazepam	Mogadon
Meprobamate group	Meprobamate	Artolon, Miltown
Diphenylmethane derivatives	Hydroxyzine	Atarax
Other groups	Chlormezanone	Trancopal
	Benzoctamine	Tacitin
	etc.	

Minor tranquillizers (ataractics) (see fig. 2). At present mostly benzodiazepine-derivatives are in use. They have a very wide margin of safety – it is hardly possible to kill anyone by overdosing –; they have sedative, sometimes hypnotic properties and cause muscular relaxation by a central mechanism on interneuronal connections. All these properties, in addition to the absence of inhibitory effects on respiration and circulation, make minor tranquillizers valuable drugs for pre-anaesthetic treatment. It is still a matter of dispute whether these drugs act selectively on the limbic system, that part of the brain consisting of amygdala, cingulum, hippocampus and adjoining regions. In this system, the integration of sensory input, emotions and central regulation of behaviour take place.

Whether or not they also act on other brain regions, minor tranquillizers *do* inhibit the limbic system. This means that they inhibit the emotional implications of experiences, while they also inhibit the *storage* of experiences in the memory. Similar effects after blocking the activity of the limbic system have been shown in many experiments in animals and in man. For instance, it has been found in man that ablation of the amygdala (for neurological reasons) decreases the affective component of pain. Or, if in cats shortly after a painful experience the amygdalae are destroyed, the unpleasant experience is momentarily forgotten. The animal may undergo the same experience as if it were all new, so without the hesitation and struggling which occur in unoperated animals when they recognize the surroundings in which they had this experience before.

Such and many similar data may be of relevance for pain therapy. Although minor tranquillizers such as Diazepam (Valium) certainly do not have any analgesic effect, it could very well be that combination with analgesics such as salicylates will bring about an analgesic effect not quite different from that of the narcotic analgesics.

As is well known, in the latter class of drugs also the affective component of pain is taken away. I am not aware of any systematic well-controlled studies in which, for instance, the analgesic effects of salicylates with or without minor tranquillizers have been compared, but I would recommend to do such a study. Also, with reference to experiments on cats which forget recent unpleasant experiences, it might well be that the quite common pre-anaesthetic administration of minor tranquillizers helps to diminish the emotional trauma which, together with somatic scars, keeps the patient's unpleasant recollection of the anaesthesiologist and surgeon vivid.

There is another recent observation which needs more confirmation but which I would like to mention here. In animal experiments it has been found that under the influence of minor tranquillizers, the brain has an improved resistance against hypoxia. If this finding could be transferred to man, it may be of importance especially for neurosurgery, but also for the prevention of sequels of shock and related conditions.

In this connection more extensive attention has to be given to a new drug with a hitherto unknown combination of effects – so new that a new name

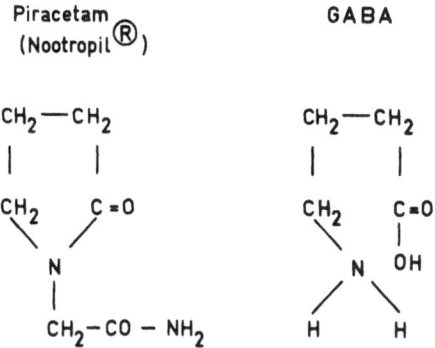

Fig. 3.

had to be coined for this category, which up till now consists of only one representative. The name of the drug is *piracetam* (see fig. 3). Chemically it is related to γ-amino-butyric acid or GABA, a substance which is supposed to be an inhibitory neurotransmitter.

Piracetam (Nootropil ®) has been developed in the laboratories of the Union Chimique Belge, under the direction of their pharmacologist, Dr. C. E. Giurgea. Clinical experience with this drug is still quite limited, but results of animal experiments, some of which I will report here, are very interesting and offer encouraging perspectives for anaesthesiological application. When given alone, the drug has hardly any effect: it is no analeptic, no sedative, does not cause motoric disturbance and does not have any antihistaminic, anticholinergic, cardiovascular or electroencephalographic effects. Its toxicity is very low, especially if compared to the dose which brings about the effects which will be mentioned now.

In many different animal tests, piracetam causes an improvement of memory and a facilitation of learning abilities such as the capacity to find the way out of a labyrinth etc. This is highly interesting as such and preliminary data indicate that especially the improvement of memory might also occur in man, especially old people; but this part of the studies is outside the domain of anaesthesiology and I will not dwell upon it. Of more importance for anaesthesiology is the finding that in animals piracetam has a marked therapeutic effect in the recovery from anoxia. This has been shown in the following experiment (see fig. 4); rabbits were put in an atmosphere consisting of 100% nitrogen. EEG recordings were made. Soon after the start of nitrogen asphyxia, the EEG waves disappeared: the EEG was silent. After 20 sec. of EEG silence, the animals were put into the air again. Such a short period of asphyxia is not lethal; animals begin to breathe

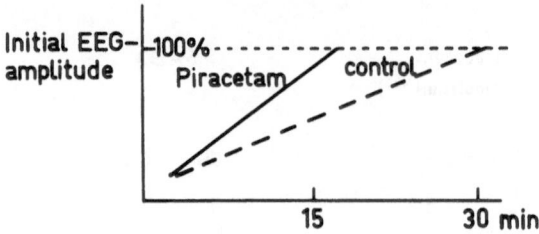

Fig. 4. Post-anoxic recuperation in rabbits (schematic, after Giurgea, 1972).

again spontaneously and after some time the EEG waves reappear. However, animals which had been pretreated with piracetam recovered more rapidly. If this would be shown to be true also for man, it might be an important drug to use in cerebral ischemia, or for conditions in which the circulation has to be interrupted during anaesthesia. The drug then should be given as a prophylactic.

Also in the related field of barbiturate intoxication, very encouraging results were obtained: two barbiturates were investigated, the quick-acting secobarbital and the longer acting allobarbital. The drugs were given intravenously. After secobarbital, in a dose of 33 mg/kg, 7 out of 10 animals died within some minutes, after a brief period of EEG silence. If, however, an hour before secobarbital 100 mg/kg piracetam had been given, none of the animals died, although they were fast asleep. In these animals, no EEG silence occurred, but the well-known barbiturate spindling was seen in the EEG (see fig. 5). It was remarkable that piracetam, when given at a shorter

Fig. 5. Piracetam protection against barbiturates in rabbits: I.

Secobarbital, 33 mg/kg i.v.		
Treatment	Number of dead animals/group total	p

1. Secobarb. + physiol. saline
   Secobarb. + Piracetam
   (1 hour before secobarb.)
	7/10
	0/10
		} < 0.01

2. Secobarb. + physiol. saline
   Secobarb. + Piracetam
   (30 min. before secob.)
	7/11
	4/11
		} non-sign.

from Moyersoons and Giurgea, 1974

interval before secobarbital, had much less protective effect. This went so far that piracetam given 15 minutes before secobarbital did not protect the animals at all. The drug thus obviously acts only after a period of latency.

This may mean that it either has to be transformed in the body into an active substance, or that it brings about some physiological alteration which needs time to develop. Whichever of the two mechanisms is involved, it means that piracetam only has *prophylactic* value for intoxications with rapidly acting barbiturates. However, since in anaesthesiological practice mostly quick-acting barbiturates are in use, the knowledge of such a prophylactic drug which apparently does not block their anaesthetic effect is important. Further experiments were performed in order to know whether piracetam also has *therapeutic* properties in intoxications with longer acting barbiturates (see fig. 6). The long-acting barbiturate allobarbital in a dose of 125

Fig. 6. Piracetam protection against barbiturates in rabbits: II.

	Allobarbital, 125 mg/kg i.v.	
Treatment	Number of dead animals/group total	p
Allobarb. + physiol. saline	11/13	
Allobarb. + Piracetam (2 min. after allobarb.)	2/13	< 0.01

from Moyersoons and Giurgea, 1974.

mg/kg i.v. killed 11 out of 13 rabbits within an hour, death being preceded by a period of EEG silence. If piracetam was given to such animals 2 minutes after the allobarbital injection – so more or less 'therapeutically' – only 2 out of 13 animals died, and no or at most short periods of EEG silence occurred.

The investigations with this drug are still in progress; no data are as yet available on possible therapeutic effects after overdosage of gaseous anaesthetics; however, the results mentioned possibly make it a valuable asset to anaesthesiology.

The mechanism of action on cellular level is not yet clear. There are some indications that the drug brings about a more extensive storage of chemical energy, in the form of ATP and phosphocreatine, in the brain. Since this accumulation of energy requires time, this may be the basis for the latent period before the drug begins to act. The drug has only very recently been made available in Holland and further clinical experiences are eagerly awaited.

Since piracetam is the first representative of a new class of drugs, the name 'nootropics' has been introduced provisionally for drugs which have an action 'directed to the mind'.

UNDESIRED EFFECTS OF PSYCHOTROPICS; THE ANTIDEPRESSANTS

Neither from a pharmacological point of view, nor from clinical data, possible useful applications of these drugs in anaesthesiology have come to my knowledge. It is not necessary to mention here that even in patients who are mentally depressed after an operation, for instance because recovery does not proceed fast enough, no antidepressant should be given: the use of these drugs is restricted to cases of endogenous depression. From the work of Van Praag in Groningen it is even getting clear that mainly a special subgroup of vital depressions will benefit by this drug treatment. In order to identify this subgroup, in addition to psychiatric symptomatology also a chemical diagnosis has to be made of the amount of metabolites of neuro-transmitters in the cerebrospinal fluid. In mentally normal but discouraged postoperative patients, no abnormalities in this respect may be expected to occur, so no antidepressant drugs should be given.

This class of drugs is noted for being a nuisance to the anaesthesiologist. Since quite a few patients are, for psychiatric reasons, under chronic anti-depressant therapy, a number of them may need surgical help for other afflictions, and in these cases the anaesthesiologist may be confronted with special problems. In order to get a clear understanding of the mechanisms involved, some basic facts about the mode of action of these drugs should be remembered. The antidepressants are divided into two distinct classes (see fig. 7): the MAO-inhibitors (with as best known examples of currently

Fig. 7. Examples of antidepressant drugs.

Group	Generic name	Trade names ® (only preparations obtainable in The Netherlands)
MAO inhibitors	Nialamide Pargyline Tranylcypromine	Niamid Eudatine (Parnate)
Tricyclic antidepr.	Imipramine Desipramine Amitriptyline Nortriptyline and about 15 others	Tofranil Pertofran Sarotex, Tryptizol Sensaval

available drugs: nialamide and mebanazide or Actomol®) and the tricyclic antidepressants (so named after their chemical structure); some examples of tricyclic antidepressants are: imipramine and amitriptyline. All in all, in Holland there are about 12 different tricyclic antidepressants available now.

Both categories of antidepressants differ considerably in their mode of action, although pharmacologically the outcome is quite similar: in both categories, more neurotransmitter is available for the specific receptor, and in both probably 2 different neurotransmitters are involved, noradrenalin (NA) and serotonin (5HT). The mechanisms by which this is brought about are different. MAO-inhibitors inhibit the enzyme MAO which is present in the axons of noradrenergic and serotonergic nerves, and, furthermore, in the liver. The enzyme is responsible for the breakdown of NA and 5HT, firstly in the neurones so that not too much transmitter accumulates there, and secondly in the liver in order to break down transmitter-like substances derived from food which may enter the bloodstream via the vena porta.

These facts are generally known, as well as the warning that persons under treatment with MAO-inhibitors should not drink French wine or eat English cheese – or such delicacies from other countries – because these contain tyramine, a sympathomimetic substance which may cause enormous increases in blood pressure if it is not destroyed in the liver. Apart from this side effect – one of many! – the antidepressant effect is probably related to an enhanced release of neurotransmitter upon arrival of a nerve impulse.

The tricyclic antidepressants have quite a different mode of action. They prevent the operation of the normal mechanism of inactivation of the neuro-transmitters, which consists of re-uptake into the nerve fibre ending. Since normally 60 to 80% of the amount released by a nerve impulse is pumped back, blockade of this re-uptake results in a large surplus of neurotrans-mitter at the level of the postsynaptic receptor. Thus, there is general agree-ment that both categories of antidepressants act by increasing the amount of NA and/or 5HT at some receptor site, although it is not known which of the many noradrenergic or serotonergic receptors in the body are specifically involved in endogenous depression.

Going into particular aspects, we may say that MAO-inhibitors have quantitatively similar inhibitory effects on the breakdown of NA and 5HT. Moreover, these drugs have many and often dangerous side effects. Of these, hypertensive crises have been mentioned already, but acute hypotension may also occur, especially if drugs like opiates, barbiturates, tranquillizers and also diuretics like chlorothiazide or furosemide are given concomitantly. The basis of this acute hypotension is unknown. Mention has to be made of the use of MAO-inhibitors as hypotensive drugs. Further-more, MAO-inhibitors often have a hepatotoxic action. It is therefore not surprising that most psychiatrists restrict the use of this category to those cases where other antidepressants do not sufficiently help. Be it as it may, it should be remembered that anaesthesia during a treatment with MAO-inhibitors is risky. It does not help much to discontinue the use of these drugs, since the decline of their action and hence of their toxicity takes many days, even some weeks. This means that, if possible, surgery on such patients should be postponed.

The *tricyclic antidepressants* are less toxic. Here we have seen some differentiation in the last few years. Whereas MAO-inhibitors hardly discriminate between NA- and 5HT-breakdown, some members of the tricyclic group have a more profound influence on re-uptake of 5HT, others on that of NA. This is connected with their chemical structure (see fig. 8): *tertiary* amines

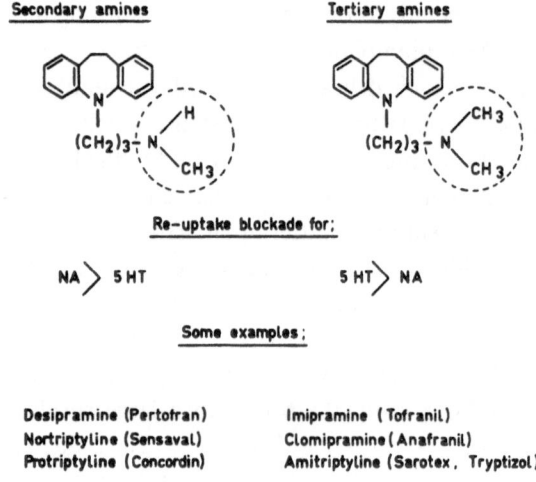

Fig. 8. Secondary and tertiary amines in tricyclic antidepressants.

such as imipramine, clomipramine, melitracen and amitriptyline have a stronger re-uptake blockade for 5HT than for NA. *Secondary* amines such as desipramine, nortriptyline and protriptyline preferentially block NA re-uptake. In the first place, this is of significance for their antidepressant effect. Although our understanding is still incomplete, it seems that increasing the amount of 5HT acting on its specific receptors is related to improvement of the mood, the general sense of well-being, whereas increasing the amount of NA has more influence on general drive and motor activity. However, since we are only at the beginning of a more selective way of drug treatment, the following statements have a provisional character. Turning our attention to points of interest for the anaesthesiologist, I would be inclined to predict that hazards of *secondary* amines (desipramine, nortriptyline, protriptyline) are greater than those of *tertiary* amines, because the secondary amines may especially cause an enhanced NA effect, with possible complications in the cardiovascular field such as increased blood pressure, increased occurrence of cardiac irregularities (especially with anaesthetics like cyclopropane), and an increased sensitivity for sympathomimetic drugs, even such widely used drugs like nasal vasoconstrictors and some common cold remedies.

No comparative studies have been performed as yet and I am well aware of the fact that the specificity mentioned is only relative: we do not have drugs yet which selectively and uniquely block either NA or DA re-uptake.

To stress the importance of cardiovascular complications of tricyclic antidepressants, mention should be made of an increasing number of reports on sudden cardiac death during chronic treatment with antidepressants. This means that we are still far away from a really satisfactory drug treatment of this important group of psychoses.

NEW NARCOTIC ANALGESICS

As a final section of this review, some new developments in the field of analgesics will be mentioned. Although, strictly speaking, these do not quite belong to the group of psychotropic drugs, the *narcotic* analgesics have such evident psychotropic effects that they should not be omitted from this paper.

Nowadays we have the disposal of many narcotic analgesics which are much more potent than the natural opium alkaloids and their semisynthetic derivatives. As an example I mention fentanyl, the usual parenteral dosage of which is about 100 times less than that of morphine. However, there would be no real advantage if the toxic dose would be equally lowered. What we need is an increased Therapeutic Index (T.I.), by which we mean the ratio between toxic and therapeutic dose. As a measure of the T.I. in animal experiments, the ratio LD50/ED50 is generally used: the larger its value is, the safer is the drug.

The T.I. of fentanyl is considerably higher than that of morphine. As usual in narcotic analgesics, the principal acute toxic effect resides in respiratory depression and it would be desirable to have drugs with a still higher T.I. Recently, improvements have been found along two lines. The first group of drugs was developed in Hungary by Prof. Knoll and associates. Starting from morphine, he developed a series of *azidomorphines* (substitu-

Fig. 9. Therapeutic index for analgesic effect in rats.

	Hot plate test	Tail flick test	Writhing test
	Therapeutic index $\dfrac{LD_{50}}{ED_{50}}$		
morphine	66	172.2	449
azidomorphine	812.5	1083	1000
azidocodeine	347.2	205	305
fentanyl	375	500	375

After Knoll et al., 1973, *J. Pharm. Pharmacol.*: 25, 929.

tion of the alcoholic OH by N-3). In figure 9 you see the T.I. of some analgesics in three commonly used analgesic tests in animals. In all three tests,
azidomorphine is 2 to 10 times as *safe* as morphine and about twice as safe
as fentanyl. This larger safety margin is of more importance than the fact
that analgesia may be obtained with dosages which are 300 times smaller
than those of morphine. In addition, animal experiments indicate that
proneness to physical dependence and abstinence is much less than with
morphine, but one has to be extra cautious in extrapolating results of such
animal tests to human conditions. Nevertheless, it seems to be a promising
new development which awaits confirmation in the field of application in
man.

Even more spectacular are recent results obtained by the group in Janssen's
Laboratories in Belgium and very recently reported on by Van Bever at the
International Congress on Pharmacology in Helsinki (see fig. 10). Starting
from the (already) very potent drug fentanyl, new derivates were synthetized
of which an example is shown in figure 10. This coded drug has an amazing

Fig. 10. Therapeutic index $\dfrac{LD_{50}}{ED_{50}}$ for the analgesic effect of the Fentanyl-derivative
R 30730 (intravenous administration).

	Mouse	Rat	Dog
R 30730	6700	25000	50000
Fentanyl	454	277	
Morphine	35	70	
Pethidine	8	5	

After Van Bever, 1975.

analgesic potency: it belongs to a group having a potency about 10.000 times higher than morphine. If these data can be transferred to man, it means that for a man of 70 kg not more than 20 *micro*grams would be required to obtain analgesia. But here too, the enormous therapeutic index is of greater importance, indicating that only in very high dosages some respiratory depression occurs.

In all, it is evident that the frontiers of analgesia research are in motion, entailing implications for anaesthesiology.

REFERENCES

1. Bever, W. F. M. van, Structure-activity relationships of a novel series of extremely potent analgesics with an unusually high safety margin. In: *Abstracts 6th Int. Congress of Pharmacology*, Helsinki, abstract no. 87, 1975.
2. Giurgea, C. E. and F. E. Moyersoons, On the pharmacology of cortical evoked potentials. *Arch. int. Pharmacodyn.* 199, 67-78, 1972.
3. Giurgea, C. E., Vers une pharmacologie de l'activité du cerveau. Tentative du concept nootrope en psychopharmacologie. In: R. Hazard & J. Cheymol (ed.), *Actualités Pharmacologiques* 25, 115-138, 1972.
4. Knoll, J., Mészáros, Z., Szentmiklósi, P. and S. Fürst, The pharmacology of 1,6 dimethyl - 3 - carbethoxy - d-oxo - 6,7,8,9 - tetrahydrohomopyrimidazol - methylsulphate (MZ-144), a new, potent, non-narcotic analgesic. I. Some basic correlations between the chemical structure and activity of homopyrimidazol analgesics. Selection of MZ-144. *Arzneimittelforschung* 21, 717-719, 1971.
5. Knoll, J., Fürst, S. and Z. Mészáros, The pharmacology of 1,6 dimethyl-3-carbethoxy--4-oxo-6, 7, 8, 9-tetrahydrohomopyrimidazol-methylsulphate (MZ-144), a new, potent, non-narcotic analgesic. II. Toxicity and analgetic effect of MZ-144 compared to narcotic and non-narcotic analgesics. *Arzneimittelforschung* 21, 719-727, 1971.
   4-oxo-6,7,8,9-tetrahydrohomopyrimidazol-methylsulphate (MZ-144), a new, potent, non-narcotic analgesic. II. Toxicity and analgetic effect of MZ-144 compared to narcotic and non-narcotic analgesics. *Arzneimittelforschung* 21, 719-727, 1971.
6. Knoll, J., Fürst, S. and K. Kelemen, The pharmacology of azidomorphine and azidocodeine. *J. Pharm. and Pharmacol.* 25, 929-939, 1973.
7. Knoll, J., S. Makleit, T. Friedmann, L. G. Harsing Jr. and P. Hadhàzy, Circulatory, respiratory and antitussive effects of azidomorphine and related substances. *Arch. int. Pharmacodyn.* 210, 241-249, 1974.
8. Knoll, J., Azidomorphines. In: *Abstracts 6th Int. Congress of Pharmacology*, Helsinki, abstract no. 172, 1975.
9. Moyersoons, F. E. and C. E. Giurgea, Protective effect of piracetam in experimental barbiturate intoxication; EEG and behavioural studies. *Arch. int. Pharmacodyn.* 210, 38-48, 1974.

10. BARBITURATES

C. M. CONWAY

The use of the intravenous route for the production of anaesthesia goes back for many years. In the early decades of this century many agents enjoyed transient popularity as intravenous anaesthetics, including paraldehyde, urethane, ethyl alcohol, bromethol, diethyl ether and chloroform. The widespread use of intravenous anaesthetics followed the introduction in 1932 of hexobarbitone (1), followed a few years later by the appearance of thiopentone (2). Since that time the use of intravenous agents to induce anaesthesia has become an almost universal practice. Whilst a large number of non-barbiturate compounds have been given trial, the rapidly acting barbiturates, especially thiopentone, still remain the most widely used drugs. To understand the reasons for this popularity it is necessary to examine the properties of rapidly acting barbiturates.

CHEMISTRY

All barbiturates used clinically are water soluble sodium salts of barbituric acid (fig. 1). Barbituric acid itself has no hypnotic activity, but substitutions of organic radicals at the 1, 2, 5 and 5' positions can produce compounds

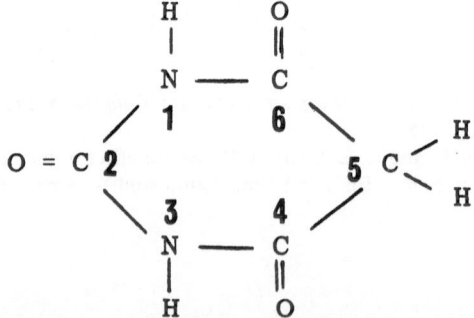

Fig. 1. Structural formula of barbituric acid. The keto form shown can convert to the enol form by transition of hydrogen attached to positions 1 or 3 to oxygen at position 2.

with hypnotic properties. Dundee and Wyant (1) have discussed at length the structure-activity relationships of these substituted compounds. The salient features which bestow useful properties as intravenous induction agents are as follows.

a. Sulphur substitution in position 2 almost invariably increases the speed of onset of drug effects. With the exceptions of hexobarbitone and methohexitone all the intravenous barbiturates are in reality thiobarbiturates.

b. Methylation at position 1 produces rapidly acting compounds, but this rapidity of action is often associated with a high incidence of excitatory phenomena.

c. Substitution of both hydrogens on C5 is essential for hypnotic activity. Whilst in general increasing the length of the sidechain at C5 causes increased potency and shortens the duration of sleep, excessively long side chain substitution produces compounds which have a reduced hypnotic effect and may have convulsant or other toxic properties. The ideal form of substitution at C5 is to have a total of between four and nine carbon atoms in the two chains with one side chain kept relatively simple.

The two most commonly used intravenous barbiturates, thiopentone and methohexitone, exemplify many of these factors. Thiopentone (fig. 2) is the

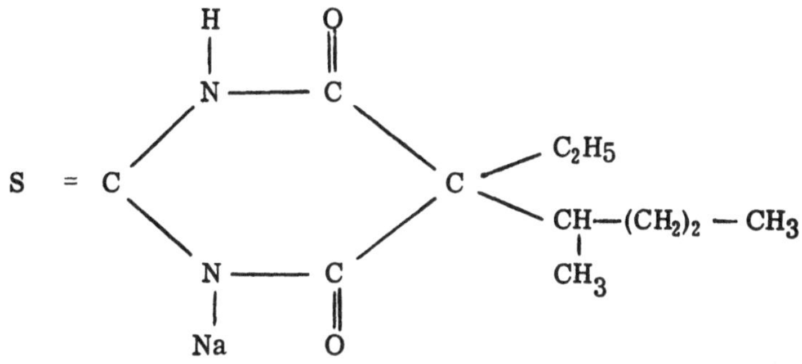

Fig. 2. Structural formula of thiopentone.

thio-derivative of pentobarbitone. Substitution of sulphur for oxygen converts the relatively slow acting parent barbiturate into a rapidly acting compound. The alkyl side chains at C5 are dissimilar and relatively simple. Methohexitone (fig. 3) is one of the few oxybarbiturates which have a rapid onset of action. Much of this rapidity of action is due to methylation at C1.

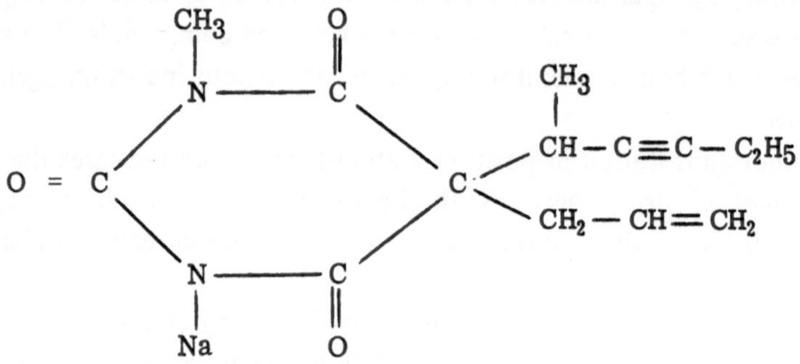

Fig. 3. Structural formula of methohexitone.

The side chains are more complex than in thiopentone and contain double and triple bonds which tend to confer shortness of action. Table 1 lists some of the commonly used intravenous barbiturates with their comparative potencies.

Table 1. Comparative potencies.

	Potency	Dose (mg/kg)
Thiopentone	1.0	5
Methohexitone	3.0	1.5
Thialbarbitone	0.5	10
Buthalitone	0.5	10
Methitural	0.7	7
Hexobarbitone	0.5	10

PHARMACOKINETICS

For a drug to produce rapid onset of unconsciousness it must reach the brain quickly and in high concentrations, and it must be able to penetrate the brain. The rapidity of action of all intravenous agents depends greatly on their mode of administration. By virtue of being injected relatively rapidly into the circulation a bolus of drug arrives at the brain within the one circulation time and produces high local concentrations. Having reached the brain, penetration of the blood brain barrier is due to two properties of rapidly acting barbiturates, their low degree of ionization and their high lipid solubility.

Ionization of barbiturates

Barbiturates are weak acids, with pKa values usually slightly higher than 7.4. Because only the unionized form of the drug can cross the blood brain barrier, the degree of ionization of a barbiturate will significantly affect its rate of action. Thiopentone has a pKa of 7.6 and is 61% unionized at pH 7.4. Methohexitone has a slightly higher pKa and is 76% unionized at normal plasma pH. By contrast phenobarbitone with a pKa lower than 7.4 is about 40% unionized at normal plasma pH.

Lipid solubility

Because rapidly acting barbiturates are largely unionized at normal plasma pH passage into the brain of these compounds will depend upon their affinity for lipid in the presence of water. Thus even though pentobarbitone is less ionized than thiopentone at pH 7.4, the low lipid solubility of the parent oxy barbiturate leads to slower brain penetration than its thiosubstituted derivative.

Protein binding

Between 65% and 75% of both thiopentone and methohexitone are bound to plasma albumin. Protein bound molecules are pharmacologically inert. The pool of protein bound barbiturate acts as a buffer maintaining the circulating level of unbound drug. Agents which interfere with the binding of barbiturates to albumin, such as sulphafurazale and meprobamate, may potentiate barbiturate induced central depression.

Distribution of intravenous barbiturates

The brevity of action of thiopentone and similar drugs is not due to their rapid breakdown. There are only slight differences in the rates of detoxification of thiopentone and pentobarbitone. The two factors which contribute to the rapid recovery of consciousness after thiopentone are dilution in blood and redistribution to other tissues.

When rapidly acting barbiturates are given intravenously they pass to the heart as a bolus and mix in the right heart with a comparatively small volume of blood. Thus the concentration of barbiturate in arterial blood is initially high. As cerebral blood flow constitutes about one sixth of the cardiac output the brain is presented within one circulation time of administration with a large mass of lipid soluble and largely undissociated drug. However blood levels fall nearly as rapidly as they have risen due to barbiturate mixing homogenously within circulating blood. As blood concentration of drug falls barbiturate passes out of the brain along a concentration gradient.

Whilst dilution of the initial bolus of barbiturate is probably the most important factor limiting the duration of cerebral action of intravenous barbiturates, redistribution of the drug to different body compartments is well known to occur with these drugs, as with all lipid soluble compounds. The initial high brain concentrations of these agents are paralleled by equally high concentrations in other well-perfused organs – liver, kidney, heart, endocrine glands. Drug concentration in muscles reaches a peak within about 15 minutes. This is achieved by redistribution from highly perfused tissues. Whilst muscle only receives about 20% of the cardiac output it constitutes about 50% of body mass. It can thus act as a reservoir for barbiturate, and as muscle drug concentration rises so does brain concentration fall. The adipose tissue of the body has an even higher capacity for barbiturates, but because of its poor blood supply drug levels in body fat do not reach a peak for several hours. Thus transfer to fat depots probably plays a negligible part in the termination of pharmacological action of intravenous barbiturates under normal clinical conditions of administration.

BARBITURATE METABOLISM

Whilst renal excretion is the major method of disposal of long acting barbiturates such as barbitone and phenobarbitone, only minimal amounts of thiopentone and methohexitone appear unchanged in urine. Metabolic transformation by hepatic microsomal enzymes is the major method of inactivation of these drugs. Oxidation of the side chains at position 5 appears to be an important step in barbiturate metabolism. Although high rates of hepatic metabolism of thiopentone have been demonstrated in both animals (2) and man (3), this method of reduction of blood thiopentone level is of much less importance than dilution and redistribution.

PHARMACOLOGICAL ACTIONS

Central nervous system
Although barbiturates are in the main used as hypnotics, intravenous administration of usual clinical doses produces central nervous depression of a depth which resembles surgical anaesthesia. The level of clinical anaesthesia produced by barbiturates is greatly related to the intensity of surgical stimu-

lation. An apparently deeply anaesthetised patient with obvious respiratory depression may respond markedly to minor stimulation. Administration of intravenous barbiturates in dosages sufficient to prevent such a response usually results in severe respiratory and cardiovascular depression. Thus barbiturates differ markedly from inhalation anaesthetics in the safety margin between effective and toxic doses.

The primary central site of action of barbiturates is on the midbrain reticular formation, depressing transmission through multisynaptic pathways and thus reducing cortical activation. Barbiturates reduce cerebral metabolic activity. Cerebral blood flow is also reduced, partly due to a loss of normal autoregulatory mechanisms in the face of a reduced perfusion pressure but also as a secondary consequence of reduced cerebral metabolism.

Respiration

Intravenous barbiturates are potent respiratory depressants. Some degree of respiratory depression is an invariable consequence of their use to produce sleep. A very transient initial respiratory stimulation may occur as central nervous effects begin to be apparent, but this is often followed by a period of apnoea. These respiratory effects of barbiturates are greatly potentiated by opiates and other respiratory depressants. The marked respiratory depressant action of barbiturates may be masked in the presence of surgical stimulation. Barbiturates reduce the sensitivity of the respiratory central system to carbon dioxide.

Laryngeal responses to stimulation are often increased during light barbiturate anaesthesia. Laryngeal spasm may occur if the respiratory tract is stimulated by irritant gases, secretions or attempted intubation.

Cardiovascular system

Myriad cardiovascular effects of intravenous barbiturates have been demonstrated in both animals and man. Direct myocardial depression can easily be demonstrated in isolated perfused heart and heart-lung preparations (4, 5). In intact animals and man the commonest haemodynamic effects of these drugs are to reduce cardiac index, stroke volume and systemic blood pressure (6). Most investigators have shown peripheral vasodilation to occur with these drugs, usually associated with an increased limb blood flow (7). Intravenous barbiturates have variable effects on heart rate and on central venous pressure. The overall effect of intravenous barbiturates in reducing cardiac output is probably related more to an effect on systemic capacitance vessels than to direct myocardial depression. Pooling of blood peripherally, by reducing diastolic filling, will reduce stroke volume (8).

In the majority of patients given clinical doses of intravenous barbiturates the initial fall in cardiac output and blood pressure is rapidly compensated for by increased sympathetic activity mediated via baroceptors. One minute after a sleep dose of these drugs heart rate, blood pressure and cardiac output may be restored to or even increased above resting levels. In patients suffering from hypovolaemia or severe cardiac disease and in subjects in whom the reflex pathways are impaired severe falls in cardiac output can follow even small doses of thiopentone and related drugs.

There have been many claims in the past that different barbiturates produced different degrees of cardiovascular depression (9). However controlled studies have shown that equivalent hypnotic doses of barbiturates produce equivalent degrees of circulatory and myocardial depression (10, 11, 12, 13). In figure 4 the relative potencies of thiopentone and methoxitone are shown

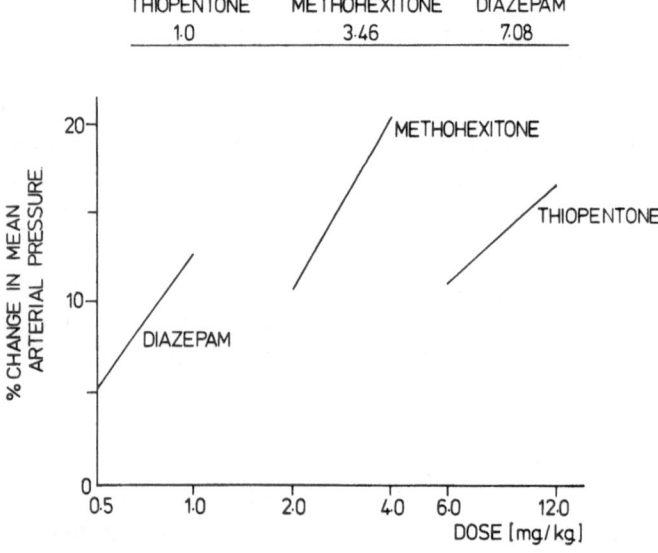

Fig. 4. Effects of thiopentone, methohexitone and diazepam on systolic blood pressure in dogs expressed as log-dose response curves. The relative potencies have been calculated from the displacements of the lines.

to differ little from the relative potencies of these drugs as hypnotics. By contrast diazepam has a lesser potency (compared to thiopentone) as a hypotensive agent than as a hypnotic. Figure 5 similarly shows that methohexitone is about three times as powerful as thiopentone as a hypotensive

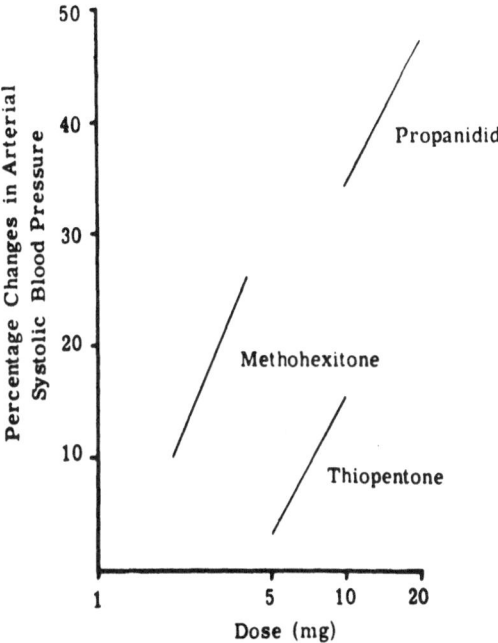

Fig. 5. Effects of thiopentone, methohexitone and propanidid on systolic blood pressure in dogs expressed as log-dose response curves (10).

agent, a figure equal to their comparative potencies as hypnotic agents. Propanidid had in these studies a hypotensive effect nearly equal to that of methohexitone whilst to produce hypnosis doses 3 to 5 times those of methohexitone are required.

Other general effects
Hepatic, renal and gastrointestinal function have all been shown to be depressed by intravenous barbiturates, but these effects are rarely of clinical significance. Both direct and indirect effects of barbiturates on neuromuscular function have been recorded, but these drugs do not affect either the intensity or duration of action of neuromuscular blocking agents.

Local effects
Venous thrombosis has not uncommonly been reported following intravenous barbiturates. It appears to have an incidence of about 3% of cases, and occurs more frequently when higher concentrations of these drugs are given (14).

Because intravenous barbiturates are highly alkaline, their injection into sites other than veins can produce severe local reactions. Subcutaneous injection may lead to tissue necrosis. Intramuscular injections usually have no deleterious local effects as absorption is rapid. Intra-arterial injection leads to intimal injury, vascular spasm and thrombosis which may result in limb gangrene. Waters (15) has suggested that intra-arterial thiopentone leads to precipitation of insoluble acid crystals which may block vessels mechanically and produce spasm by local noradrenaline release.

Abnormal reactions

Sensitivity to intravenous barbiturates is extremely rare. Dundee and Wyant (1) have reviewed 13 cases reported in the world literature up to 1974. All the patients they detail had known allergies or had previously had thiopentone.

Patients with porphyria are particularly susceptible to barbiturates. These drugs may cause an acute relapse in cases of acute intermittent porphyria and porphyria variegata. Porphyriac patients who are given intravenous barbiturates commonly develop postoperative paralysis which may be fatal. Barbiturates are not the only drugs which aggravate porphyria. They and other drugs which do so have been shown to induce the hepatic enzyme delta-aminolaevulic acid synthetase (ALA synthetase). This enzyme which limits synthesis of haem and porphyrin is increased in porphyria.

CONTRAINDICATIONS

The indications for the use of intravenous barbiturates are very wide, and the world wide popularity of these drugs is a tribute to their safety. The only absolute contraindication to their use is porphyria. In many situations intravenous barbiturates should be used with caution. These drugs are better avoided in patients with known sensitivity to barbiturates, and prolonged central depression can occur after use in cases of dystrophia myotonica. Patients with a low or fixed cardiac output, hypovolaemia, respiratory obstruction or greatly reduced hepatic or renal function may all be given intravenous barbiturates safely if suitable adjustments are made to the dosage and rate of administration.

SUMMARY

The great popularity of barbiturates, especially thiopentone, as intravenous induction agents, owes much to the large body of experience attained during forty years of their use. The choice between individual intravenous barbiturates depends only slightly upon real pharmacological differences between these agents. Used intelligently these drugs have a wide margin of safety. None of the non-barbiturate agents as yet available seems likely to rival their world wide popularity.

REFERENCES

1. Dundee, J. W. and G. M. Wyant, *Intravenous Anaesthesia.* London, Churchill Livingstone (1974).
2. Saidman, L. J. and E. I. II. Eger, The effect of thiopental metabolism on duration of anesthesia. *Anesthesiology*, 27, 118 (1966).
3. Mark, L. C., L. Brand, S. Hamvyssi, R. C. Britton, J. M. Perel, M. A. Landran and P. G. Dayton, Thiopental metabolism by human liver in vivo and in vitro. *Nature*, 206, 1117 (1965).
4. Gordh, J., Postural, circulatory and respiratory changes during ether and intravenous anaesthesia. *Acta. chirurg. Scand.* Suppl. 102, 92 (1945).
5. Cotten, M. de V. and E. Bay, Comparison of the cardiovascular properties of a new non barbiturate intravenous anesthetic agent with those of thiopental. *Anesthesiology*, 17, 103 (1956).
6. Johnson, S. R., The effect of some anaesthetic agents on the circulation in man. *Acta. chirurg. Scand.* Suppl. 158 (1951).
7. Prime, F. J. and T. C. Gray, Effect of certain anaesthetic and relaxant agents on circulatory dynamics. *Br. J. Anaesth.*, 24, 101 (1952).
8. Conway, C. M. and D. B. Ellis, The haemodynamic effects of short acting barbiturates. *Br. J. Anaesth.*, 41, 534 (1969).
9. Barron, D. W., J. W. Dundee, W. R. Gilmore and P. J. Howard, Clinical studies of induction agents, XVI: a comparison of thiopentone, buthalitone, hexobarbitone and thiamylal as induction agents. *Br. J. Anaesth.*, 38, 802 (1966).
10. Conway W. M., D. B. Ellis and N. W. King, A comparison of the acute haemodynamic effects of thiopentone, methohexitone and propanidid in the dog. *Br. J. Anaesth.*, 40 736 (1968).
11. Whitwam J. G. and D. S. Young. Observations on dental anaesthesia induced with methohexitone, III. Blood pressure changes. *Br. J. Anaesth.*, 36, 237 (1964).
12. Lyons, S. M. and R. S. J. Clarke, A comparison of different drugs for anaesthesia in cardiac surgical patients. *Br. J. Anaesth.*, 44, 575 (1972).
13. Blackburn, J. P., C. M. Conway, J. M. Leigh, M. J. Lindop and J. A. Reitan, The effects of anaesthetic induction agents upon myocardial contracility. *Anaesthesia*, 26, 93 (1971).
14. O'Donnell, J. F., J. C. Hewitt and J. W. Dundee, Clinical studies of induction agents XXVIII: A further comparison of venous complications following thiopentone, methohexitone and propanidid. *Br. J. Anaesth.*, 41, 681 (1969).
15. Waters, D. J., Intra-arterial thiopentone (a physico-chemical phenomena). *Anaesthesia*, 21, 346 (1966).

11. ALTHESIN

LEO STRUNIN

Althesin, a potent intravenous anaesthetic agent (1), is a mixture of two steroids, alphaxalone and alphadalone acetate in a ratio of 3:1, dissolved in an aqueous vehicle containing 20% polyoxyethylated castor oil (Cremophor EL). Alphadalone acetate has only about half the anaesthetic activity of alphaxalone but is necessary to enhance the solubility of alphaxalone. Therefore 1 ml of Althesin contains 9 mg of alphaxalone, 3 mg of alphadalone acetate, has a pH of 7 and the protein binding varies between 20 and 40% dependant on the respective steroids.

Carson and his colleagues (2) have determined the comparative potency, taking speed of onset measured by counting, of Althesin against thiopentone and methohexitone. They found that 60-80 µl/kg Althesin was equivalent to 4 mg/kg thiopentone and 1.2 mg/kg methobexitone. Therefore an induction dose of Althesin in a 70 kg patient would be some 4-5.5 ml.

METABOLISM AND EXCRETION

Studies in the rat (3, 4) using Althesin labelled with carbon-14 alphaxalone, showed that the plasma half-life of carbon-14 alphaxalone was 6-8 min and the liver was the main site of metabolism. There was no redistribution in fat and approximately 70% of the radio-activity was excreted in the bile in the first three hours after administration. Further excretion studies over 5 days showed that 60-70% appeared in the faeces and only 20-30% in the urine.

Recently the metabolism and excretion of carbon-14 alphaxalone has been studied in man (5, 6). Patients with normal hepatic and renal function (controls), chronic liver disease, renal disease and anuria and one patient with acute liver disease were given carbon-14 labelled Althesin as part of their anaesthetic. The results show that there is rapid clearance of radio-activity from the plasma probably as a result of uptake by the liver. Radio-activity was apparent in the bile within ten minutes but the actual amount excreted was very small. Radio-activity was detected in the urine within thirty minutes. In the the control patients and those with chronic liver disease 80% of the administered radioactivity was excreted in the urine over five days. In the anuric patients the plasma clearance curve was similar to the controls. In the patient with acute liver disease plasma clearance was delayed. It is concluded that, in normal man, Althesin is rapidly taken up by the liver, metabolised to a more polar compound and then excreted in the urine. Plasma clearance is diminished in the presence of poor liver function.

CARDIOVASCULAR AND RESPIRATORY EFFECTS

Several studies have been carried out both in unpremedicated and premedicated patients (7, 8, 9). After induction of anaesthesia with Althesin in doses up to 100 µl/kg there was a fall in peripheral resistance, stroke volume, central venous pressure and arterial blood pressure (both systolic and diastolic). There was a compensatory tachycardia and cardiac output was maintained or even rose. These changes are similar to those seen after administration of thiopentone.

Characteristically after induction of anaesthesia with Althesin the patient takes a few deep breaths, then there may be a short period of apnoea followed by rapid shallow breathing. Arterial oxygen tension falls initially, but then tends to recover to the pre-induction level. There was little change in pH or arterial carbon dioxide tension.

Administration of the solvent (Cremophor EL) to unpremedicated volunteers had no significant cardiovascular effect (10).

In summary, Althesin produces cardio-respiratory changes similar to those seen after administration of barbiturates.

CLINICAL USAGE

With the exception of hyoscine, which causes an increased incidence of involuntary muscle movements, all the commonly used premedicant drugs are compatible with Althesin – as are the common gaseous and volatile anaesthetic agents and neuro-muscular blocking drugs.

Althesin is a more viscous solution than thiopentone and onset of anaesthesia is usually smooth but slightly slower. Recovery after single doses is similar to thiopentone and there is little cummulative effect. Nevertheless, Althesin as a sole anaesthetic has serious limitations. Intubation is not possible, and analgesia is poor. If large doses are given there is an appreciable incidence of involuntary muscle movements and cardio-respiratory depression will occur.

Althesin has been used as a continuous infusion (11). 5 ml of Althesin are added to 25 ml of 5% dextrose solution and the mixture infused using a calibrated infusion pump. Two uses have been suggested for this technique. Firstly it may be used for general anaesthesia in combination with an analgesic, a neuro-muscular blocking drug and intermittent positive pressure ventilation with an oxygen/air mixture. This form of anaesthesia is, of course, pollution free. Secondly an Althesin infusion may be used to sedate patients in the Intensive Care Unit. The advantages being that 'light sleep' is provided, there can be rapid variation of the level of sedation and since there is no effect on the pupil reflexes the central nervous system can be assessed easily. However, there is no analgesia with an Althesin infusion and there may be cardio-respiratory depression. Furthermore, if hiccups or involuntary muscle movements occur these may confuse diagnosis.

Althesin appears to be acceptable for Caesarian section, but crosses the placental barrier. The effects on the foetus have not yet been established. Theoretically Althesin is not contra-indicated in the patient with porphyria, but in the rat Althesin, like the barbiturates, activates ALA synthysase the enzyme involved in the metabolism of porphyrins. The safety of Althesin in patients with malignant hyperthermia has yet to be established. Althesin is suitable for patients with chronic renal or hepatic desease (5, 6). Unlike the barbiturates, Althesin lowers intracranial pressure (ICP) due to a reduction in cerebral blood flow and volume. Althesin may be the drug of choice for induction of anaesthesia in patients with raised ICP (12).

UNWANTED EFFECTS

Undesirable local venous sequelae after injection of Althesin are similar to those seen after 2.5% thipentone but less than after propanidid (Epontol). As Althesin solution is isotonic and pH 7, intra-arterial injection is probably harmless. As yet no vascular damage has been reported associated with intra-arterial injection.

The more serious unwanted effects related to Althesin concern those of an allergic nature. Clarke and his colleagues (13) have followed up 100 reported reactions to intravenous agents. 82 of these followed administration of Althesin. The reactions were classified as histaminoid, histaminoid with bronchospasm, bronchospasm only and cardiovascular collapse. There were no deaths associated with Althesin, whereas 4 of 14 reactions to thiopentone were fatal. The most likely explanation of these unwanted reactions is that histamine release occurs related to some immunological mechanism or as a direct effect on mast cells. In the case of Althesin suspicion has fallen on its solvent (Cremophor EL) which is a noted histamine releaser in certain strains of dog. However in man this does not seem to be the case and it is likely that the two steroids themselves are the antigenic substances. Clarke and his colleagues (13) inferred that the incidence of reactions to Althesin in Great Britain was 1:11,000-19,000 injections.

Treatment of the unwanted effects of Althesin is symptomatic. An obvious first step is to avoid using the drug if there is any previous history of an adverse reaction. Bronchospasm has responded to oxygen therapy, aminophylline and hydrocortisone intravenously, cardiovascular collapse to fluid infusion. Pre-medication with antihistaminic drugs may be of prophylatic value.

ADVANTAGES AND DISADVANTAGES COMPARED WITH THE BARBI-TURES

a. Advantages
Althesin is a stable, isotonic, non-irritant (pH 7) solution. It is a potent agent with a good therepeutic ratio. The drug is rapidly metabolised by the liver and there is little cummulative effect. Intracranial pressure is reduced.

b. Disadvantages
Althesin is a complex drug, its main constituent is not water soluble and as a result the solution as supplied is viscous. There are no clear advantages with respect to cardio-respiratory effects over barbiturates. The incidence of unwanted effects (hiccups, involuntary muscle movements and allergic phenomena) is higher than the barbiturates.

On balance, there is a place for Althesin in current anaesthetic practice, although it is not the 'ideal intravenous agent'. However many steroids are now known to have anaesthetic activity and perhaps further development may remove the limitations currently seen with Althesin.

ACKNOWLEDGEMENTS

The author would like to thank his colleagues for the discussions of their views on Althesin and Miss Amanda Shaw for secretarial tolerance.

REFERENCES

1. Child, K. J., J. P. Currie, B. Davis, M. G. Dodds, D. R. Pearce and D. J. Twissel, The pharmacological properties in animals of CT 1341 – a new steroid anaesthetic. *Brit. J. Anaesth.* 43, 2 (1971).
2. Carson, I. W., J. W. Dundee, R. J. S. Clarke, The speed of onset and potency of Althesin. *Brit. J. Anaesth.* 47, 512 (1975).
3. Card, B., P. J. McCulloch and D. A. H. Pratt, Tissue distribution of CT 1341 (Althesin) in the rat: an autoradiographic study. *Postgrad. med J.* 2 (Suppl.), 34 (1972).
4. Child, K. J., W. Gibson, G. Harnby and J. W. Hart, Metabolism and excretion of CT 1341 (Althesin) in the rat. *Postgrad. med. J.* 2 (Suppl.), 37 (1972).
5. Strunin, L., J. M. Strunin, K. M. Knights and M. E. Ward, Metabolism of ^{14}C alphaxalone in man. *Brit. J. Anaesth.* 46, 319 (1974).
6. Ward, M. E., Y. Adu-Gyamfi and L. Strunin, Althesin and pancuronium in chronic liver disease. *Brit. J. Anaesth.* 47, 1199 (1975).
7. Savege, T. M., E. I. Foley, R. J. Coultas, B. Walton, L. Strunin, B. R. Simpson and D. F. Scott, CT 1341: Some effects in man. *Anaesthesia* 26, 402 (1971).
8. Savege, T. M., E. I. Foley, L. Ross and M. P. Maxwell, A comparison of the cardio-respiratory effects during induction of anaesthesia with Althesin, thiopentone and methohexitone. *Postgrad. Med. J.* 2 (Suppl.), 66 (1972).
9. Clarke, R. J. S., J. W. Dundee and I. W. Carson, A new steroid anaesthetic – Althesin. *Proc. Roy. Soc. Med.* 66, 1027 (1973).
10. Savege, T. M., E. I. Foley and B. R. Simpson, Some cardiorespiratory effects of Cremaphor EL in man. *Brit. J. Anaesth.* 45, 515 (1973).
11. Ramsay, M. A. E., T. M. Savege, B. R. J. Simpson and R. Goodwin, Controlled sedation with alphaxalone – alphadalone. *Br. Med. J.* 2, 656 (1976).
12. Pickerodt, V., D. G. McDowall, N. J. Coroneos and N. P. Keaney, Effects of Althesin on cerebral perfusion, cerebral metabolism and intra cranial pressure in the anaesthetised baboon. *Brit. J. Anaesth.* 44, 751 (1972).
13. Clarke, R. J. S., J. W. Dundee, R. T. Fanett, F. R. McArdle and J. A. Sutton, Adverse reactions to intravenous agents. *Brit. J. Anaesth.* 47, 575 (1975.

12. DIAZEPAM – LORAZEPAM AND FLUNITRAZEPAM

G. ROLLY

The first clinically useful benzodiazepine, chlordiazepoxide (Librium®), introduced in 1958 into clinical use, (1), was rapidly followed by diazepam (Valium®) in 1961 (2). Lorazepam (Temesta®) became available in 1971 and flunitrazepam (Rohypnol®) still more recently. The structural formulae are shown in figure 1.

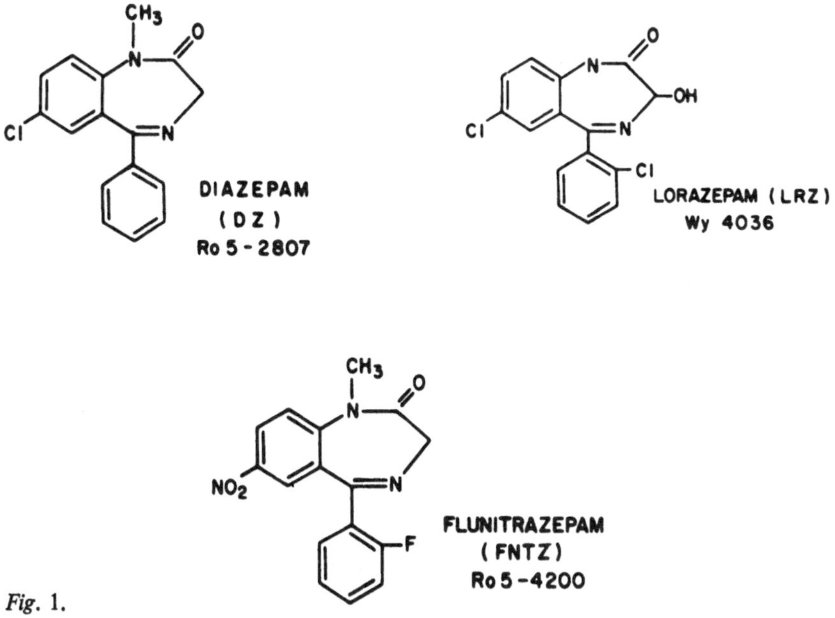

Fig. 1.

DIAZEPAM

Pharmacological properties
Diazepam is a colorless, crystalline compound, insoluble in water. It is available in tablets (2.5 and 10 mg) and in solution (5 mg/ml) with a pH of

6.4 to 6.9. The organic solvents employed consist of 40% propylene glycol, 10% ethyl alcohol, 5% sodium benzoate and 5% benzoic acid, with 1.5% benzyl alcohol as a preservative. This solution causes visible precipitation and cloudiness in water, but this does not seem to decrease potency.

Diazepam is lipid soluble and probably circulates strongly bound to serum albumin (95%) over a wide range of concentrations (3). Bioavailability of diazepam is influenced by the mode of administration (4). Intramuscular administration in the thigh gives higher plasma levels than injection of the same doses in the buttock, and oral administration gives a slow rise in plasma levels.

After oral administration, diazepam is fairly rapidly absorbed and peak levels occur within 2 to 4 hours. Clearance from blood can be represented as a double exponential function, with a half life of 7 to 10 hours for the fast component and more than 2 days for the slow component (5). The initial rapid disappearance represents redistribution; thereafter the drug is slowly biotransformed and excreted. This biphasic elimination pattern is still more marked after I.V. administration. A 10 to 20 mg dose produces a level of about 1 μg/ml at 4 min., coincident with profound clinical sedation and a short period of anterograde amnesia. Blood-levels fall rapidly to 0.25 μg/ml within 1 hour, accompanied by clinical 'recovery'. The rate of elimination then slows. Baird and Hailey noted a 'resurgence' of blood levels at approximately 6 hours following the dose, at which time subjects again become drowsy (6). This can be related either to mobilisation of diazepam from lipid storage sites or to release of diazepam or its active metabolites from the enterohepatic circulation.

The highest levels of diazepam in the tissues have been found in the liver, with high levels in the adipose tissue and low levels in the brain. Diazepam 10 to 20 mg I.V. given during labor is distributed equally in maternal and fetal blood (7).

Diazepam is exclusively excreted in urine in the form of its metabolites, principally oxazepam. It is demethylated and then slowly hydroxylated to oxazepam. Of a 10 mg dose of radioactive diazepam, 71% was found in urine and 10% could be detected in the faeces.

Actions
Diazepam, like other benzodiazepines, has important psychopharmacologic properties. Relief of anxiety is an important feature. Low doses cause sedation and higher ones induce an hypnotic state. The mechanism of action of benzodiazepines is different from that of the barbiturates. While the barbi-

turates produce depression of the brainstem reticular formation, and enhancement of the thalamic recruiting responses, the benzodiazepines produce much less of the former and none of the latter.

The central muscle relaxant effect of diazepam is pronounced and its site is principally the gamma motor system. It affects principally polysynaptic, rather than monosynaptic, reflexes (8). The site of action is thought to be at the supraspinal level, probably at the reticular formation of the brainstem.

Diazepam potentiates and prolongs the paralysing effects of non depolarising muscle relaxants, but does not potentiate the effects of succinylcholine. Although experimental evidence suggests that benzodiazepines are predominently central muscle relaxants, observations imply that diazepam may in addition have a more distal effect which is not yet well understood.

Diazepam is very effective in antagonizing generalized seizures induced by systemic administration of various analeptic drugs. Its effect upon focal seizure activity is somewhat different. Diazepam is 5 to 10 times as active as chlordiazepoxide as an anticonvulsant.

Side effects

Benzodiazepines affect blood pressure and myocardial function through both direct and neurogenic mechanisms, the result depending on the interaction of the two influences. After large doses, diazepam produces a depression of the cardiovascular system with a moderate decrease of heart rate, contractile force, blood pressure and cardiac output. In healthy subjects doses up to 0.2 mg/kg produced no clinically important changes in blood pressure or cardiac output (9). Some ASA Class IV cardiac patients have shown transient episodes of bradycardia and hypotension. Knapp and Dubow found after 0.2 mg/kg diazepam I.V. that in less than 1% of subjects was there a reduction of cardiac output of more than 15%, and in no subjects did blood pressure fall by more than 15% (10).

All benzodiazepines are potential respiratory depressants. In healthy individuals diazepam produces no clinically important respiratory depression and does not potentiate the depressant effects of opiates. Following I.V. use, it has negligible effects on respiration, as shown by blood gas analysis. In some studies a 10% decrease in tidal volume was noticed after 0.2 mg/kg I.V. diazepam, compared to 15% decrease after 2 mg/kg thiopental (11). Some cases of apnoea were recorded after I.V. administration (12). A 34% increase in VD/VT rates has been reported together with a depression of the ventilatory response to carbon dioxide in 50% of the patients (13).

Intramuscular diazepam produces an elevation of serum creatinine phosphokinase (CPK) activity (14).

Clinical uses

In anesthetic practice, diazepam is useful by mouth as a tranquillizing drug before surgery, or as a sedative or hypnotic drug. For some observers REM sleep is not influenced, but for others it is depressed in a dose related manner (15). For premedication 10 mg I.M. is found to be effective in producing a quiet, tranquil patient without sedation, free from anxiety and with no untoward disturbances of vital function. A useful degree of amnesia is provided by 10 to 30 mg diazepam I.V. (16), but neither anterograde or retrograde amnesia is found with I.M. diazepam (17).

Because of minimal circulatory effects, diazepam is advocated as an intravenous induction agent, but the dose is difficult to assess. Dose ranges of 0.2 to 0.8 mg/kg have been suggested. Anesthesia is induced more slowly than with barbiturates. The duration of sleep is usually 20 to 30 minutes, and recovery from general anesthesia is prolonged as compared to recovery from short acting barbiturates. A high incidence (22%) of burning at the site of injection and venous thrombosis in the smaller peripheral veins is noticed with diazepam, unless it is diluted (18). Diazepam has no analgesic or anti-emetic properties. It reduces the M.A.C. of volatile anesthetics (19, 20).

Diazepam is also frequently used for facilitating endoscopy and for cardioversion in a dose of 15 to 20 mg I.V. The anticonvulsant properties are used in treatment of status epilepticus and convulsions due to overdose of local anesthetics, but high doses are needed.

Diazepam is frequently given as a sedative in small I.V. doses during regional anesthetic techniques. It is also popular as a sedative during prolonged artificial ventilation and in hypnotic doses for the treatment of tetanus, where its muscle relaxant effect is highly beneficial, although it has not been shown to reduce overall mortality (21).

Diazepam can be used to decrease the psychomimetic reactions after ketamine anesthesia (22, 23).

Whether diazepam is used as premedicant or as induction agent, a delay in emergence from general anesthesia is frequently reported and ambulatory recipients of diazepam are to be advised not to drive for 10 to 24 hours (24).

LORAZEPAM

Pharmacological properties
Lorazepam (Temesta ®) is one of the newer and highly active benzodiazepines. It is 2 to 4 times more potent than diazepam. It is a white powder,
almost insoluble in water. It is presented in tablets of 1 and 2.5 mg. Recently
for experimental purposes an injectable form is available and each ml contains 5 mg lorazepam, in 80% propylene glycol, 18% polyoxyethylene glycol,
and 2% benzylalcohol. It is painless when injected into small veins (25).
After oral administration of 7.5 mg lorazepam, peak plasma values are
found between 1 and 6 hours, barely exceed 0.05 μg/ml of free drug, and
subside over 24 hours (26). In plasma both free lorazepam and a glucuronide
bound form exist. Four hours after administration, the drug is mainly in the
conjugated form. Excretion takes place almost exclusively as the glucuronide
in urine. Less than 1% is found in faeces.

Actions
Lorazepam has good anxiolytic and tension relieving effects, inducing a
quiet, calm patient. An interesting phenomenon is the lack of recall found
with this drug (27, 28), which is in pronounced contrast with diazepam.
Intravenous injections of both diazepam and flunitrazepam are followed
immediately by a short period of amnesia. Lorazepam 4 mg I.V. has a slow
onset of action for anterograde amnesia and only produces pronounced
effect after 75 minutes, but this action persists for a period of several hours
(29).

Side effects
Cardiovascular functions are not influenced even at higher dosages. Comer
et al. found 9 mg lorazepam I.V. caused no changes in blood pressure,
cardiac output or total peripheral resistance in healthy male volunteers (30).
Double-blind studies proved that 5 mg lorazepam administered I.M. had no
marked effect on the cardiovascular parameters, measured 90 minutes later
(31).
    Respiratory effects are negligible. 90 minutes after I.M. injection of 5 mg
lorazepam, a decrease of peak flow, FEV_1, FEV_3 and V.C. have been demonstrated, but are probably attributable to diminished perseverance on
the part of the patient (32). After I.V. injection of 2 mg, the CO_2 response is
unaffected, but it is depressed after 5 mg I.M. (30).

Clinical use

In anesthetic practice, lorazepam can be used by mouth the evening before surgery in a dose of 2 to 2.5 mg. In older or arteriosclerotic patients, the dose must be reduced to 1 mg or even 0.5 mg. It can also be given in a dose of 5 mg I.M. for premedication, but the injection has to be given at least 90 minutes before surgery to obtain favourable results. It considerably diminishes the recall of events of the operative day.

Lorazepam can be used I.V. for anesthetic induction. Very high doses (up to 13 mg) are needed for induction, and agitation and disorientation are common in the postoperative period. Lorazepam 0.1 mg/kg, with O_2-N_2O and muscle relaxation is not a satisfactory technique, as high doses of muscle relaxants are needed, and adverse cardiovascular effects are commonly seen.

It has been combined with analgesics in a technique called 'amnanalgesia' (0.05 mg/kg lorazepam, 0.005 mg/kg fentanyl, O_2-N_2O and curarisation), combining the properties of lorazepam with those of an analgesic drug. Although used as an induction agent, lorazepam does not induce loss of consciousness as barbiturates do. A total lack of recall of events beginning around 75 minutes after I.M. injection of lorazepam and lasting 6 to 8 hours after surgery is noticed. This is considered by most patients as a useful effect. Slight restlessness in the postoperative period is occasionally encountered, but can be prevented by providing good analgesia.

Lorazepam is more active than diazepam in inhibiting convulsions induced by metrazol. In man a dose of 5 mg has been used I.V. for terminating pentylenetetrazol induced abnormal discharge activity. The same dose has also been used I.V. to suppress an epileptic attack (33).

FLUNITRAZEPAM

Pharmacological properties

The first fluorinated benzodiazepine used in clinical practice was flurazepam (Dalmadorm®), recently followed by flunitrazepam (Rohypnol®). Flunitrazepam is a crystalline substance, readily soluble in alcohol, but only sparingly in water. It is available in tablets of 2 mg and in ampoules containing 2 mg, to be dissolved in organic solvent composed of propylene glycol, ethylalcohol, sodium benzoate and benzoic acid. It causes pain when given directly into a small vein and sometimes thrombophlebitis occurs (34). Animal experiments have shown that this drug possesses sedative, hypnotic and anticonvulsant properties, which are superior to those of diazepam.

Actions

In man the I.V. hypnotic dose varies between 1 to 3 mg with a mean dosage of 2 mg. Sleep usually occurs in less than one minute after the end of injection (34). After a short period of slurred speech, the patient goes to sleep in a relaxed mood. The major drawback, as with diazepam, is the large individual dosage variation as compared with other induction agents. Resistance to induction is found in patients already taking tranquillizing agents and in chronic alcoholics. Flunitrazepam does not possess any analgesic properties.

Side effects

In contrast to diazepam, flunitrazepam has not been found to reduce the requirements for muscle relaxants.

Although some authors report the absence of respiratory depression, others have observed a depressant effect on respiration with $PaCO_2$ increases (35). A small shortlived decrease of PaO_2 is noticed after I.V. injection of 1 mg of flunitrazepam (36).

The cardiovascular effects are minimal. Sometimes a slight decrease of arterial blood pressure and heart rate can be observed, of little significance. In hypertensive or hypovolemic patients this can be more pronounced (34). In induction studies for orthopedic surgery, flunitrazepam 0.03 mg/kg was without significant influence on cardiac output and stroke volume (37). 2 to 3 mg I.V. has been shown to cause slight decrease of cardiac output, stroke volume, blood pressure and central venous pressure (38, 39).

Flunitrazepam possesses a marked synergetic action with barbiturates and analgesics. When these drugs are combined, emergence from anesthesia may delayed. Flunitrazepam in a dose of 0.03 mg/kg impaired flicker fusion discrimination and co-ordination for up to 10 hours, so that patients should not drive or operate machinery for at least 24 hours (24).

Clinical use

Flunitrazepam has been used by mouth as sedative the evening before surgery (40), or intramuscularly as a premedicant (40). It can be used as an I.V. induction agent, but due to its prolonged effect, it is best reserved for long lasting surgery (41), and has been combined with some form of neuroleptanalgesic technique (42). The future use of this drug may be as a prolonged sedative agent.

REFERENCES

1. Tobin, J. M. and N. D. Lewis, New psychotherapeutic agent, chlordiazepoxide. *J.A.M.A.*, 194, 1242 (1960).
2. Sussex, J. N., P. A. Linton and C. D. Herliby, Anxiety and depression in borderline schizophrenic states – treatment with Valium, a Librium analog. *Psychosomatics*, 2, 256 (1961).
3. Van der Kleijn, E., J. M. Van Rossum, E. T. Muskens, N. V. M. Rijntjes, Pharmacokinetics of diazepam in dogs, mice and humans. *Acta Pharmacol. Toxicol.* 29 (suppl. 3), 109-127 (1971).
4. Gamble, J. A. S., J. W. Dundee, R. A. Assaf, Plasma diazepam levels after single dose oral and intramuscular administration. *Anaesthesia*, 30; 164-169 (1975).
5. DeSilva, J. A., M. Schwarts, V. Stefanovic, J. Kaplan, L. D'arconte, Determination of diazepam (Valium) in blood by gas liquid chromatography. *Anal. Chem.* 36, 2099 (1964).
6. Baird, E. S. and D. M. Hailey, Delayed recovery from a sedative: correlation of the plasma levels of diazepam with clinical effects after oral and intravenous administration. *Brit. J. Anesth.*, 44, 803-808 (1972).
7. Cavanagh, D. and C. S. Condo, Diazepam-pilot study of drug concentrations in maternal blood, amniotic fluid and cord blood. *Curr. ther. Res.*, 6, 122 (1964).
8. Ngai, S. H., D. T. C. Tseng, S. C. Wang, Effect of diazepam and other central nervous system depressants on spinal reflexes in cats; a study of site of action. *J. Pharmacol. Exp. Ther.* 153, 344 (1966).
9. Healy, T. E., J. S. Robinson, M. D. Vickers, Physiological responses to intravenous diazepam as a sedative for conservative dentistry. *Brit. Med. J.*, 3, 10-13 (1970).
10. Knapp, R. B. and H. Dubow, Comparison of diazepam with thiopental as an induction agent in cardiopulmonary disease. *Anesth. Analg.*, 49, 722-726 (1970).
11. Knapp, R. B. and H. Dubow, Diazepam as an induction agent for patients with cardiopulmonary disease. *South. Med. J.*, 63, 1451-1453 (1970).
12. Doughty, A., Unexpected danger of diazepam. *Brit. Med. J.*, 2, 239 (1970).
13. Catculove, R. F. and E. R. Kafer, Effects of diazepam on the ventilatory response to carbon dioxide and a steadystate gas exchange. *Anesthesiology*, 341, 9 (1971).
14. Kuster, J., Increased creatine-kinase concentrations after intramuscular injection of diazepam. *German Med.*, 2, 154-155 (1972).
15. Lanoir, J. and E. K. Killam, Alteration in the sleep-wakefulness patterns by benzodiazepines in the cat. *Electroenceph. Clin. Neurophysiol.*, 25, 530-542 (1968).
16. Keilty, S. R. and S. Blackwood, Sedation for conservative dentistry. *Brit. J. Clin. Pract.*, 23, 365 (1969).
17. Dundee, J. W. and S. R. Keilty, Diazepam. In Clarke R. S. (ed.). The New Intravenous Anesthetics. *Int. Anesthesiol. Clin.*, 7, 91 (1969).
18. McClish, A., Diazepam as an intravenous induction agent for general anesthesia. *Can. Anaesth. Soc. J.*, 13, 562 (1966).
19. Perisho, J. A., D. R. Buechel, R. D. Miller, The effect of diazepam (Valium ®) on minimum alveolar anaesthetic requirement (MAC) in man. *Can. Anaesth. Soc. J.*, 18, 536-540 (1971).
20. Tsunoda, Y., Y. Hattori, E. Takatsuka, T. Sawa, T. Hori, E. Ikezo, Effects of hydroxyzine, diazepam, and pentazocine on halothane minimum alveolar anesthetic concentration. *Anesth. Analg.*, 52 390-394 (1973).

21. Hendrickse, R. G. and P. M. Sherman, Tetanus in childhood: report of a therapeutic trial of diazepam. *Brit. Med. J.*, 2, 860 (1966).
22. Lean, T. H., S. S. Ratnam, R. Sivasamboo, Use of benzodiazepines in the management of eclampsia. *J. Obstet. Gynaecol. Br. Commonw.*, 75, 856 (1968).
23. Lebowitz, W., Electrical conversion of arrhythmias under diazepam sedation. *Conn. Med.*, 33, 173 (1969).
24. Korttila, K. and M. Linnoila, Skills related to driving after intravenous diazepam, flunitrazepam or droperidol. *Brit. J. Anesth.*, 46, 961 (1974).
25. Verschraegen, R. and G. Rolly, Amn-Analgesia: preliminary results. *Acta Anaesth. Belg.*, 25, 340-349 (1974).
26. Knowles, J. A., W. H. Comer, H. W. Ruelius, Disposition of 7-chloro-5-(o-chloro-5-(o-chlorophenyl)-1,3-dihydro-3-hydroxy-2H-1,4-benzodiazepin-2-one (lorazepam) in humans and four animal species. *Arzneim Forsch*, 21, 1059-1065 (1971).
27. Wilson, J., Lorazepam as a premedicant for general anaesthesia. *Curr. Med. Res. Opin.*, 1, 308-316 (1973).
28. Turner, D. J., Lorazepam as a premedicant in anaesthesia: a pilot study. *Curr. Med. Res. Opin.*, 11, 302-307 (1973).
29. Dundee, J. W., The amnesic action of Diazepam, Flunitrazepam and Lorazepam in man. *Acta Anaesth. Belg.*, presented for publication (1975).
30. Comer, W. H., N. Nomof, G. Navarro, H. W. Ruelius, Pharmacology of parenterally administered lorazepam in man. *J. Int. Med. Res.*, 1, 216 (1973).
31. Verschraegen R. and G. Rolly, Intramuscular premedication with lorazepam (Temesta ®). *Acta Anaesth. Belg.*, 25, 68-81 (1974).
32. Verschraegen, R. and G. Rolly, The influence of lorazepam (Temesta ®) on anesthesia. *Acta Anaesth. Belg.*, 24, 256-264 (1973).
33. Waltregny, A. and J. Dargent, Preliminary study of parenteral lorazepam in epileptic states in man. *Acta Neurolog. Belg.*, 75, fasc. 5, 219-229 (1975).
34. Stovner, J., R. Endresen, A. Osterud, Intravenous anaesthesia with a new benzodiazepine RO 5-4200. *Acta Anaesth. Scand.*, 17, 163-170 (1973).
35. Pearce, C., A clinical trial of RO 5-4200 (flunitrazepam) used to supplement spinal anaesthesia in elderly patients. *Brit. J. Anaesth.*, 46, 877-880 (1974).
36. Van de Walle, J., P. Lauwers, H. Adriaensen, Clinical experimentation with flunitrazepam (RO 05-4200). *Acta Anaesth. Belg.*, 25, 350-359 (1974).
37. Rolly, G., P. Lamote, P. Cosaert, Hemodynamic studies of flunitrazepam or RO 05-4200 injection in man. *Acta Anaesth. Belg.*, 25, 359-370 (1974).
38. Coleman, A. U., J. W. Downing, D. G. Moyes, A. O'Brien, Acute cardiovascular effects of RO 5-4200: a new anaesthetic induction agent. *South Afr. Med. J.*, 47, 382-384 (1973).
39. Rifat, K. and M. Bolomey, Les effets cardiovasculaires du Rohypnol ® utilisé comme agent d'induction anesthésique. *Ann. Anesth. Franç.*, 16, 135-145 (1975).
40. Schwander, D., A. Sirvysw, R. Marco, A. Bart, Emploi du RO 5-4200 chez les patients à resque élevé. *Proc. Europ. Congres Anaesth. Madrid*, 5-11 Sept. (1974).
41. Geens-Bastenier, J., C. Genicot, J. Primo-Dubois, Utilisation du RO 5-4200 comme agent hypnotique dans la neuroleptanalgézie. Comparaison avec le méthohexital et le diazépam. *Anesth. Analg. Réanim.*, 51, 687-699 (1974).
42. Kurka, P., Klinische Erfahrungen mit RO 5-4200 in der Anästhesie. *Der Anaesthesist*, 23, 375-381 (1974).

13. KETAMINE TODAY

W. K. HAMILTON

The remarks in this paper will be somewhat different from others presented here. We have been presented with good discussions of pharmacokinetics and clinical pharmacology of many popular intravenous anaesthetic agents. This discussion will therefore not be a consideration of either of these areas. It will rather be an overview of the phenomenon of Ketamine, its introduction and its current status. The remarks are largely philosophical in nature and are in no way to be considered exact and precise data. Personal opinions are however plentiful.

Ketamine was introduced into clinical anaesthesia with almost unprecedented promotion. This was to be an entirely new ERA in anaesthesia. This was not just another barbiturate or tranquilizer – this was a dissociative anaesthetic which would separate the patients' senses from the painful environs of surgery in a new – yet unexplained – way. This new form of anaesthesia would be so revolutionary that the most common problems of anaesthesia would be banished. This is perhaps an over-statement of the claims, but at least the common problems would be minimized.

The circulation would be depressed little, if at all. Blood pressure and pulse rate and cardiac output would be maintained or even increased! Everybody knows that big numbers are good numbers and therefore the situation resulting from Ketamine anaesthesia would be a happy one for patients and anaesthesiologists. The hearts that would be asked to work at higher rates, outputs and pressures were not consulted.

Respiration would also escape bad effects when Ketamine was used. Not only was there minimal, if any, depression of the respiratory centre and its neuromuscular connections, but airways *would be maintained!* The 'protective reflexes' were also to remain unviolated and this happy combination of beneficial effects was awaited with anxiety. Imagine the carefree life of anaesthesia practice with minimal circulatory and respiratory depression and self-maintained airways.

In addition to the above, it was tempting to consider the so-called advantages of intravenous drugs as opposed to inhaled agents. Anaesthesia personnel could stay out of the surgeon's way. There were no noxious vapours to breathe and fewer instruments would be needed to maintain airways.

I recall vividly the very first day Ketamine was to be released for clinical use. Very early in the morning, I was met at the door of the hospital by a representative of the company handing out free samples of this promising new product.

What has happened now a few years after this promotional introduction? What do we see when Camelot is revisited? I can only report my own impressions – they result, however, from experiences in two medical centres 6,000 miles apart and lesser experiences as points in between are visited.

We saw an initial flurry and enthusiasm which faded rapidly. A search of anaesthesia journals in 1975 reveals Ketamine to be far from popular. It is reasonable to inquire concerning the reasons for this. This cannot be answered with data or measurements at this time. Some likely causes for failure of Ketamine to assume a leading role can be identified however.

One of the more notable reasons was bizarre post-operative behaviour. Whether this is properly called hullucinations, delirium or 'bad trip' is not important. There were undesirable episodes of not infrequent occurrence which were not liked by doctors, nurses, patients and relatives. The abnormal behaviour ellicited fears as to permanent or long-lasting changes in central nervous system function which persist – unproven – in some minds today. The abnormal behaviour could be prevented – or treated – by keeping patients quite isolated or by adding other depressant drugs. Neither of these seemed desirable – or, at least, advantageous. The companies which dispensed the drug provided printed signs which announced 'This patient had Ketamine – please do not disturb'. One could argue that absolute quietude is not part of a desired post-operative routine.

The drug was often found to be unsatisfactory when used alone. It is of course non-volatile and it therefore lacked flexibility so prolonged sleeping time – or recovery time – was experienced by many. Movement of arms, fingers, legs and head during surgery made surgeons restless and even prevented performance of surgery in some instances. Again, supplemented drugs were needed and the proposed advantages were not readily identified.

Airways did obstruct. The first day we used Ketamine, we selected a patient for relatively minor surgery in the prone position. He rapidly developed complete upper airway obstruction requiring temporary termination of the surgery and establishing airway control by conventional methods. It is likely that airway problems are an inherent accompaniment of unconsciousness and finding obstruction and aspiration in patients anaesthetised with Ketamine was not surprising to older observers.

The announced circulatory advantages were perhaps more proposed than real. There is now much question as to beneficial effect from maintained output, blood pressure and heart rate during anaesthesia – especially in ischemic heart disease. Internists and many anaesthetists believe reduction of after-load, reduction in oxygen demand and an accompanying decrease in myocardial contractility, work and oxygen consumption are appropriate. At least Ketamine has demonstrated no proven advantage over halothane for instance in management of patients who have ischemic heart disease.

In summary, the new approach did very little that available drugs did not already do and introduced new complications of its own.

Ketamine is certainly *not* a useless drug. There are many instances where it is a fine and perhaps preferred induction agent. It also provides excellent anaesthesia for many procedures requiring little 'depth' of anaesthesia. Perhaps the future holds a greater place for Ketamine as an adjunct to nitrous oxide. This role certainly was the eventual niche for thiopental.

Perhaps the greatest lesson for us now to harvest from this experience is in evaluation of anaesthetic agents. The final role of these agents is more likely to be determined by overall patient well-being rather than a few rather isolated pharmacologic facts.

14. DROPERIDOL

W. SOUDIJN

Droperidol, a neuroleptic drug of the butyrophenone type is widely used, together with a potent analgesic like e.g. fentanyl in neuroleptanalgesia.

It is one of the most potent members of the series, but has a much shorter duration of action in animal experiments than e.g. haloperidol. In a typical experiment for the estimation of antipsychotic potency, the amphetamine test in rats, pretreatment with an effective neuroleptic protects the rat against the stereo-typed behaviour and agitation evoked by an injection of amphetamine. The lowest ED_{50} of haloperidol in this test is 0.038 mg per kg and of droperidol 0.025 mg per kg. For 4 hours protection the dose of haloperidol needed is 1.9 times higher than the lowest effective dose (1.9 × 0.038 = 0.07 mg per kg). However, droperidol has a much shorter duration of action, since for 4 hours protection 23 times the lowest ED_{50} is required. Droperidol is therefore also one of the shortest acting neuroleptics known.

Amphetamine induced stereotyped behaviour is also seen in monkeys and in man. Monkeys stare and grab at nonexistent objects and the head or limbs often move in a stereotyped manner. Man may perform actions, which by their monotonous repetition become pointless, or may continuously repeat sentences, words or parts of a song. Hallucinations may also occur.

The amphetamine syndrome is caused by stimulation of dopaminergic neurones in the striatum and in the limbic system through the mobilisation of dopamine by amphetamine. Neuroleptics are effective blockers of dopaminergic receptors and abolish the amphetamine evoked symptoms. Although droperidol is a neuroleptic with a fairly rapid onset of action it is not used in psychiatry because of its short duration of action.

In neuroleptanalgesia it is used for pre-medication in a dose of 2.5-5 mg i.m. together with fentanyl 0.05-0.1 mg i.m., in induction a dose of 15-20 mg i.v. is used with fentanyl in a dose of 0.4-0.6 mg i.v. This treatment results in the majority of patients in an indifference to the surroundings and complete mental detachment. In a minority of cases however, agitation, anxiety, fear, depersonalization syndromes and refusal of surgery following premedication has been observed. The cause of this phenomenon is not known and controlled data are not available yet.

A similar phenomenon is known in psychiatry as a paradoxal syndrome of neuroleptics. In some schizophrenic patients, sudden and dramatic exacerbations of psychosis, experiences of abject terror and restlessness occur after treatment with neuroleptics. Dose increases lead to a more florid psychosis. When the dose is lowered, the patient may be well controlled. The paradoxal syndrome is promptly reversed by an anticholinergic drug like biperiden. Whether both paradoxal phenomena have a common cause is a matter of speculation. Schaer and Jenny (1) showed in surgical patients that droperidol is eliminated very rapidly from human plasma. It is bound extensively (85-90%) but apparently only weakly to plasma proteins. Five minutes after intravenous administration (0,31 mg per kg) only 7.5 percent of the administered dose was detectable in the plasma. The rapid tissue penetration of the drug correlates with the fast onset of action.

Cressman and his coworkers (2) studying the pharmacokinetics of droperidol in healthy male volunteers also found a rapid initial distribution phase. They also showed that following intramuscular administration, absorption is so rapid that the response to droperidol is likely to be almost equivalent to that observed following intravenous administration.

The cardiovascular stability of the patient undergoing surgery under neuroleptanaesthetic conditions with droperidol and fentanyl or phenoperidine is well documented, but much less satisfactory understood.

In animal experiments droperidol is an effective alpha adrenergic blocking agent, protecting rats against death caused by cardiovascular collapse due to a lethal dose of epinephrine or norepinephrine.

The lowest effective ED_{50}'s of droperidol, haloperidol and chlorpromazine are 0.1, 3 and 0.6 mg per kg respectively. In 'in vitro' experiments droperidol appeared to be as potent as phentolamine in alpha blocking activity and devoid of any beta-1 or beta-2 blocking properties (van Nueten, personal communication). The effect of droperidol on cardiac tissues like auricular preparations of guinea-pig, papillary muscles of dog and cat, and Purkinje fibers of dog, cow and sheep was studied by Carmeliet, Xhonneux and their coworkers (3) and by Wojtczak and Beresewics (4). Low doses, well in the therapeutic range, decreased pacemaker activity and prolonged the effective refractory period, explaining the antiarrhythmic properties of the drug. It appeared that droperidol had no deleterious effect on Ca^{++} mediated action potentials and that the effects can be explained by a reduction in sodium conductance. It seems that droperidol has a membrane stabilizing

effect in cardiac tissue, which is unrelated to adrenergic receptor blocking
properties, but which might protect the cardiac tissue against a sudden rise
in the blood level of catecholamines, caused by surgical stress, inhalation
anaesthetics, shock or postmyocardial infarctation conditions. Tammisto
and his coworkers (5) showed that droperidol does not inhibit the liberation
of catecholamines provoked by surgery.

It is conceivable that alpha blockade, membrane stabilization of cardiac
tissue and central nervous system effects of droperidol all play a role in the
maintenance of cardiovascular stability.

Another characteristic property of droperidol is the blocking of dopaminergic neurones in the chemoreceptor triggerzone (zone of Borison and
Wang) caudally situated in the floor of the fourth ventricle. The zone is
stimulated by narcotic agonists, apomorphine, dihydroxyphenylalanine
(DOPA) etc. This stimulation is transmitted to the cholinergic vomiting
centre; the diaphragm and abdominal muscles contract and emesis occurs.
At very low doses neuroleptics inhibit the stimulation of the chemoreceptor
triggerzone without inducing behavioural changes in man and in the dog.
The anti-emetic potency of neuroleptics is tested by estimating the effective
dose for the inhibition of emesis of dogs challenged by a standard dose of
apomorphine. The lowest ED_{50}'s of droperidol, haloperidol and chlorpromazine are 0.001, 0.018 and 0.70 mg per kg respectively, when administered
subcutaneously, showing that droperidol is a potent anti-emetic drug. The
toxicity of the drug is very low indeed, and the therapeutic-ratio very high,
in the order of 21000-25000. The LD_{50}'s of droperidol, haloperidol and
chlorpromazine, when administered subcutaneously in the rat are > 640,
63, and 137 mg per kg.

The duration of action in man has been estimated by Edmonds-Seal and
Prys-Roberts (6) to be between 6 and 12 hours, and is conditioned by the
rate of metabolism and excretion and by the retention time of the drug in
chemoreceptor triggerzone and in the limbic system. In fact, it was shown
that neuroleptics like haloperidol and pimozide, chemical congeners of
droperidol are selectively taken up and retained by these brain structures
(Janssen and coworkers (7), Soudijn and van Wijngaarden (8)).

The rate and route of excretion and the metabolic fate of tritium labeled
droperidol in the rat was studied by Soudijn, van Wijngaarden and Allewijn
(9). The drug is extensively metabolized by a pathway common to most
neuroleptics of the butyrophenone type (fig. 1).

In man the majority of these drugs are degraded by the same pathway.
The metabolites are pharmacologically inactive. In the rat ^{3}H-droperidol is

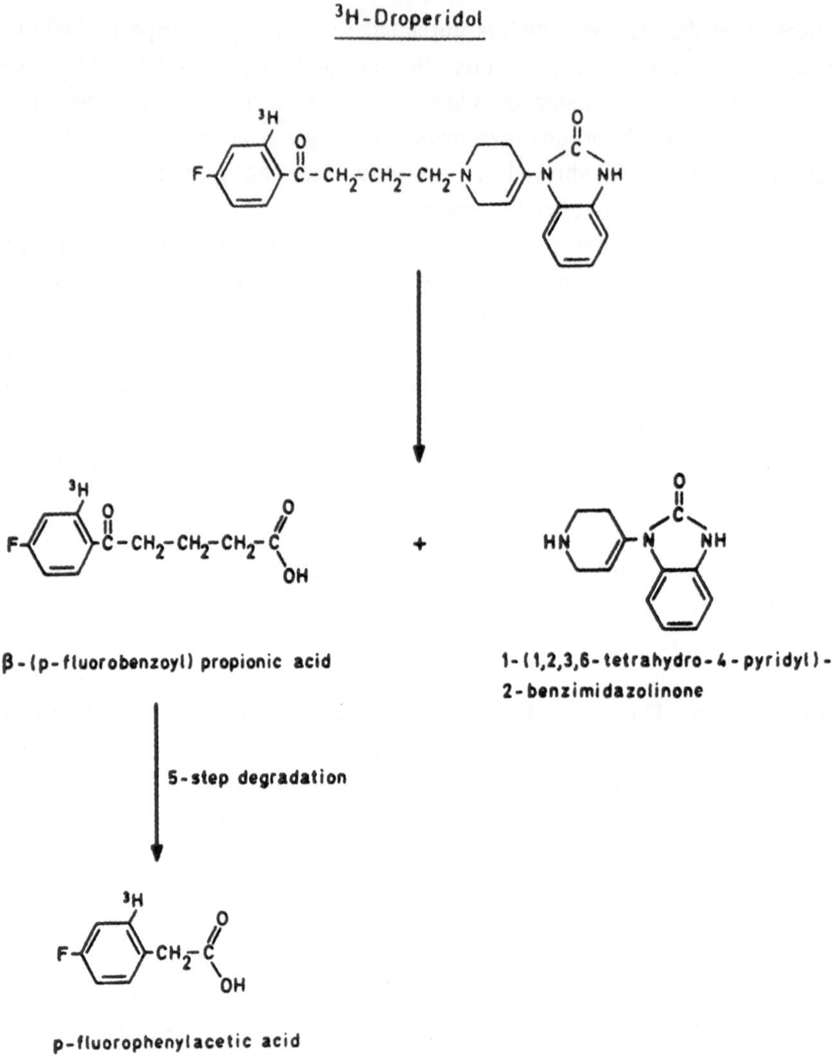

Fig. 1. Metabolic pathway of tritium-labeled droperidol in the male adult Wistar rat.

rapidly metabolized and excreted, 30 percent in urine and 62 percent in feces. The major part (83%) was excreted within the first 24 hours. Fifteen minutes after injection about 60 percent of the total radioactivity in liver and 35 percent in blood and brain was found to originate from metabolites of droperidol. The brain level of unchanged droperidol correlates well with its neuroleptic activity as tested in the antiamphetamine test in the rat (Heykants, unpublished data). The kinetic data account for the short duration of action of droperidol in the rat. Cressman (2) has shown that in man the kinetics of droperidol follow a two compartment open model. After an initial rapid distribution phase with a half-life of 10 minutes droperidol is eliminated from the plasma with a half-life of 2.2 hours. The drug is rapidly metabolized and the major route of excretion is in the urine. Seventy-five percent of the dose (5 mg i.m.) is excreted in the urine, the major part within 24 hours. Only 1% of the excretion products is unaltered droperidol. Twenty-two percent of the dose is excreted in feces, 50 percent as unchanged droperidol. It is feasible that higher doses of droperidol may have a prolonged action caused by recirculation of the drug through an entero-hepatic shunt.

Concerning the interactions of droperidol with other drugs frequently used in neuroleptanalgesia, it may be stated that droperidol potentiates the analgesic effect of narcotic analgesics, but there is neither interaction with anticholinergic drugs nor with muscle relaxants.

There is no clinical evidence of toxicity or impairment of liver function caused by droperidol or its metabolites following several administrations. Droperidol and fentanyl or phenoperidine are used in the specialized treatment of severely burned patients requiring frequent changing of dressing, often on alternate days (10, 11).

Sensitization of the very ill patient does not occur and toxic effects after repeated administration are not observed.

Vogel (12) using large doses of fentanyl and droperidol in prolonged therapy requiring artificial respiration for long periods because of tetanus, chest injuries, or post-operative respiratory deficiency, did not report toxic effects or sensitization of the patients.

REFERENCES

1. Schaer, H. and E. Jenny, Plasmakonzentration und Plasma-eiweiszbindung von Droperidol und Fentanyl während der Neuroleptanästhesie beim Menschen. In W. F. Henschel (ed.), *Neue klinische Aspekte der Neurolept-analgesie*. Stuttgart and New York: Schattauer (1970).
2. Cressmann, W. A., J. Plostnieks and P. C. Johnson, Absorption, Metabolism and Excretion of Droperidol by human subjects following intramuscular and intravenous administration. *Anesthesiology* 38, 363 (1973).
3. Carmeliet, E., R. Xhonneux, van A. Glabbeek and R. Reneman, Electrophysiological effects of Droperidol in different cardiac tissues. *Naunyn-Schmiedebergs Arch. of Pharmacol.* In press (1975).
4. Wojtczak, J. and A. Beresewicz, Electrophysiological effects of neuroleptanalgesic drugs on the canine cardiac tissue. *Naunyn-Schmiedebergs Arch. of Pharmacol.* 286, 211 (1974).

5. Tammisto, T., S. Takki, P. Nikki and A. Jäättelä, Effect of operative stress on plasmacatecholamine levels during neuroleptanalgesia. *Anaesthesist* 22, 158 (1973).
6. Edmonds-Seal, J. and C. Prys-Roberts, Pharmacology of drugs used in neuroleptanalgesia. *Brit. J. Anaesth.* 42 207 (1970).
7. Janssen, P. A. J., W. Soudijn, I. van Wijngaarden and A. Dresse, Pimozide, a chemically novel, highly potent, and orally long-acting neuroleptic drug. *Arzneim. Forsch.* 18 282 (1968).
8. Soudijn, W. and I. van Wijngaarden, Localization of ^{3}H-pimozide in the rat brain in relation to its anti-amphetamine potency. *J. Pharm. Pharmacol.* 24 773 (1972).
9. Soudijn, W., I. van Wijngaarden and F. Allewijn, Distribution, excretion, and metabolism of neuroleptics of the butyrophenone type. *Eur. J. Pharmacol.* 1 45 (1967).
10. Barry Smith, G. and D. A. Hollis, The use of dehydrobenzperidol and phenoperidine for repeated burn dressings. *Brit. J. Anaesth.* 38 471 (1966).
11. Baskett, P. J. F., J. Hyland and M. Deane, Analgesia for burns'dressing in children. In W. F. Henschel (ed.), *Neue klinische Aspekte der Neuroleptanalgesie.* Stuttgart and New York, Schattauer (1970).
12. Vogel, W. Über die Langzeitbehandlung mit Fentanyl und Dehydrobenzperidol. In M. Gemperle, *Anaesthesiology and Resuscitation* Vol. 18. Berlin and New York; Springer (1966).

15. ETOMIDATE, A NEW, SAFE, SHORT-ACTING INTRAVENOUS HYPNOTIC-EXPERIMENTAL PHARMACOLOGY AND INTERACTIONS

R. S. RENEMAN

CHEMISTRY

Etomidate (R-(+)-ethyl-1-(1-phenylethyl)-1H-imidazole-5-carboxylate), is a new, potent, short-acting and safe intravenous hypnotic, with the following structural formula:

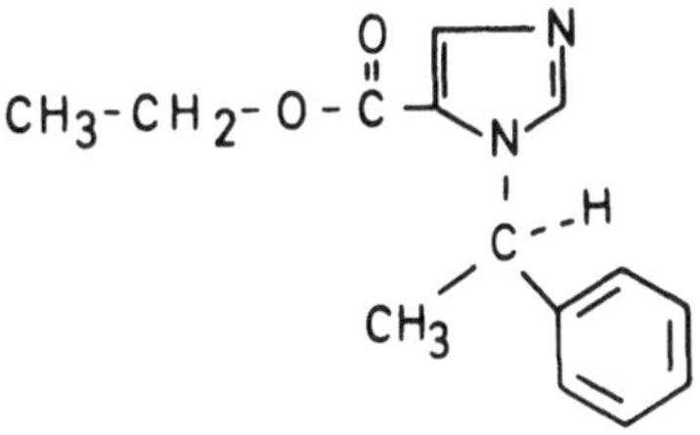

$$CH_3-CH_2-O-C \qquad\qquad R-(+)$$

Fig. 1.

Etomidate is supplied as the sulphate (molecular weight: 342, 36) and is dissolved in 1.8 mg $Na_2 HPO_4 \cdot 12 H_2O$ and 2.2 mg $Na H_2 PO_4 \cdot 1 H_2O$ with 4.2% glucose in a concentration of 1.5 mg etomidate base per ml (pH about 3.4).

GENERAL PHARMACOLOGY

On rapid (2 sec) intravenous injection in rats, etomidate (ED_{50} = 0.57 mg/kg) is approximately 6 times more potent than methohexital (ED_{50} = 3.51 mg/kg) and about 25 times more potent than propranidid and thiopental (ED_{50}'s = 13.4 mg/kg). The safety margin (LD_{50}/ED_{50}) in rats is, for etomidate 26.0, for methohexital 9.5, for propranidid 6.7 and for thiopental 4.6. The potency and toxicity of etomidate increase slightly with increasing injection rates without affecting the safety margin significantly (1,2).

Etomidate is a pure hypnotic and has no analgesic activity. It has a rapid onset of action and induces hypnosis within one min. In rats, guinea pigs and dogs, the duration of hypnosis with etomidate is dose-dependent; the duration of the hypnotic effect being doubled when the dose is doubled. With lower body weights higher doses in mg/kg are required for inducing hypnosis of comparable duration. No tolerance is observed after repeated administration. The time needed to recover from hypnosis is short and related to the duration of the hypnosis. The recovery-time is approximately 4 to 5 times the duration of the hypnotic effect at low doses and about 1.5 times the duration of the hypnotic effect at high doses (1,2).

TOXICOLOGY AND TERATOLOGY

ECG, haematological and biochemical analyses, urinanalysis and histopathology fail to reveal any drug-related adverse effects after the daily intravenous injection of etomidate for 3 weeks in rats (highest dose 5.0 mg/kg) and 2 weeks in dogs (highest dose 1.5 mg/kg).

Etomidate is devoid of any teratogenic effect in rats and in white rabbits of the New-Zealand strain. The highest dose of etomidate given to rats was 5.0 mg/kg i.v. daily from day 6 through day 15 of pregnancy and to rabbits 4.5 mg/kg i.v. daily from day 6 through day 18 of pregnancy (2).

DISTRIBUTION AND METABOLISM

During the first 30 min after administration in humans, the plasma level of unchanged etomidate decreases rapidly and then more slowly with a half-life time of 75 min (3). During transport etomidate is bound to the plasma-proteins (4). Directly after intravenous injection in rats the plasma level of etomidate drops quickly and the hypnotic penetrates the brain rapidly since the levels are maximal within one min after administration. This finding corresponds to the fast onset of the hypnotic effect as observed in animals and humans. In rats, the minimum level of etomidate sufficient to induce hypnosis can be estimated at 1.5 ± 0.35 µg/g brain tissue. Elimination from the brain is also very rapid. A rapid uptake of etomidate is also found in lung, kidney, muscle, heart and spleen. In these tissues maximum levels are reached within 2 min after injection. A significantly slower uptake of etomidate is seen in fat, in the testicles and in the stomach. Levels in these tissues are maximal between 7 and 28 min after administration (5).

Since the breakdown of etomidate mainly occurs in the liver (see below), the concentration of the metabolite in this organ is higher than that of etomidate, even 3 min after administration. In rats the biological half-life of etomidate is approximately 40 min.

The distribution of both optical isomers of etomidate (R-(+) and S-(−)) does not differ substantially in blood, brain and liver. In spite of almost equal brain concentrations for both isomers, the S-(−) form has considerably less hypnotic acitivity, suggesting the presence of a stereo-specific receptor for etomidate in the brain (5).

Etomidate is rapidly metabolized, mainly in the liver, by hydrolysis of the ester group whereby the carboxylic acid of etomidate, which is the main metabolite, is formed. Smaller amounts, provided by lower doses are metabolized more rapidly than larger amounts, provided by higher doses. The metabolite is pharmacologically inactive (5). In rats approximately 77% (5) and in humans approximately 75% (3) of the intravenously injected dose is excreted with the urine during the first 24 hours after the administration, mainly as the metabolite. Over the same period of time about 13% of the administered dose is found in the faeces.

IN VITRO PHARMACOLOGY

In *in vitro* studies etomidate, 2.5 mg/1, was found to have no effect on the Ca^{2+} response-curves in papillary muscles isolated from cats. Besides a weak anti-nicotinic activity no anti-spasmogenic action is produced by etomidate on such tissues as guinea-pig ileum, rabbit duodenum, rabbit spleen and rat fundus (6). No overt effect of the hypnotic was observed on the vasoconstriction in isolated peripheral arteries induced by KCl or sympathetic stimulation.

In studies involving intracellular microelectrode techniques, etomidate, 2.5 mg/l, was found to be devoid of any effect on the electrophysiological variables determined in Purkinje fibres and papillary muscles isolated from dog hearts and in papillary and auricular muscles isolated from guinea-pig hearts. Methohexital, 10 mg/l, and propranidid, 50 mg/l, have no significant effect on the variables determined in papillary muscles, but significantly reduce the amplitude and the rate of rise of the action potential and the conduction velocity, and significantly prolong the effective refractory period in Purkinje fibres isolated from dog hearts. In addition propranidid significantly decreases the spontaneous activity in guinea-pig auricles. These findings demonstrate that at comparative doses, selected on the basis of sleep duration (7), methohexital and propranidid depress the fast sodium conductance in Purkinje fibres, while etomidate is devoid of this side effect (8).

CARDIOVASCULAR PHARMACOLOGY IN DOGS

Experiments on unpremedicated, non-anaesthetized labradors reveal that the cardiovascular effects of etomidate, 1.25 and 2.5 mg/kg i.v., are minimal as compared with those of methohexital, 10 mg/kg i.v., and propranidid, 50 mg/kg i.v. (9). In this study comparative doses of the various hypnotics are selected on the basis of sleep duration (7). The doses of etomidate, methohexital and propranidid, required for adequate sleep durations, are respectively about 5, 6 and 10 times higher in dogs than in man.

At 1.25 mg/kg i.v., etomidate slightly but significantly decreases systolic and diastolic aortic blood pressure, while at 2.5 mg/kg i.v. this decrease in aortic blood pressure is associated with a slight but significant increase in heart rate. The decrease in aortic blood pressure probably results from a direct vasodilatory property of the compound and the increase in heart rate is likely to be secondary to the decrease in aortic blood pressure since etomidate has no effect on the spontaneous activity in auricular muscle. Etomidate, 1.25 and 2.5 mg/kg i.v., has no significant effect on the maximum first derivative of left ventricular pressure, at constant heart rate, and on mean aortic and mean coronary blood flow.

On the contrary, methohexital, 10 mg/kg i.v., markedly increases heart rate and systolic and diastolic aortic blood pressure and, therefore the oxygen demand of the left ventricle, while the changes in the maximum first derivative of left ventricular pressure indicate that this hypnotic has some negative inotropic properties (9).

Propranidid, 50 mg/kg i.v., has shown to have pronounced negative inotropic properties in this study, as demonstrated by the marked decrease in the maximum first derivative of left ventricular pressure and mean aortic blood flow, in the presence of a pronounced increase in heart rate. Systolic and diastolic aortic blood pressure also decrease after intravenous injection of propranidid.

At doses of 1.25 and 2.5 mg/kg i.v., etomidate does not induce histamine release in unpremedicated, non-anaesthetized beagles. A significant increase in plasma histamine levels, however, is found after intravenous injection of propranidid, 50 mg/kg. An increase, which is not seen after injection of Cremophor, the solvent of propranidid (10).

THE EFFECT OF ETOMIDATE ON RESPIRATORY RATE, pH, Po_2, Pco_2 AND BASE EXCESS IN DOGS

In unpremedicated and non-anaesthetized labradors, etomidate, 2.5 mg/kg i.v., has some depressant effect on the respiratory system as indicated by the significant decrease in respiratory rate and arterial Po_2 after injection of the hypnotic. A significant decrease is also observed in arterial pH. Arterial Pco_2 slightly increases and arterial base excess slightly decreases after the intravenous administration of 2.5 mg/kg etomidate, but these changes are not significant (11).

INTRA-ARTERIAL INJECTION OF ETOMIDATE

The effect of intra-arterial injection of etomidate on the structures of skeletal muscle and arterial wall was studied in rabbits (12). In this study thiopental, which is known to induce tissue necrosis after intra-arterial injection (13, 14, 15), was used as a reference substance. In the model used intra-arterial thiopental leads to necrosis and fibrosis in skeletal muscle and to intimal proliferation and intimal oedema in the intramuscular arteries. In several of these arteries, the proliferation and oedema result in total occlusion of the vessel. In the clinically used concentration of 1.5 mg base/ml, etomidate, 2.5 mg/kg, is devoid of these side effects (12).

INTERACTIONS

A. Interference of etomidate with anti-hypertensive agents
Anti-hypertensive treatment is fairly common in patients who are submitted to surgical procedures. Several anti-hypertensive agents are known to potentiate the hypotensive effects of anaestics and hypnotics (16, 17) and/ or to prolong the duration of sleep induced by these compounds (17, 18). The interaction between etomidate, 2.5 mg/kg i.v., and the antihypertensive agents propranolol and α-methyl-dopa (oral treatment with 10 mg/kg and 100 mg/kg, respectively, for 3 days) was studied in unpremedicated, non-anaesthetized labradors (19). No interference was found between these anti-hypertensive drugs and etomidate, at least as far as the effect on heart rate, systolic and diastolic aortic blood pressure, respiratory rate and duration of sleep is concerned.

B. Interference of etomidate with fentanyl and droperidol
In unpremedicated, non-anaesthetized labradors both droperidol (0.5 mg/kg i.v.) and fentanyl (50 µg/kg i.v.) significantly prolong the duration of sleep induced by etomidate 2.5 mg/kg i.v. The effect of fentanyl is more pronounced when etomidate is injected one min after the administration of the morphinomimetic than when the hypnotic is injected after 10 min (11).

SUMMARY

In the present paper a survey is given of the chemistry, pharmacology, toxicology, teratology, distribution and metabolism of etomidate, a new, safe and potent intravenous hypnotic. The interference of etomidate with fentanyl, droperidol and the anti-hypertensive agents propranolol and α-methyl-dopa is described as well. Both fentanyl and droperidol significantly prolong the duration of sleep induced by etomidate. No interaction is present between the anti-hypertensive drugs and etomidate, at least as far as the effect on heart rate, aortic blood pressure, respiratory rate and duration of sleep is concerned.

REFERENCES

1. Janssen, P. A. J., C. J. E. Niemegeers, K. H. L. Schellekens and F. M. Lenaerts, Etomidate, R-(+)-ethyl-1-(α-methyl-benzyl) imidazole-5-carboxylate (R 16659), a potent, short-acting and relatively atoxic intravenous hypnotic agent in rats. *Arzneimittelforsch.* 21, 1234-1243 (1971).
2. Janssen, P. A. J., C. J. E. Niemegeers and R. P. H. Marsboom, Etomidate, a potent non-barbiturate hypnotic. Intravenous etomidate in mice, rats, guinea-pigs, rabbits and dogs. *Arch. int. Pharmacodyn.* 214, 92-132 (1975).
3. Heykants, J. J. P., J. Brugmans and A. Doenicke, *On the pharmacokinetics of etomidate (R 26490) in human volunteers: plasma levels, metabolism and excretion.* Clinical Research Report R 26490/1. Janssen Research Products Information Service, Beerse, Belgium (1973).
4. Meuldermans, W. E. G. and J. J. P. Heykants, The plasma protein binding and distribution of etomidate in dog, rat and human blood. A comparative study between commonly used methods for the determination of protein-drug interaction. Arch. int. Pharmacodyn. In press.
5. Heykants, J. J. P., W. E. G. Meuldermans, L. J. M. Michiels, P. J. Lewi and P. A. J. Janssen, Distribution, metabolism and excretion of etomidate, a short-acting hypnotic drug, in the rat. Comparative study of (R)-(+) and (S)-(−)-etomidate. *Arch. int. Pharmacodyn.* 216, 113-129 (1975).
5. Van Nueten, J. M., *Etomidate, a short-acting non-barbiturate hypnotic. Study on cardiac tissues and on smooth muscle preparations in vitro.* Biological Research Report R 26490/6. Janssen Research Products Information Service, Beerse, Belgium (1974).
7. Jageneau, A. H. M., R. Xhonneux and R. S. Reneman, *Cardiovascular effects of the intravenously injected short-acting hypnotics etomidate, methohexital and propranidid*

in unanaesthetized dogs. Biological Research Report R 26490/3. Janssen Research Products Information Service, Beerse, Belgium (1973).

8. Xhonneux, R., E. Carmeliet and R. S. Reneman, *The electrophysiological effects of etomidate (R 26490), a new, short-acting hypnotic, in various cardiac tissues.* In: *Recent progress in anaesthesiology and resuscitation* 157-161. Excerpta Medica, Amsterdam – London. (1975).

9. Reneman, R. S., A. H. M. Jageneau, R. Xhonneux and P. Laduron, *The cardiovascular pharmacology of etomidate (R 26490), a new, potent and short-acting intravenous hypnotic agent. Recent progress in Anaesthesiology and resuscitation* 152-156 Excerpta Medica, Amsterdam – London. (1975).

10. Laduron, P. and P. Janssen, *Histamine release in dogs after intravenous injection of hypnotic agent.* In: *Recent progress in anaesthesiology and resuscitation* 152-156. Excepta Medica, Amsterdam – London. (1975).

11. Reneman, R. S., W. Van Gerven and R. Xhonneux and R. Kruger, *The interaction between etomidate, and fentanyl and droperidol.* In preparation.

12. Reneman, R. S., F. Verheyen, R. Kruger, W. Van Gerven and M. Borgers, The effect of intra-arterial injection of etomidate and thiopental on the skeletal muscle- and arterial wall-structures. In: *Anaesthesie und Wiederbelebung.* Springer Verlag. In press.

13. Cohen, S. M., Accidental intra-arterial injection of drugs. *Lancet* 2, 361-371 (1948).

14. Kinmonth, J. B. and R. C. Stepherd, Accidental injection of thiopentone into artery. Studies of pathology and treatment. *Brit. Med. J.* 2, 914-918 (1959).

15. Burn, J. H., Why thiopentone injected into an artery may cause gangrene. *Brit. Med. J.* 2, 414-416 (1960).

16. Stump, J. M. and W. W. Fleming, The effects of guanethidine, cocaine and reserpine on the hypotensive action of thiopental. *J. Pharmacol. Exp. Ther.* 147, 298-302 (1965).

17. Kienlen, J., Interférences des médicaments de l'hypertension artérielle avec l'anesthesie (en dehors des beta bloquants). *Ann. Anesth. Franç.* 15, 45-60 (1974).

18. Malhotra, C. L., P. K. Das and N. S. Dhalla, Investigations on the mechanism of potentiation of barbiturate hypnosis by hersaponin, acurus oil, reserpine and chlorpromazine. *Arch. int. Pharmacodyn.* 138, 537-547 (1962).

19. Reneman, R. S., W. Van Gerven and R. Kruger, Interaction between etomidate and the antihypertensive agents propranolol and α-methyl-dopa. In: *Anaesthesie und Wiederbelebung.* Springer Verlag. In Press.

16. CLINICAL EXPERIENCE WITH ETOMIDATE

D. T. POPESCU

Clinical experience with this new non-barbiturate shortacting hypnotic is still limited. Doenicke was the first, in March 1972, to use etomidate clinically; he found that as an induction agent it was superior to barbiturates and to flunitrazepam (1).

In May 1973, at the Postgraduate course in Vienna the administration of etomidate to a total of 2500 patients was reported by Doenicke (2). He stated that the administration of a dose three times larger than the effective one did not lead to more side effects. He also mentioned that if 5 mg diazepam is included in the premedication, the occurrence of myoclonia is significantly reduced.

Publications began to appear in 1973 indicating that etomidate has no adverse effect on the ventilation even in patients with pulmonary dysfunction (3). The effective sleep dose lies between 0.15 and 0.30 mg/kg for young non-premedicated volunteers, the duration of sleep then being about 3 minutes; a slower injection (lasting 60 seconds) reduced the incidence of myoclonia (4). The drug was demonstrated to have no histamine-releasing properties (5).

Between 1973 and 1974, four theses were published in Munich concerning etomidate and its effects on blood gases (6), on lipid metabolism (7), on myocardial inotropism (8) and a clinical comparison with propanidid (9). All of these publications demonstrated that etomidate is superior to other induction agents.

Further publications in 1974 showed that in comparison with methohexitone and propanidid, etomidate has the least depressant effect on myocardial function and circulation (10). Even in patients premedicated with a combination of pethidine-promethazine-atropine, induced with thiopentone-suxamethonium and maintained on nitrous-oxide-oxygen, alcuronium and 0.3% halothane or on neuroleptanaesthesia, the administration of 0.3 mg/kg etomidate led only to nonsignificant modifications of cardio-vascular parameters, which returned to normal within 10 minutes (11).

Etomidate compared favourably with ketamine, methohexitone, propanidid and Althesin, all of which had a greater effect on the circulation under the same conditions. Kettler (12) used 0.30 mg/kg etomidate for the induction of 5 patients and maintained them on a continuous infusion of 0.12 mg/kg/min. He measured a variety of cardiovascular parameters plus blood gases, electrolytes and coronary perfusion. He found that the pulse rate is raised minimally, stroke volume is maintained, cardiac index is slightly increased, blood pressure is barely influenced, coronary perfusion is lightly increased and the oxygen consumption of the left ventricle is reduced. This last effect is a very useful property of etomidate, especially for patients with a low myocardial reserve.

In 42 patients scheduled for cardiac surgery, Hempelman et al. (13, 14) found a significant decrease in the arterial PO_2 (but following 0.3 mg/kg in 15 sec), and significant alterations of cardiac parameters; they concluded that etomidate is extremely valuable for patients with myocardial insufficiency.

Morgan et al. (15) in the first 100 patients they induced on etomidate found a significant drop in systolic blood pressure with a mean dose of 0.28 mg/kg, 12% of patients showing apnoea (5-90 seconds), 4% hiccups, 25% involuntary muscle movements (tremor) but only 4% convulsion-like movements. 15% of patients had pain upon injection and 1% trombophlebitis.

Experience with etomidate started in Leiden in May 1974 and up to July 1975 a total of 162 patients have received the drug. Details of the patients and the type of anaesthetic are given in Table 1.

Table 1. Clinical material – anaesthetic techniques.

162 Males	60 Females
18 not intubated	
142 intubated	< 131 succinylcholine
	11 pancuronium

Maintenance	
$N_2O - O_2$ – droperidol – fentanyl – relaxant	64
$N_2O - O_2$ – fentanyl – relaxant	39
$N_2O - O_2$ – halothane	30
$N_2O - O_2$ – enflurane	27
Spinal block	1
No added anaesthetic	1

Figure 1 shows the age distribution of these patients, whilst Table 2 indicates the type of surgery performed. Nine patients were in a state of shock at the time of surgery.

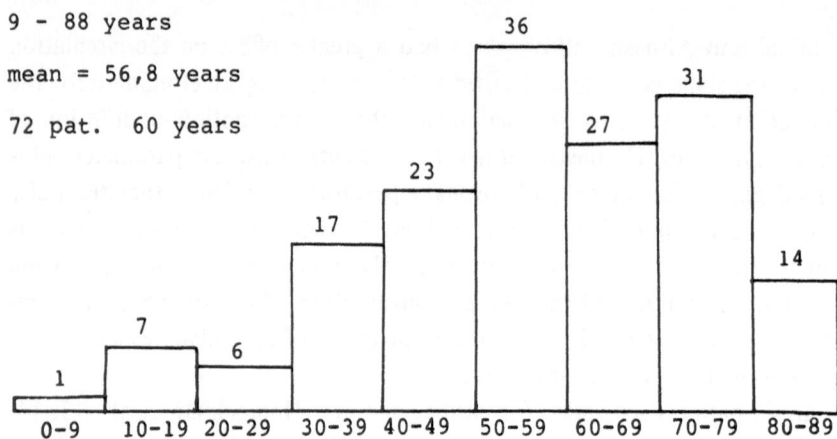

9 - 88 years

mean = 56,8 years

72 pat. 60 years

Fig. 1. Age of the patients: mean 56.8 years; range 9-88 years; 72 patients older then 60 years.

Table 2. Clinical material – surgery performed.

Urological (including endoscopies)	38
Neurosurgery	36
Intra-abdominal – gastro intestinal	25
Intra-abdominal – vascular	14
Extremities	18
Breast	10
Lumbar sympathectomy	5
Haemorrhagic shock	4
Septic shock	5
Others	7

The associated pathology is shown (fig. 2) as the distribution of risks: 13% of the patients were in risk groups 4 and 5 and 4% of these two groups were emergencies.

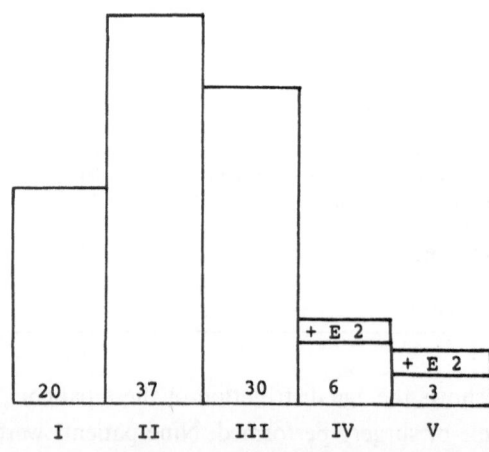

Fig. 2. Anaesthetic risk (N.A.V. classification) arabic numbers represent percentages.

Table 3. Clinical material – premedication.

None	4
Atropine	8
Analgesic-atropine	6
Psychotropic – atropine	6
Droperidol – Fentanyl – atropine	138
+ Euphyllin suppository	11

The premedication is listed in Table 3. It varied from none to our routine Thalamonal-atropine. In 11 of the patients a suppository of 360 mg. Euphyllin was also considered necessary by the anaesthetist.

The induction dosage is given in figure 3. The mean is 0.21 mg/kg. Higher

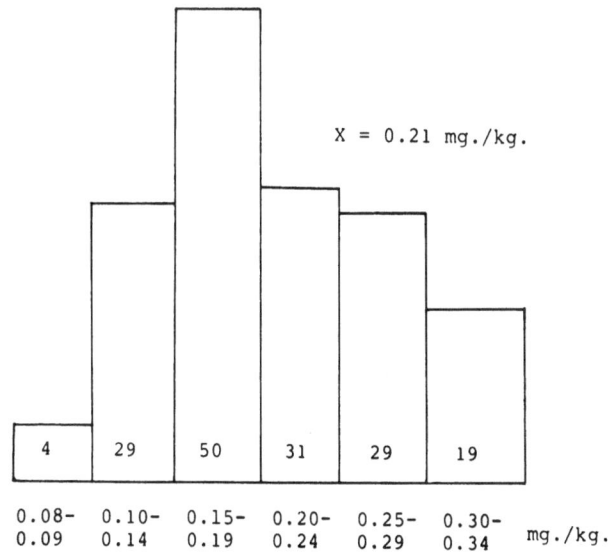

Fig. 3. Frequency distribution of doses: mean = 0.21 mg/kg. Numbers in the bars represent number of patients in each dose range.

doses were used in young strong patients in an attempt to obtain a deeper degree of hypnosis in order to decrease the hypertensive response to intubation. It appears that old and high-risk patients sleep and lose the palpebral reflex on about 0.10 mg/kg. The average premedicated adult requires a mean of 0.15 mg/kg while more resistant patients need up to 0.25 mg/kg. Higher doses more resistant patients need up to 0.25 mg/kg. Higher doses are generally unnecessary even if they are innocuous (2).

SIDE EFFECTS

In the literature the side effects cited are hypoventilation and apnoea, hiccups, pain at the injection site and involuntary movements. In this series we encountered the following side effects:

1. Pain at the injection site
Etomidate was always administered in an infusion of glucose and saline. Pain was mentioned by 10 patients (6.2%). Five of these patients already had chronic symptoms of pain.

In addition to the pain, three patients also showed an elevated arterial pressure which could be interpreted as a sympathetic reaction to pain. Three patients also exhibited involuntary movements which could be a possible motor reaction to pain.

Occurrence of pain was mentioned much more frequently during the early use of the drug (2, 11, 12). The incidence has decreased since the manufacturer changed the solvent and added a buffer.

2. *Hypoventilation*, was noted in 7 patients (4.3%). No special measurements were carried out, the 'clinical impression' of the anaesthetist was recorded usually without indicating whether rate or amplitude changed. In two cases apnoea was seen and the duration listed (2 and 4 minutes). Four of the patients showing respiratory depression received succinylcholine and were intubated, six were premedicated with Thalamonal-atropine and the seventh with opiate-atropine.

We have concluded that hypoventilation is seldom seen but that it can occur as with all induction agents in premedicated patients.

3. *Involuntary movements* were observed in 14 patients (9.3%). They varied from light tremor and/or some slight movements in 12 patients, to severe myoclonia in two patients (1.2%).

One patient who presented with severe myoclonia during induction of anaesthesia had the same symptoms upon awakening; at that point laboratory results were received which indicated hypocalcaemia. 1.5 g of calcium lactobionate was slowly administered and the myoclonia disappeared.

The significance of these movements is not yet known. They are observed with many of the newer anaesthetic drugs (methohexitone, Althesin, enflurane) but they seem to be harmless, which explains the wide acceptance of methohexitone, at least by anaesthetists in Great Britain (15).

4. Influence on heart rate

Bradycardia was noted in two patients. Both were neurosurgical patients and 0.23 or 0.3 mg/kg etomidate had been administered immediately after 0.3 mg fentanyl. Bradycardia is a recognized side effect of fentanyl.

Tachycardia occurred in two patients. In one of these administration of 0.25 mg/kg etomidate produced a 19% drop in the systolic pressure and 31% increase in the pulse rate. None of the patients with preoperative ventricular extrasystoles, atrial fibrillation, bundle branch block, hypertension, anaemia or shock showed alterations in their ECG (which was continuously monitored) nor significant modifications of the heart rate.

5. Other side effects

Hiccups and venous thrombosis were not seen.

One patient became *nauseated* during the administration of 0.2 mg/kg which did not induce sleep; another 0.06 mg/kg induced sleep and awakening was without troubles. Arterial hypotension and hypertension were listed regularly by the anaesthetists but since there was no reliable data for these patients, a prospective study was planned. (See below)

COMBINATIONS

We have distinguished here between patients who were being treated with various drugs preoperatively and various anaesthetic combinations.

No adverse effects were seen in any of the patients who were receiving one or more of the 26 drugs listed in table 4.

As mentioned previously (table 1), during anaesthesia we combined etomidate with nitrous-oxide, droperidol, fentanyl, halothane, enflurane and once with a spinal anaesthetic (mepivacaine 4%). In 35 patients the muscle relaxant was pancuronium; in 131 patients succinylcholine was used for the intubation of the trachea. No adverse effects were seen as a result of the combinations with the exception of the combination with succinylcholine (which produced a tendency toward hypotension and tachycardia which was of a much lesser degree than the combination of succinylcholine and other induction agents).

Table 4. Clinical material – concommitant drug therapy.

Anticonvulsants		Antidiabetic	
Diphantoin	4	Insulin	
Luminal	3	Tolbutamide	
Psychotropics		Circulatory drugs	
Diazepam	8	Digitalis	
Librium	3	Euphyllin	
Neuleptil	1		
Haloperidol	1	Anti-arrhythmic agents	
		Beta blockers	
Analgesics	5	Quinidine	
Corticosteroids	7	Antihypertensives	
Diuretics		Aldomet	
Frusemide	13	Hydergine	
Hygroton	8	Dihydralazine	
		Reserpine	
Dytaurese	2	Coronary dilaters	
Aldactone	1	Nitroglycerine	
Esidrex	1	Anti Parkinsonian drugs	
		Orphenadrine	
		Levodopa	

PROSPECTIVE STUDIES

A. Clinical study

This study included 45 patients in risk groups 1 or 2 who were scheduled for short operations; the induction agent was thiopentone. Althesin or etomidate chosen on the basis of a statistical random table (16).

All the patients were premedicated with Thalamonal according to an age table; up to 65 years: 2 ml, 65-75 years: 1.5 ml and more than 75 years: 1 ml, plus 0.5 mg atropine in all cases. Blood pressure by oscillotonometry and pulse rate were noted before induction of anaesthesia, after administration of the induction agent, after administration of succinylcholine and immediately after intubation of the trachea.

Induction was considered complete when the palpebral reflex disappeared. The comparable induction doses of the three agents are shown in table 5.

The systolic arterial pressure was influenced least by etomidate (-1.4% versus -3.1% and -3.8%). The administration of 1 mg/kg succinylcholine

Table 5. Effects of comparable doses of induction agents on systolic presure.

	Etomidate	Thiopentone	Althesin
Equipotent dose	0.19 mg/kg	3.01 mg/kg	52.3 microl/kg
Systolic pressure changes			
On induction	− 1.4%	− 3.1%	− 3.8%
After succinylcholine	− 3.2%	− 4.4%	− 4.8%
After intubation	+ 20%	+ 25%	+ 28%

reduced the systolic pressure even more and intubation of the trachea was followed by a maximum systolic pressure which varied between 120% and 128% of the initial value. In order to have a more detailed picture of the action of induction drugs we planned a more elaborate study.

B. CARDIAC OUTPUT STUDY

Material and methods
We were interested in studying the effect of the induction agents on the circulation, under clinical conditions. Thus, patients scheduled for transurethral resection of bladder tumors or for a graft of the aortic bifurcation (risk groups 2-4) and premedicated as mentioned above were included in this study. After performing an Allen test, a radial artery was cannulated with a 18 G teflon cannula and coupled through a P 37 Statham pressure transducer to a TNO cardiac output computer (17). This apparatus recognizes on the arterial pressure curve the moment of closure of the aortic valves and integrates the area under the systolic curve, expressing the result in ml/stroke or when it is multiplied by the heart rate in 1/min as cardiac output. Previous experience with this equipment both in animals and in man (18, 19, 20, 21, 22) demonstrated a close correlation with the dye-dilution methods of determining cardiac output. Since it is not possible to make dye-dilution determinations in a busy surgical department we compiled the data for the Fick method, for dye-dilution, and for thermal-dilution determinations from 39 authors (23) and constructed a nomogram for the cardiac index (cardiac output/square meter of body surface) based on the patient's age. We accepted the inaccuracies of this method as we were more interested in trends than in absolute values of cardiac output.

In the initial studies, the arterial pressure and the cardiac output were recorded. Later, the digital plethysmogram, lead I of the ECG, arterial and central venous pressures, heart rate, stroke volume, cardiac output and, following intubation, the capnogram, were registered on an 8-channel writer (Elema-Schönander).

Premedicated patients were brought to the operating theatre and monitoring was commenced. An I.V. infusion of glucose-saline was started and after the parameters became stable, induction was started with one of the 3 drugs chosen at random (16).

Up to July 1975, nine patients had been induced on thiopentone, eight on Althesin and ten on etomidate. Induction was again considered complete when the palpebral reflex disappeared; the patients then received 1 mg/kg succinylcholine, the trachea was intubated with a cuffed tube and anaesthesia was continued with nitrous-oxide-oxygen plus other anaesthetics.

Results have been expressed as changes from control values. In the wards preoperatively blood pressure was measured by auscultation. For the group as a whole, direct measurement gave systolic pressures which were 6.5 mmHg higher than those measured in the ward and diastolic pressures which were 9.5 mmHg lower. For each patient the directly measured pressure is considered as 100% and the variations are expressed as percentage deviations from the initial value. The same procedure has been used to express changes in other parameters measured. The statistical studies were carried out by Dr. J. M. H. Hermans (Medical Statistics Department Leiden) and consisted of comparison of means, standard deviations and Student's t test for determination of significance.

RESULTS

Figure 4 shows the behaviour of the arterial systolic pressure in 10 patients who received a mean of 0.20 mg/kg etomidate preceded by 0.15 mg fentanyl. In two patients the systolic pressure remained virtually constant; in all others it decreased, the mean reduction being 9.03% ± 3.69.

Changes in diastolic pressure are shown in figure 5. It increased in two patients, remained constant in two and was diminished in the other six. Statistical calculation gives a mean and standard deviation of −5.53 ± 4.47 which indicates the large range of the variations and the lesser correlation of diastolic pressure with the clinical condition of the patient.

The variable influence of etomidate on the heart rate is shown in figure 6. The mean heart rate decrease was by 2.75 ± 1.93%.

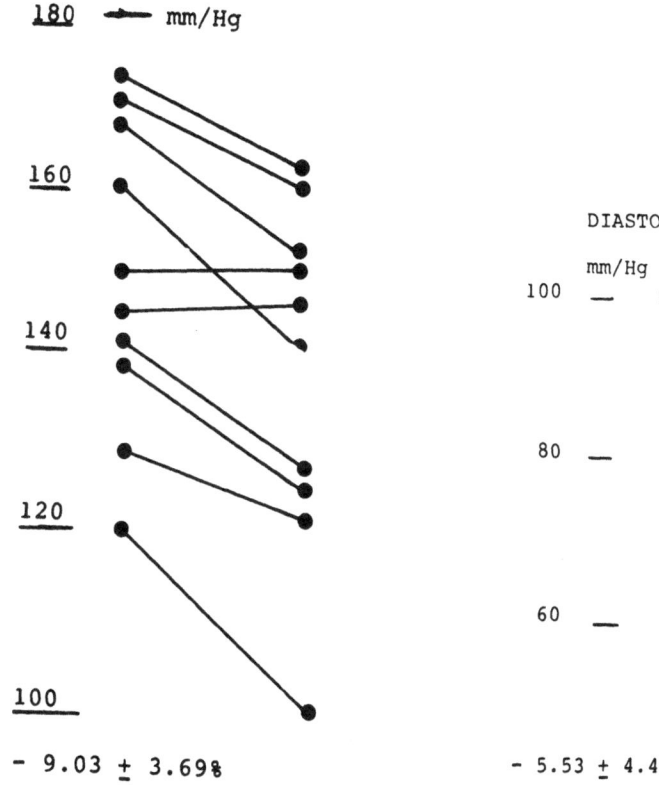

- 9.03 ± 3.69%

Fig. 4. Evolution of the systolic
pressure after the etomidate administration, individual cases and mean
reduction 9.03% ± s. deviation 3.69.

- 5.53 ± 4.47%

Fig. 5. Evolution of the diastolic
pressure after etomidate administration, individual cases and mean
reduction 5.53% ± s. deviation 4.47

The stroke volume was noted for five patients (fig. 7). It shows the same
trend as the pulse rate: in one patient it remained constant, in another it
increased slightly and in three the value was lower. The mean and standard
deviation expressed in percentages are −14.4 ± 7.3%.

The influence of the drug on the cardiac output is seen in figure 8. Of the
eight patients included in this measurement two showed no change; in six
patients there was a slight reduction of the output. Calculations demonstrated
a reduction with a mean of −14.57 ± 8.78%.

The influence of etomidate on the central venous pressure and on the
peripheral circulation (finger plethysmogram) are shown in figure 9.

Comparisons of the effects of etomidate with other induction agents gave
interesting results. Figure 10 illustrates the changes in the systolic pressure

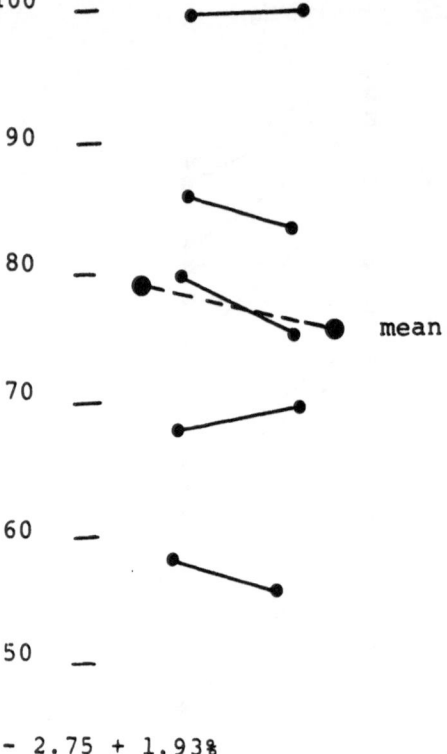

Fig. 6. Evolution of the heart rate, individual cases and representation of the mean $(-2.75 \pm 1.93\%)$.

mean

$-2.75 \pm 1.93\%$

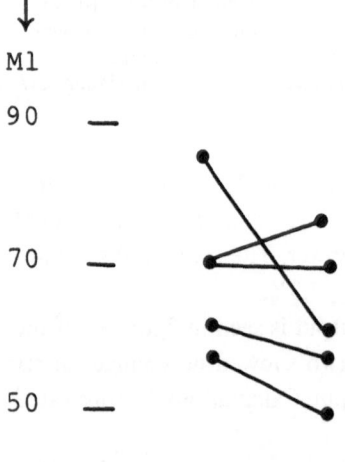

Fig. 7. Evolution of the stroke volume, individual cases and mean reduction 14.4% ± s. deviation 7.3.

$-14.4 \pm 7.3\%$

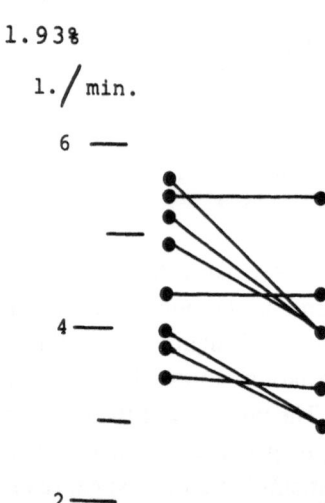

l./min.

$-14.57 \pm 8.78\%$

Fig. 8. Evolution of the cardiac output, individual cases and mean reduction 14.57% ± s. deviation 8.78.

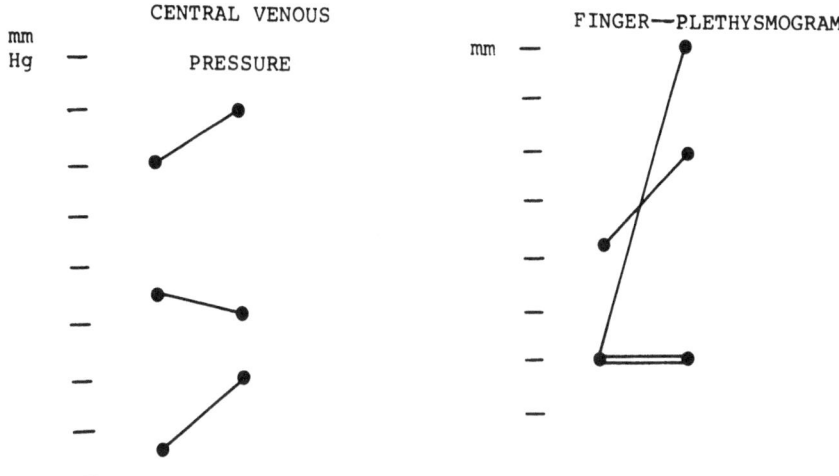

Fig. 9. Modification of the central venous pressure and of the finger plethysmogram (individual cases).

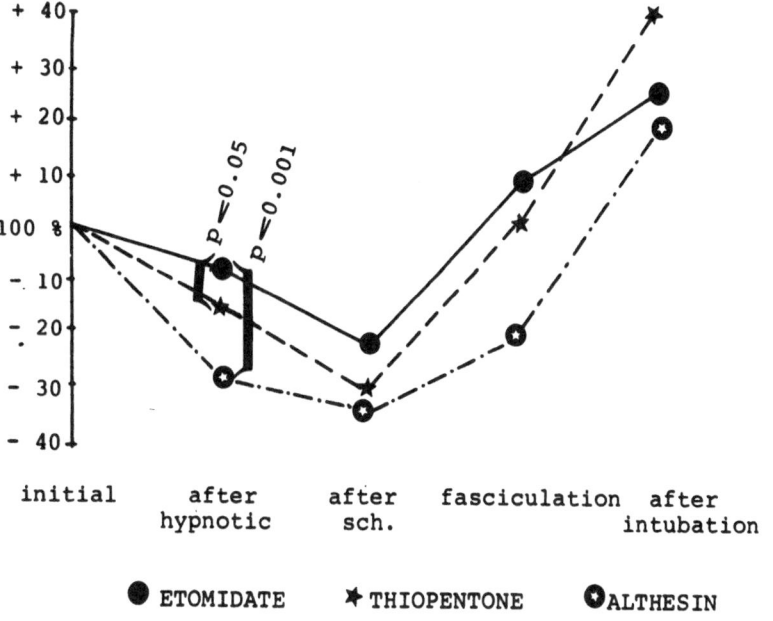

Fig. 10. Comparative sequence of the evolution of the systolic pressure during induction and intubation under etomidate, thiopentone and alphadione (Althesin). Significant difference between etomidate and thiopentone and highsignificant difference between etomidate and Althesin.

as a result of the sequence: hypnotic drug, succinylcholine and intubation. We saw a just significant difference ($p < 0.05$) between etomidate and

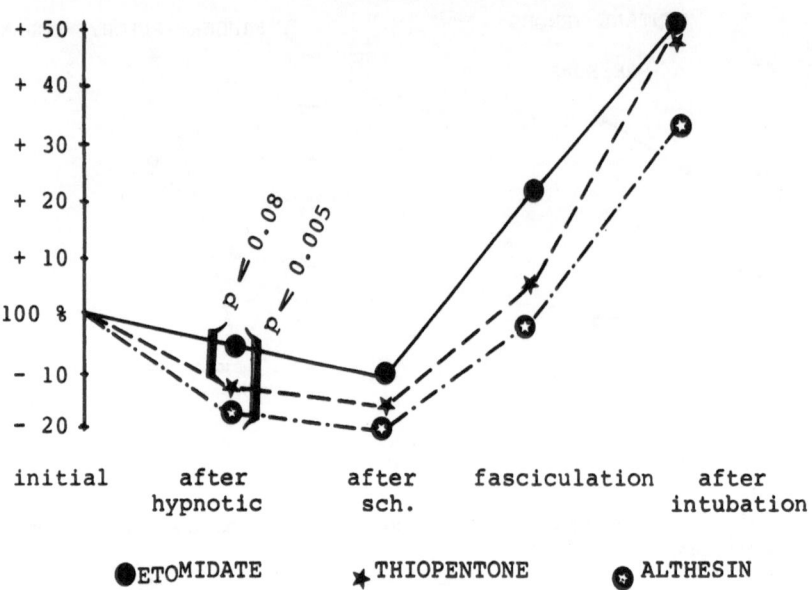

Fig. 11. Comparative sequence of the evolution of the diastolic pressure. High significant difference only between etomidate and Althesin.

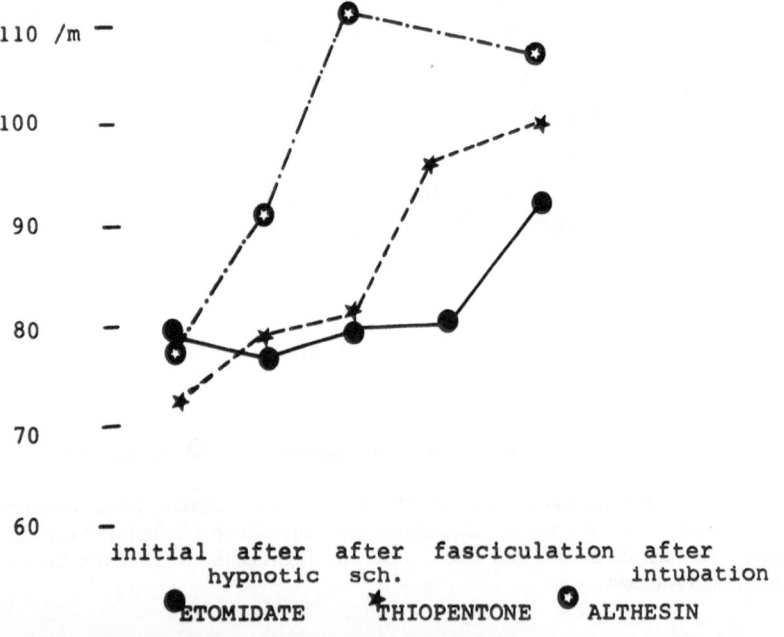

Fig. 12. Comparative evolution of the heart rate during induction and intubation under the three drugs.

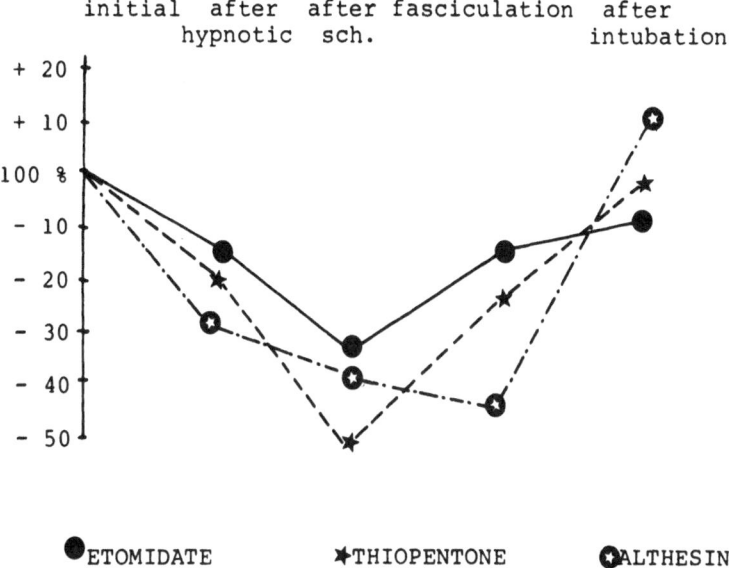

initial   after   after fasciculation   after
          hypnotic   sch.   intubation

Fig. 13. Comparative evolution of the stroke volume under the three drugs (no statistical significant difference).

thiopentone, a highly significant difference ($p < 0.001$) between etomidate and Althesin and no significant difference between thiopentone and Althesin. It is of interest to note the mean pressure drop of 34% for the combined effect of Althesin and succinylcholine, and the peak seen with all three drugs after the intubation of the trachea.

Figure 11 shows the modification of the diastolic pressure: a just significant difference ($p < 0.05$) was found between etomidate and Althesin and no significant difference between etomidate and thiopentone. Here again a hypertensive peak is seen after intubation.

Figure 12 shows the influence of the three drugs on the heart rate: etomidate is the only one which causes a slight reduction of the rate; thiopentone produces a slight rise and Althesin an important increase which is aggravated even further by the administration of succinylcholine.

Figure 13 shows the changes in the stroke volume and figure 14 demonstrates the modifications of the cardiac output.

There are no significant differences between the three drugs and their combination with succinylcholine until after the intubation of the trachea when a just significant difference ($p < 0.05$) between etomidate and thiopentone is observed. There is a higher peak with Althesin (+ 103%) but be-

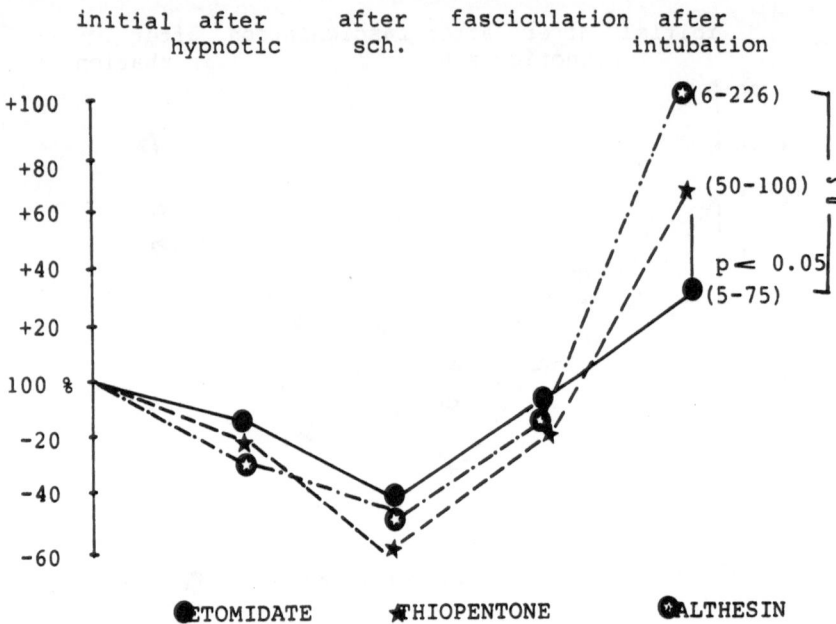

initial after   after   fasciculation after
        hypnotic   sch.   intubation

●ETOMIDATE   ★THIOPENTONE   ◉ALTHESIN

Fig. 14. Evolution of the cardiac output during induction with the three drugs and intubation. Significant difference between etomidate and thiopentone, no significant difference with Althesin (very big range by patients on Althesin).

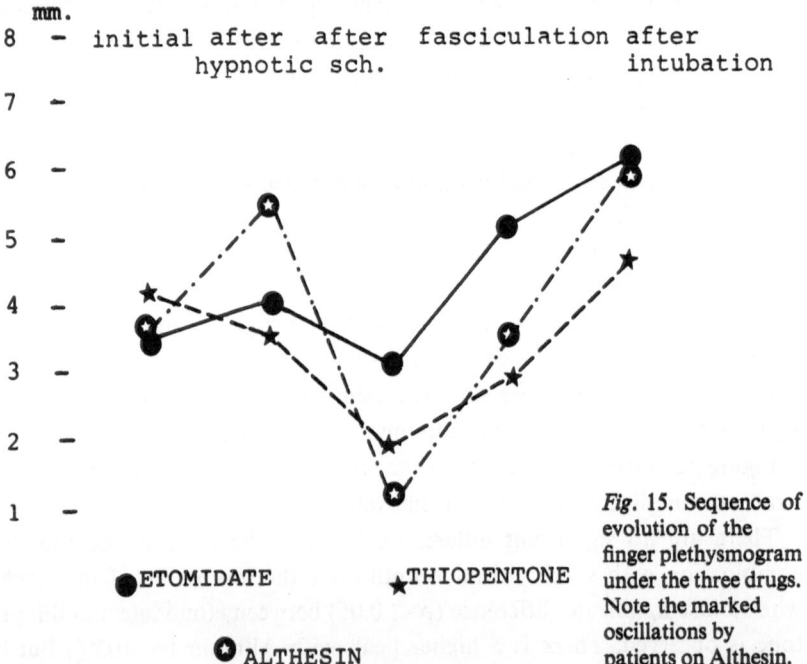

mm.

initial after   after   fasciculation after
        hypnotic   sch.   intubation

●ETOMIDATE   ★THIOPENTONE

○ ALTHESIN

Fig. 15. Sequence of evolution of the finger plethysmogram under the three drugs. Note the marked oscillations by patients on Althesin.

cause of the enormous range (6-226%) there is no statistically significant difference.

Figure 15 shows the minimal effect of etomidate on the finger plethysmogram compared to the pronounced increase produced by Althesin.

CONCLUSIONS

We have compared etomidate under clinical conditions as an induction agent for high-risk patients with a known (thiopentone) and a new (Althesin) hypnotic. These early results demonstrate that due to its minimal effect on chronotropism and because peripheral vasodilatation is only slight, etomidate is at the moment the drug of choice for induction of cardiac-risk patients.

We have also started a comparative trial with neuroleptanaesthesia (droperidol-fentamyl) but the number of patients observed is still too small for presentation and conclusions.

In view of the results of this investigation we are also trying to determine the best combination for the induction of patients who are exposed to considerable risk as a result of large oscillations in the arterial pressure (cerebral aneurysms, aortic aneurysms, obstructions of the carotic arteries and coronary patients) produced by the usual drugs and methods.

REFERENCES

1. Doenicke, A., Etomidate, a new intravenous hypnotic. *Acta Anaesth. Belg.*, 25: 3: 307 (1974).
2. Doenicke, A., *Klinisch-experimentele Untersuchungen und Klinische Erfahrungsbericht über ein neues i.v. applizierbares Narkoticum.* Proceedings of the 6th International Anaesthesia Postgraduate Course, Vienna Mai (1973).
3. Doenicke, A., E. Wagner, K. H. Betz, Blutgasanalysen nach drei kurzwirkenden i.v. Hypnotica. *Der Anaesth.* 22: 353 (1973).
4. Doenicke, A., J. Kugler, G. Penzel, M. Laub, L. Kalmar, J. Killian and H. Bezecny, Hirnfunktion und Tolleranzbreite nach Etomidate, einem neuen barbituratfreien i.v. applizierbaren Hypnoticum. *Der Anaesth.* 22: 357 (1973).
5. Doenicke, A., W. Lorenz, R. Beigl, H. Bezecny, G. Uhlig, L. Kalmar, B. Practorius and G. Mann, Histamine release after intravenous application of short-acting hypnotics. *Brit. Journ. Anaesth.* 45: 1097 (1973).
6. Beetz, K. H., *Blutgasanalysen nach drei kurzwirkenden i.v. Hypnotica.* Thesis, München 1973.
7. Kruis, K. J., *Fettstoffwechsel nach Propanidid, Methohexital, Etomidat.* Thesis, München 1973.

168 D. T. POPESCU

8. Gabanyi, D., *Kreislaufverhalten und Myokardfunction nach drei kurzwirkenden i.v. Hypntoika: Etomidate, Methohexital, Propanidid.* Thesis, München 1974.
9. Büchner, G., *Einleitung der Algemeinanaesthesie mit Propanidid oder Etomidate.* Thesis, München 1974.
10. Doenicke, A., D. Gabanyi, H. Lemce and M. Schürk-Bulich, Kreislaufverhalten und Myocardfunktion nach drei kurzwirkende i.v. Hypnotica: Etomidate, Propanidid, Methohexital. *Der Anaesth.* 23: 108 (1974).
11. Brückner, J. B., J. W. Genthmann, D. Patschke, J. Tarnow, A. Weymar, Untersuchungen zur Wirkung von Etomidate auf den Kreislauf des Menschen. *Der Anaesth.* 23: 322 (1974).
12. Kettler, D., H. Sonntag, U. Donath, D. Regensburger and H. D. Schenk, Hämodynamic, Myokardmechanik, Sauerstoffbedarf und Sauerstoffversorgung der menschlichen Herzens unter Narkose-einleitung mit Etomidate. *Der Anaesth.* 23: 116 (1974).
13. Hempelmann, G., W. Hempelmann, S. Piepenbrock, W. Oster, G. Karliczek, Die Beinflussung der Blutgase und Hämodynamik durch Etomidate bei Myocardial vorgeschädigten Patienten. *Der Anaesth.* 23: 423 (1974).
14. Hempelmann, G., S. Piepenbrock, W. Hempelmann, G. Karliczek, Influence of Althesin and Etomidate on blood gases and hemodynamics in man. *Acta Anaesth. Belgica.* 25: 3: 402 (1974).
15. Morgan, M., J. Lumley, J. G. Whitwam, Etomidate, a new water-soluble nonbarbiturate intravenous induction agent. *The Lancet* 7913 (26 April): 955 (1975).
16. Moses, L. E., R. V. Oakford, *Tables of random permutations.* Stanford Univ. Press., Stanford (1963).
17. Wesseling, K. H., N. T. Smith, W. W. Nickols, H. Weber, B. de Wit, J. E. V. Beneken, *Beat to beat cardiac output from the arterial pressure pulse contour. In: Measurement in Anaesthesia.* Boerhaave series no. 9 Leiden. University Press p. 150 (1974).
18. Wesseling, K. H., B. de Wit, J. A. P. Weber, Computer zur Ermittlung des Herzminutenvolumens aus der Pulskontur. *Med. Technik.* 94: 3: 64 (1974).
19. Remington, J. W., Estimates of stroke volume by E.M.F. compared with two calculations from control pressure contour. *Amer. Journ. Physiol.* 224: 2: 405 (1973).
20. Purschke, R., E. Pütz, J. O. Arndt, Studies on the reliability of stroke volume determinations from the aortic pressure curve Part I. Results in animal experiments. *Der Anaesthesist* 22: 11: 483 (1974).
21. Wesseling, K. H., N. T. Smith, W. W. Nickols, B. de Wit, J. A. P. Weber, A small beat-to-beat cardiac output computer. *Proceedings Bio-Medical Symposium San Diego.* 13: 107 (1974).
22. Smith, N. T., K. H. Wesseling, J. A. P. Weber, B. de Wit, Preliminary evaluation of a pulse contour cardiac output computer in man. Feasability of brachial or radial arterial pressures. *Proceedings Bio-Medical Symposium San Diego.* 13: 113 (197?).
23. Wade, O. L., Ch. Ferencz, in: *Handbook of circulation* p. 72-73. Saunders, Philadelphia (1959).

PART FOUR

DRUGS USED IN INDUCED HYPOTENSION

17. THE PHYSIOLOGY AND PHARMACOLOGY OF INDUCED HYPOTENSION

I. R. VERNER

Induced hypotension is now accepted as a technique to aid surgery and as a measure to relieve the demands on an overstressed heart. Though the cardiovascular state of a patient can be altered radically and swiftly, the monitoring processes at our disposal trail far in the wake of our power to cause physiological change.

In the absence of simple and reliable methods of determining pressure, flow, or metabolism in vital organs, the conduct of controlled hypotension must be based on currently accepted physiological and pharmacological concepts, and it is proposed to review some of the basic and some of the novel tenets of the present time.

CARDIOVASCULAR PHYSIOLOGY

Acceptable hypotension rests on the concept of tissue perfusion being sufficient to satisfy tissue metabolic needs despite a lowered perfusion pressure, a state that demands a suitable cardiac output. The latter is determined by the relationship between the cardiac potential difference and the overall vascular resistance. The cardiac potential difference (the differential between the mean aortic and mean right atrial pressures) is normally 90-100 mmHg in man. Cardiac output will be reduced either if mean aortic pressure falls or if mean right atrial pressure rises, provided the peripheral resistance remains unchanged. Vascular resistance is generated mainly by the arterioles, but severe venoconstriction may also increase the left heart afterload. By combining cardiac output and peripheral resistance some estimate of whole body perfusion may be made, using the Poiseuille (1) formula:

$$\text{Flow} = \left(\frac{\pi P_{\text{aortic}} - P_{\text{r atrial}} \ r^4}{8 \ 1 \ \eta} \right)$$

where r is the radius of the vessels, 1 their length, and η the viscoscity of the blood. Since the viscoscity of the blood, the calibre of the larger vessels and the length of the arterioles are, by and large, constant, and since the length of the capillaries is negligible, the peripheral resistance is determined mostly by the radius of the arterioles. During hypotension, when right atrial pressure is lowered through venous dilatation and posture, overall tissue perfusion can be maintained through dilated arterioles provided that cardiac output does not fall unduly. Tissue oxygen availability is ensured provided there is an adequate haemoglobin concentration and well arterialised blood.

Since the circulation of most vital organs is autoregulatory, during hypotension there may be regional variations in blood flow. Some estimate of organ resistance to blood flow may be made by using peripheral resistance units (PRU's), where PRU_{100} is the resistance to flow generated by 100g of tissue, according to the formula:

$$PRU_{100} = \frac{\text{mean pressure head}}{\text{flow/100g/min}}$$

The distribution of blood to vital organs with varying weights and metabolisms leads to clear differences of perfusion between the organs, and a precise account of these problems has been made by Neil (2). Tissue oxygen utilisation may be assessed by organ $A\text{-}V_{O_2}$ measurements, most studies indicating that any decrease in organ perfusion during controlled hypotension is compensated for by an increased tissue extraction of oxygen from the blood. It should be noted that such studies measure tissue oxygen utilisation, which does not necessarily reflect tissue oxygen need.

VASCULAR CONTROL

The vasomotor centre effects vascular and cardiac control through the autonomic nervous system, and receives feedback from the vasculature largely via the aortic, subclavian and carotid sinus baroreceptors. Rising arterial pressures stimulate the baroreceptors, which then restore normotension through vasomotor centre inhibition (fig. 1).

Activity within the sympathetic nervous system ranges between 1 impulse/ sec. at rest and 16 impulses/sec. during high activity. Variations in activity of as little as 1-2 impulses/sec. give rise to noticeable changes in blood pressure, implying a control system that is highly susceptible to pharmacological interference.

Currently, much interest is centred on the baroreceptors. Pressure/activity plots of both the aortic and carotid sinus baroreceptors show a sigmoid

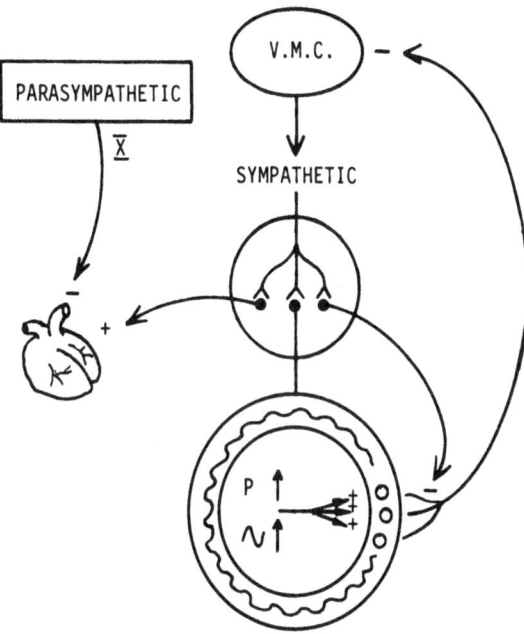

Fig. 1. The vasomotor centre-baroreceptor control system. Increasing pressure or the amplitude of pulsations in the great vessels stimulates the baroreceptors in the vessel wall, leading to negative feedback on the vasomotor centre (V.M.C.). Sympathetic stimulation augments cardiac performance and desensitises the baroreceptors.

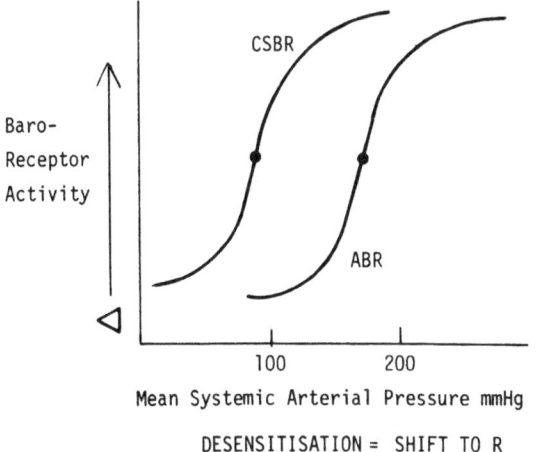

Fig. 2. Pressure/activity relationships of the carotid sinus (CSBR) and aortic (ABR) baroreceptors. Note the relationship between the centres of the plots, and that desensitisation of the baroreceptors shifts the plots to the right.

distribution. For the carotid sinus the centre of the curve lies midway between normal systolic and diastolic pressures, but the aortic receptor centre is displaced to the right (fig. 2). The carotid sinus receptors appear to respond to pulsatile flow at normal pressure, and are probably responsible for the day-to-day maintenance of normotension. The aortic receptors are more sensitive to a sustained, raised pressure, being recruited if the carotid sinus receptors are overtaxed, and possibly playing little role during hypotension (3). The baroreceptors themselves have a rich sympathetic innervation which, when stimulated, desensitises the receptors, perhaps to preserve blood flow during defence reactions.

CLINICAL IMPLICATIONS OF THE CARDIOVASCULAR PHYSIOLOGY

During hypotension, tissue perfusion and oxygenation are best preserved by using techniques which maintain cardiac output and dilate both resistance and capacitance vessels. Hypotension stimulates 'regulating reflexes', and these may make the maintenance of low pressure difficult. The inhibition of baroreceptors which follows low great vessel pressures may evoke a tachycardia, which may itself be augmented by the vagal inhibitory action of ganglion blockers. Finally, it is possible that the sympathetic system overactivity of hypertensive subjects may explain their marked sensitivity to hypotensive drugs and techniques.

PULMONARY PHYSIOLOGY

The effective filling pressure of the heart, upon which cardiac output depends, is determined by the differential between pulmonary arterial and intrathoracic pressures. Raising intrathoracic pressure reduces the effective filling pressure, but since the pulmonary vascular bed acts as a smoothing network, cardiac output does not fall proportionately. Rapid inflation and deflation of the lungs and a 1:2 inspiratory/expiratory ratio minimises the circulatory effects of intermittent positive pressure ventilation (IPPV) in healthy subjects (4), and the shape of the respiratory waveform is largely unimportant (5, 6). During induced hypotension however, when right atrial pressures are lower than normal and the venous capacitance vessels accomodate more blood, increased intrathoracic pressures rapidly oppose the return of blood to the heart. In this situation, a marked respiratory effect on cardiac output and systemic blood pressure may be observed (fig. 3).

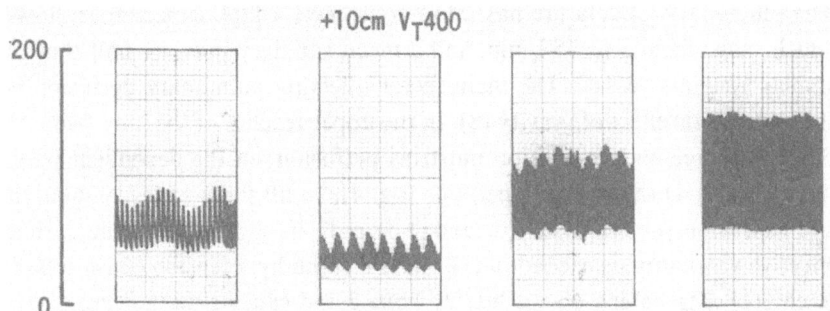

Fig. 3. The effects of IPPV on various levels of systemic arterial pressure. Ventilatory effects are most marked during hypotension, and virtually absent with normotension. Left hand recording at faster paper speed to show arterial waveform.

Additionally, certain methods of producing hypotension (notably deep halothane anaesthesia, ganglion blockade, and beta-blockade) alter the normal responses to the Valsalva manoeuvre. Under these conditions, prolonged inspiratory positive pressure is followed by a progressive fall in both stroke volume and blood pressure, no change in pulse rate, and a much slower return to normal values in phase IV of the manoeuvre (7). Such effects will be accentuated when postural pooling of blood produces a relative hypovolaemia.

PULMONARY BLOOD FLOW EFFECTS OF HYPOTENSION AND IPPV

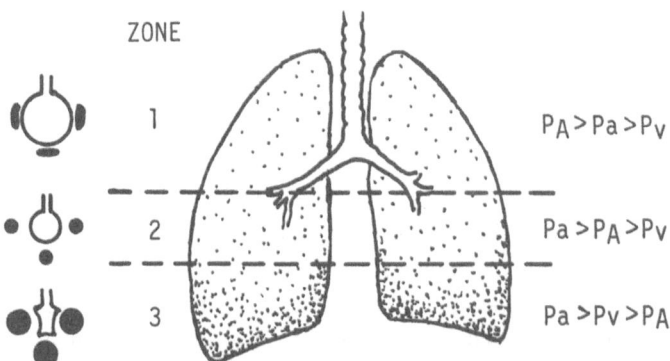

Fig. 4. Ventilation/perfusion relationships in the lung (after West *et al.*). At the left, the relative sizes of the alveoli and vessels are shown diagramatically. To the right, the relative pressures between the alveoli (PA), the arteries (Pa) and the veins (Pv) in the various zones are indicated.

The pulmonary vasculature has a low resistance, a high capacitance, flows which range from 3 to 25 l/min, and a mean capillary pressure half that of similar systemic vessels. The main factor affecting pulmonary perfusion is the hydrostatic effect of gravity (8). In the upper reaches of the lung (zone 1) blood is scarce and ventilation outstrips perfusion; in the dependent parts (zones 3 and 4) the opposite pertains (fig. 4). In all these zones ventilation and perfusion are mismatched, and it is only in the central zone 2 that effective ventilation is carried out. Both IPPV and hypotension cause zone 1 to enlarge, enroaching on the 'useful' zone 2 and causing an increase in the physiological deadspace (V_D/V_T ratio). Normal ratios of 0.3 (9) were observed to increase to 0.8 during induced hypotension with IPPV by Eckenhoff et al. (10).

CLINICAL IMPLICATIONS OF PULMONARY PHYSIOLOGY

There are two important considerations to be taken into account during induced hypotension. Firstly, to minimise the adverse effects of IPPV on cardiac output, inspiratory pressures should be the minimum needed to achieve effective ventilation. Obviously, when a return to normotension is needed, spontaneous ventilation should be re-instated. Secondly, to avoid the consequences of the inevitable increase in the V_D/V_T ratio that accompanies induced hypotension, ventilation must be sufficient to clear carbon dioxide and inspired oxygen fractions should be at least 50 per cent. to ensure a Pa_{O_2} of at least 100 mmHg. There is much to commend frequent determinations of blood gases during induced hypotension.

CEREBRAL PHYSIOLOGY

Over a mean arterial pressure range of 60-150 mmHg the cerebral circulation is autoregulatory. Normal cerebral blood flow (CBF) is 53-55ml/100g/min, and when induced hypotension is not severe vascular adaptation returns the CBF to normal values once the pressure head has fallen. This adaptation fails when the mean arterial pressure falls to a critical value of one third below normal (11).

Every increase in the Pa_{CO_2} of 1 mmHg leads to a rise in CBF of 1ml/ 100g/min, and a falling Pa_{CO_2} evokes a decrease in CBF of like magnitude. Hypotension accompanied by hypocapnia can be deadly, and it is unwise to let arterial carbon dioxide levels fall below 25 mmHg during anaesthesia and induced hypotension. Anaesthetic agents may partially annul the vasoconstriction produced by hypocapnia.

High arterial oxygen tensions cause cerebral vasoconstriction. It is worth remembering that the increased inspired oxygen levels that are needed to counteract the augmented physiological deadspace may, if overdone, lead to a reduction in CBF.

A raised intracranial pressure resulting either from an elevation of cerebrospinal fluid pressure or from jugular venous congestion will, by opposing CBF, reduce cerebral oxygenation. It is for these reasons that Eckenhoff (12) has cautioned against induced hypotension in the 'head down' position. Lowering the arterial pressure in the presence of large space-occupying intracranial lesions is similarly hazardous.

Anaesthetic agents are known to affect the cerebral circulation profoundly. Halothane dilates the cerebral vessels, the effect being marked when strong inspired concentrations are employed. Lately, Smith (13) has postulated that the primary action of halothane in this context is metabolic. He theorises that halothane primarily reduces the cerebral metabolism ($CMRO_2$), cerebral venous oxygen content is then reflexly adjusted to give a favourable cerebral tissue oxygen tension, and that CBF alters passively to follow these changes. Thiopentone and neuroleptic drugs depress the $CMRO_2$, giving them a 'sparing' effect on cerebral tissues that are hypoxic. For this reason they have a place in the anaesthesia given for induced hypotension during neurosurgery.

RENAL EFFECTS OF HYPOTENSION

Renal blood flow (RBF) has two control mechanisms, extrinsic (humoral) and intrinsic. RBF is autoregulatory over a mean renal arterial pressure range of 80-180 mmHg, but the autoregulation is abolished by general anaesthesia. Below a renal artery systolic pressure of 80-90 mmHg. RBF decreases, glomerular filtration slows and urine production may stop (14). A further reduction in renal arterial pressure to a systolic value of 70 mmHg or less may, through the release of renin, angiotensin I and II, lead to a fall in renal perfusion. It is true to say that the lowest 'safe' renal artery pressure is not known, but practical experience shows that a reduced or absent urine flow during general anaesthesia is not to be equated with renal tissue death. Indeed, most studies of renal function following induced hypotension (15, 16), have failed to show any evidence of renal damage.

CORONARY ARTERY BLOOD FLOW AND HYPOTENSION

The coronary circulation is autoregulatory, control being mainly dependent on myocardial demands. Lowering arterial pressure with ganglion blocking drugs leads to a reduction in cardiac work, cardiac output, left ventricular oxygen consumption and coronary blood flow. Coronary blood flow is sustained by the mean aortic blood pressure which, in each individual, has a lower limit for effective myocardial oxygen supply. Rollason and Hough (17) suggest that the limiting pressure is best determined by observing the ECG, the appearance of arrythmia signalling that the limit has been over-stepped.

Blood carbon dioxide levels can effect cardiac output, a Pa_{CO_2} in the range 40-55 mmHg. raising output, and in the 55-70 mmHg. level causing an age-related reduction (18). Prys-Roberts et al. (19) showed that deep halothane reduced myocardial contractility, a property shared, on occasion, by both ganglion and beta-blocking drugs.

Nevertheless, hypotension can be helpful to the myocardium, Franciosa et al. (20) being able to demonstrate that mild hypotension applied to patients with recent acute coronary occlusion led to a fall in left ventricular filling pressure and an augmented cardiac output. They concluded that the hypotension did not embarrass the coronary circulation. Currently there is an increasing use of mild hypotension to reduce left heart afterload in the period immediately following cardiac surgery.

THE LIVER AND HYPOTENSION

The blood supply of the liver is both hepatic and portal in origin, neither system being autoregulatory. Liver blood flow (LBF) from the hepatic supply is reduced whenever the systemic arterial pressure falls. If the Pa_{CO_2} rises or the Pa_{O_2} falls, the evoked catecholamine release will lead to splanchnic vessel constriction and a further fall in LBF.

As with renal function, it is the combination of hypotension and hypoxia which appears to harm liver tissue, and not hypotension per se.

Pharmacology

For the anaesthetist, the pharmacology of induced hypotension concentrates upon drugs whose primary action is to reduce either cardiac output or peripheral resistance. Many other techniques produce hypotension as a secondary effect (e.g. spinal and epidural anaesthesia, deep general anaesthesia, and hypothermia), but it is not proposed to discuss such methods in this article.

Adequate tissue perfusion is all-important during induced hypotension, and a bloodless surgical field achieved primarily by curtailing cardiac output is not advocated. However, attempts to lower arterial pressure by reducing only peripheral vascular tone are frequently accompanied by a reflex increase in cardiac output through a tachycardia. This may be so marked as to make it impossible to produce a satisfactory surgical field, and it is in this situation that the judicious addition of agents which depress cardiac output is often justified. Drugs that lower cardiac output act either by slowing the heart rate or by reducing the force of myocardial contraction. Without exception they are long-acting, and have no specific antagonists. If they are used, the return to cardiovascular normality in the patient will depend on the rate of biotransformation of the particular agent, and it follows that they should always be given in their minimum effective dosage.

In contrast, some drugs which lower peripheral resistance are both transient in action and extremely powerful. This combination is confined to those agents (e.g. phentolamine, sodium nitroprusside) which act on the periphery of the vasomotor control system. Such drugs demand a high degree of attention whilst they are being administered, but are not accompanied by copious unwanted side-effects. Blood pressure returns rapidly to normal once their administration is stopped, and inadvertent overdosage can be swiftly counteracted by withdrawing the agent and infusing intravenous fluids.

The peripheral resistance may also be lowered by centrally acting agents which diminish transmission in autonomic ganglia or the central nervous system. Frequently the actions of such drugs are both slow in onset and prolonged, and the hypotension they produce is accompanied by side effects which persist for as long as 48 hours after the active induction of hypotension has ceased.

Many routinely used general anaesthetic drugs will influence the course of induced hypotension, notably induction agents, neuro-muscular blocking drugs and their antagonists, parasympatholytics, catecholamines and diuretics. A suitable anaesthetic technique to accompany induced hypotension will always take into account the actions of such drugs, and adjust their dosage and timing to favour the required cardiovascular state at any moment. Similarly, concurrent medication which influences the patient's cardiovascular status profoundly alters the choice and dosage of hypotensive agents. Many review articles on induced hypotension exist (21, 22) which discuss in more detail the interplay between hypotensive and other drugs.

GANGLION BLOCKING AGENTS

It should be remembered that these agents paralyse parasympathetic as well as sympathetic ganglia. This gives rise to unpleasant and undesireable side effects, including pupillary cycloplaegia, paralytic ileus and urinary bladder atony. These actions may persist long after sympathetic blockade has apparently worn off, and make the use of ganglion blocking agents hazardous in patients suffering from prostatic enlargement and incipient or developed glaucoma.

Hexamethonium bromide
After the intravenous administration of this drug, the onset of hypotension is seen in under one minute (23). Its action lasts for 10-15 minutes, but tachyphylaxis is frequently seen in young, fit patients (24). Initial dosage is 10-25 mg, with subsequent doses of the same order. Pallister (25) has described a technique using only one initial dose of hexamethonium followed by meticulous positioning of the patient to achieve a bloodless field with only minimal hypotension, for which he has adopted the name of 'rheostasis'.

Trimetaphan camsylate (Arfonad)
This drug has similar actions to hexamethonium, but is more powerful, has a swifter onset of action and an intravenously administered action of 3-5 minutes. Parasympathetic blockade clearly persists for several hours after the drug has been stopped. Trimetaphan also relaxes the smooth muscle of arterioles, releases histamine (26) and can reduce both cardiac output and stroke volume (27, 28). Trimetaphan is given intravenously either as a 0.1 per cent. infusion or by intermittent injections of a 10 per cent. solution, 5-10 mg doses being reccomended.

Pentolinium tartarate (Ansolysen)
Pentolinium is more potent than hexamethonium and when given intravenously its actions are slow to appear (2-5 minutes), and very slow (45 minutes) to wear off. After an initial dose, 0.5 mg/kg being advised by

Bennett and Dalal (29), a progressive and controllable hypotension can be achieved by posturing the patient. Subsequent doses of pentolinium are frequently not as effective as the initial administration (tachyphyllaxis).

Postural hypotension can be seen in patients who have received pentolinium for up to 48 hours post-operatively, and attention must be paid to this during their recovery. Pentolinium is not a suitable agent for the aged and frail in view of the possibility of a prolonged and profound hypotension after its use in these subjects.

ALPHA-ADRENERGIC BLOCKERS

Phenoxybenzamine and *phentolamine* have both been used to produce hypotension a priori, but their main application for the anaesthetist lies in the management of patients with phaeochromocytoma undergoing operation. Both are powerful drugs, with a blocking action confined to the periphery of the efferent sympathetic nerves. Both can induce profound hypotension, the actions of phenoxybenzamine lasting for up to 48 hours whilst those of phentolamine may be as transient as 5 minutes. Phenoxybenzamine is given orally in doses of 5-10 mg up to four times daily, whereas phentolamine is administered intramuscularly or intravenously at a similar dosage level. In the pre-operative management of phaeochromocytoma, phenoxybenzamine is given up to 48 hours before operation, when phentolamine is then substituted in the immediate preoperative and operative periods. In this way, the tissues are cleared of long-acting alpha blockade before the tumor is removed. Since the advent of sodium nitroprusside its use has been reccomended instead of phentolamine for the control of blood pressure whilst operating on phaeochromocytomata (30). Concurrent medication with alpha-adrenergic blockers will drastically reduce the required dosage of other hypotensive agents.

SODIUM NITROPRUSSIDE

In the next chapter Stamenkovic will give a detailed review of this drug. For the sake of completeness I will briefly summarize my views on the subject. This newly revived hypotensive agent has aroused considerable interest and controversy. In the author's opinion it is the best available hypotensive by virtue of its extreme power and controllability and the complete absence of side effects when intelligently used.

The relevant moiety of the sodium nitroprusside molecule is an iron atom, to which are attached one nitrosyl (NO) and five cyanide (CN) radicals; the iron-nitrosyl grouping is believed to be the active fraction, acting directly (in an unknown way) on the muscle coat of the arterioles to produce relaxation. The resulting hypotension has been shown (32, 33) to have the favourable characteristics of a reduced peripheral resistance and a maintained cardiac output. In use, freshly prepared 0.01 per cent. solutions of the drug in 5 per cent. dextrose are infused intravenously, hypotension commencing immediately the infusion is started, and normotension returning 2-5 minutes after the infusion is terminated. The depth of hypotension is directly proportional to the rate of infusion, and tachyphylaxis is rare, though resistance to the agent is seen on occasion. The clinical management of sodium nitroprusside hypotension has been described in detail (34).

The metabolism of sodium nitroprusside has given rise to some concern. By weight, 45 per cent. of the nitroprusside is cyanide, which is normally converted to thiocyanate by enzymatic combination with free sulphydryl (SH) groups in red cells. The thiocyanate is slowly excreted by the kidneys, but it is thought possible to overload the SH combining mechanism by fast infusions of sodium nitroprusside, leading to raised cyanide levels in red cells and other tissues (35, 36). To avoid excess cyanide in the body, the rate of infusion of sodium nitroprusside should never exceed 0.07 mg/kg/min. In practice, long before such rates of infusion are reached, the nitroprusside induced hypotension should be augmented by other drugs which lower arterial pressure; in this way, the rate of nitroprusside administration can be slowed to acceptable (0.005-0.02 mg/kg/min) values. Further aspects of nitroprusside therapy exist, notably the protection conferred by hydroxycobalamin against CN poisoning, and the possible thyroid depressant and metabolic acidotic actions of nitroprusside itself.

If used with caution, sodium nitroprusside is an attractive hypotensive agent, and it can be adapted to suit either short periods of hypotension in the operating theatre or longer therapy in the intensive care or medical disciplines. The author believes that it can be used to help all types of surgical problems where hypotension is apposite, but its extreme controllability makes it especially valuable in the sphere of neurosurgery (37).

DRUGS REDUCING CARDIAC OUTPUT

Halothane and the *beta-adrenergic blocking agents* are the currently favoured drugs in this category. Though halothane, especially when vapourised within a closed circuit, can produce deep hypotension, the concentrations required are usually sufficient to place the patient far to the right on the halothane dose/response curve. This ensures that the hypotension is inevitably accompanied by deep general anaesthesia, that intra-operative arrythmias are common, and that, post-operatively, recovery is slow, rigidity, tremors, respiratory and metabolic acidosis, and prolonged myocardial depression are frequent. The myocardial actions of halothane have been investigated by Prys-Roberts (19).

However, halothane given in low (0.5-1.0 per cent) inspired concentrations is a valuable adjunct to hypotension induced by peripheral vascular relaxing drugs; in such concentrations it lowers cardiac output only fractionally, need not delay recovery from either anaesthesia or hypotension, but does considerably reduce the required dosage of ganglion blockers and peripheral vascular relaxants.

BETA-ADRENERGIC BLOCKING AGENTS

The anaesthetist uses these drugs as an adjunct to hypotension. Enderby (38) advocates that propanolol (0.035 mg/kg) or practolol (0.14 mg/kg) be given intravenously before attempting hypotension in those patients with a high sympathetic tone, usually children and young adults. An alternative is to give small (0.5-1.0 mg) increments of either drug until a reduction of cardiac rate begins to be apparent. When administered intravenously, the effects of these drugs take up to five minutes to appear, and the duration of action of propanolol (45 min) is considerably shorter than practolol (2-3 hours). After they have been employed there may be a noticeable delay in the return to normotension, and a post-operative reduction in cardiac reserve. Patients on concurrent medication with beta- blockers in excess of 150-200 mg daily are extremely sensitive to other hypotensive agents, being unable to counteract any drop in peripheral resistance by increasing their cardiac output.

REFERENCES

1. Poiseuille, J. L. M., Recherches expérimentales sur le mouvement des liquides dans les tubes de très petits diamètres. *Mémoires Savant Étrangers*, 9, 433 (1846).
2. Neil, E., Principles of vascular control. *Postgrad. Med. J.*, 50, 557 (1974).
3. Kidd, C. and R. J. Linden, Recent advances in the physiology of cardiovascular reflexes, with special reference to hypotension. *Brit. J. Anaesth.*, 47, 767 (1975).
4. Cournand, A., H. L. Motley, L. Werko and D. W. Richards, Physiological studies on

the effects of intermittent positive pressure breathing on cardiac output in man. *Am J. Physiol.*, 152, 162 (1948).

5. Bergman, N. A., Effects of varying respiratory waveforms on gas exchange. *Anesthesiology*, 28, 390 (1967).

6. Adams, A. P., A. P. Economides, W. E. I. Finlay and M. K. Sykes, The effects of variations of inspiratory flow waveform on cardiorespiratory function during controlled ventilation in normo-, hypo- and hypervolaemic dogs. *Brit. J. Anaesth.*, 42, 818 (1970).

7. Conway, C. M., Haemodynamic effects of pulmonary ventilation. *Brit. J. Anaesth.*, 47, 761 (1975).

8. West, J. B., *Regional differences in blood flow and ventilation in the lung.* Advances in Respiratory Physiology. London 1966.

9. Campbell, E. J. M., J. F. Nunn and B. W. Peckett, A comparison of artificial ventilation and spontaneous respiration with particular reference to ventilation-blood flow relationships. *Brit. J. Anaesth.*, 30. 166 (1958).

10. Eckenhoff, J. E., G. E. H. Enderby, A. Larson, A. Edridge and D. E. Judevine, Pulmonary gas exchange during deliberate hypotension. *Brit. J. Anaesth.*, 35, 750 (1963).

11. Finnerty, F. A., L. Witkin and J. F. Fazekas, Cerebral hemodynamics during cerebral ischemia induced by acute hypotension. *J. Clin. Invest.*, 33, 1227 (1954).

12. Eckenhoff, J. E., J. M. Leigh, E. Neil and R. Shanks, Panel discussion. *Postgrad. Med. J.*, 50, 568-571 (1974).

13. Smith, A. L., The mechanism of cerebral vasodilatation by halothane. *Anesthesiology*, 39, 581 (1973).

14. Larson, C. P., R. I. Mazze, L. H. Cooperman and H. Wollman, Effects of anaesthetics on cerebral, renal and splanchnic circulations: recent developments. *Anesthesiology*, 41, 169 (1974).

15. Evans, B. and G. E. H. Enderby, Controlled hypotension and its effect on renal function. *Lancet*, 1, 1045 (1952).

16. Hugosson, R. and S. Högström, Factors disposing to morbidity in surgery of intracranial aneurysms with special regard to deep controlled hypotension. *J. Neurosurg.*, 38, 561 (1973).

17. Rollason, W. N. and J. M. Hough, An examination of some electrocardiographic studies during hypotensive anaesthesia. *Brit. J. Anaesth.*, 41, 985 (1969).

18. Eckenhoff, J. E., G. E. H. Enderby, A. Larson, R. Davies and D. E. Judevine, Human cerebral circulation during deliberate hypotension and head-up tilt. *J. Appl. Physiol.*, 18, 1130 (1963).

19. Prys-Roberts, C., J. W. Lloyd, A. Fisher, J. H. Kerr and T. J. S. Patterson, Deliberate profound hypotension induced with halothane: studies of haemodynamics and pulmonary gas exchange. *Brit. J. Anaesth.*, 46, 105 (1974).

20. Franciosa, J. A., N. H. Guiha, C. J. Limas, E. Rodriguera and J. N. Cohn, Improved left ventricular function during nitroprusside infusion in acute myocardial infarction. *Lancet*, 1, 650 (1972).

21. Larson, A. G., Deliberate hypotension: a review. *Anesthesiology*, 25, 682 (1964).

22. Adams, A. P., Techniques of vascular control for deliberate hypotension during anaesthesia. *Brit. J. Anaesth.*, 47, 777 (1975).

23. Van Bergen, F. H., J. J. Buckley, L. A. French, A. B. Dobkin and I. A. Brown, Physiologic alterations associated with hexamethonium induced hypotension. *Anesthesiology*, 15, 507 (1954).

24. Enderby, G. E. H. and J. F. Pelmore, Controlled hypotension and postural ischaemia to reduce bleeding in surgery: review of 250 cases. *Lancet*, 1, 663 (1951).

25. Pallister, W K., Rheostasis. The use of ganglion blockade to reduce operative bleeding without sustained hypotension. *Ann. R. Coll. Surg.* (In press).

26. Payne, J. P., *Histamine release during controlled hypotension with Arfonad.* Proc. World Cong. Anesthesiologists, Scheveningen, The Netherlands, September 1955. Minneapolis (1956).

27. Didier, E. P., O. T. Clagett and R. A. Theye, Cardiac performance during controlled hypotension. *Anesth. Analg.* (Cleve.), 44, 379 (1965).

28. Jordan, W. S., C. L. Graves, W. A. Boyd, I. Ueda and T. S. Roberts, Cardiovascular effects of three techniques for inducing hypotension during anesthesia. *Anesth. Analg.* (Cleve.), 50, 1059 (1971).

29. Bennett, E. J. and F. Y. Dalal, Hypotensive anaesthesia for coarctation. A method of prevention of postoperative hypertension. *Anaesthesia*, 29, 269 (1974).

30. Katz, R. L. and C. E. Wolf, *Highlights of Clinical Anesthesiology.* New York (1971).

31. Taylor, T. H., M. Styles and A. J. Lamming, Sodium nitroprusside as a hypotensive agent in general anaesthesia *Brit. J. Anaesth.*, 42, 859 (1970).

32. Styles, M., A. J. Colemann and W. P. Leary, Some haemodynamic effects of sodium nitroprusside. *Anesthesiology*, 38, 173 (1973).

33. Wildsmith, J. A. W., R. L. Marshall, J. L. Jenkinson, W. R. MacRace and D. B. Scott, Haemodynamic effects of sodium nitroprusside during nitrous oxide/halothane anaesthesia. *Brit. J. Anaesth.*, 45, 71 (1973).

34. Verner, I. R., Sodium nitroprusside: theory and practice. *Postgrad. Med. J.*, 50, 576 (1974).

35. McDowell, D. G., N. P. Kearney, J. M. Turner, J. R. Lane and Y. Okuda, The toxicity of sodium nitroprusside. *Brit. J. Anaesth.*, 46, 327 (1974).

36. Vesey, C. J. and P. V. Cole, Nitroprusside and cyanide. *Brit. J. Anaesth.*, 47, 1115 (1975).

37. Siegel, P., P. P. Moraca and J. R. Green, Sodium nitroprusside in the surgical treatment of cerebral aneurysms and arteriovenous malformations. *Brit. J. Anaesth.*, 43, 790 (1971).

38. Enderby, G. E. H., Pharmacological blockade. *Postgrad. Med. J.*, 50, 572 (1974).

18. THE PLACE OF SODIUM NITROPRUSSIDE

L. STAMENKOVIĆ

A potent, rapidly-acting agent which would lower blood pressure on intra-venous administration has long been needed. Sodium nitroprusside (S.N.P.) causes an immediate, potent and highly evanescent hypotensive response when given intravenously. For a sustained hypotension continuous infusion of the drug is required. Oral administration does not produce this dramatic decrease in blood pressure, the effects being similar to those obtained with oral potassium thiocyanate therapy (1). During the last decade a steadily increasing number of reports have attested to the safety and effectiveness of S.N.P. in clinical practice.

HISTORY

The nitroprussides were first synthesized in 1849 by Playfair (2). Familiar as a sensitive reagent in qualitative chemical analysis, S.N.P. is used to detect the presence of sulphur and of alkaline solutions of sulphites and acetone by colour reactions. The effect on animals was first described in 1886 by Hermann (3), who erroneously attributed the toxic effects to the liberation of cyanogen. In 1929, Johnson (4) differentiated the low-dose hypotensive action from the toxic potential of larger doses. He also demonstrated that the systemic action is effected by the nitrous group, which though similar is 50 to 1,000 times more potent than the closely related nitrite group, which has a much shorter action on vascular smooth muscle (4). He described the hypotensive effect of the drug in three subjects and suggested therapeutic possibilities. This aspect was largely ignored until the early 1950s, when Page and colleagues reported on the therapeutic and cardiovascular actions of S.N.P. (5, 1), having demonstrated that decomposition of the compound was not essential for its depressor activity. In 1959, Gifford (6-9) published the first of several reports on the therapeutic value of S.N.P. during hypertensive emergencies. He considered it the most potent and consistently effective agent when other antihypertensive drugs had failed to produce a satisfactory response. Interest in S.N.P. gradually increased after subsequent clinical trials confirmed its safety and effectiveness.

Currently, the drug is used to produce hypotension during hypertensive emergencies (6-9), during anaesthesia for many kinds of surgical procedures (10-28), in the treatment of acute myocardial infarction (29, 30), chronic heart disease (31-33), diagnostic procedures (18-20, 34), and ergot poisoning (35). S.N.P. was first employed in anaesthesia in 1962 by Moraca (18).

CHEMISTRY

S.N.P. dihydrate (sodium nitroferricyanide dihydrate) Na_2Fe (NO) $(CN)_5$ · $2H_2O$ is a hydrated nitrosylpentacyanoferrate compound. The ruby-red transparent crystals dissolve readily in water, forming a brownish solution unstable upon standing and exposure to light. Decomposition leads to a change of ferric into ferrous ion, the colour changing from brown to blue.

PHARMACOLOGICAL ACTIONS

The cellular mode of action of S.N.P. is still only partly understood. Studies in the intact animal have shown that the major site of action of the drug is on the vascular smooth muscles of the resistance and capacitance vessels. Action is independent of autonomic innervation. There is no direct effect on the heart nor on isolated cardiac muscle at concentrations 100 times those required to relax the aorta (36). Markedly hypotensive doses of S.N.P. have no effect on uterine, duodenal or bladder smooth muscle (1). Coronary artery flow is increased (37, 38) without impairing myocardial contractility (39, 40). In fact, there is an improvement in left ventricular function as left ventricular end-diastolic pressure (L.V.E.D.P.) and myocardial oxygen consumption is reduced (28, 29, 32, 33, 39-41). Total peripheral resistance is enormously reduced, with an increasing venous return. These beneficial effects reflect the reduction of the after-load and pre-load respectively on the heart. In hypotension induced with S.N.P. central venous pressure (C.V.P.) is considerably reduced, cardiac output (C.O.) is increased 20-30%, whereas the total peripheral resistance, pulmonary vascular resistance, and right atrial pressure are all reduced (23, 24, 27, 40, 42-45). Heart rate changes are variable. Usually there is a 16-20% increase, which is most likely to occur in young fit patients even under complete beta-adrenergic receptor blockade

(26). Tachycardia is probably the effect of the intrinsic action on the pacemaker tissue of the heart (39). Renal vascular resistance is markedly reduced. Renal blood flow and natriuresis are increased in the isolated dog kidney (46) and in patients (28, 32, 33). A definite increase in renal venous and systemic venous renin activity in response to acute reductions of arterial pressure by S.N.P. shows a significant correlation with the degree of hypotension in normotensive and renovascular hypertensive patients (47). The response is more striking in the latter, without a significant release of renin in the contralateral, uninvolved kidney. Cerebral oxygenation remains normal at low perfusion pressures induced with S.N.P., with no evidence of hypoxia. Autoregulation of cerebral blood flow continues to function even below its minimal normal range of 60 torr (25).

The hypotensive effects of S.N.P. are due to the parent molecule itself, because they occur promptly within 90 seconds and long before the appearance of any metabolic product such as thiocyanate or cyanogen (1, 4, 5). Hypotension is more marked in elderly and hypertensive subjects and the action of ganglion blockers is potentiated.

BIOCHEMISTRY

Discontinuing an infusion of S.N.P. causes the blood pressure to rise within seconds, pre-infusion levels being reached within 1 to 5 minutes. The evanescence of the hypotensive effect is due to the destruction of the active radical which is converted slowly in the body to cyanogen (1, 48) by interaction of the ferrous ion in the nitroprusside with sulfhydryl groups (SH) in the tissues and erythroxytes (1, 49, 50) producing cyanmethemoglobin (51). The hepatic enzyme rhodanase (transsulfurase) converts S.N.P. to thiocyanate (52). The cyanogen produced in this way is then altered by the tissue rhodanase and endogenous thiosulphate to thiocyanate. Some of the latter is oxidized back to cyanide by a thioxyanate oxidase present in erythrocytes (49, 50, 53). There is a dynamic equilibrium between the two compounds, although strongly favouring thiocyanate (54). This keeps the pool of free cyanide very low even in the face of relatively large loads of cyanide or their precursors. The cyanide-thiocyanate pathways must be intact, i.e. there must be adequate amounts of normal tissue rhodanase and endogenous thiosulphate available which is the rate limiting factor in the pathway (55). Consequently, the blood cyanide levels are well below those of thiocyanate. This may not be so in patients with Leber's optic atrophy or tobacco amblyopia, since they have high cyanide and low thiocyanate levels in their blood (56).

The conversion of S.N.P. to cyanide is rather slow. It takes 90 minutes in blood incubated at 38°C. Therefore the hypotensive action cannot be dependent on its conversion to cyanide. As a result, toxicity may become apparent some time after the start or even after the termination of the injudicious intravenous administration of an overdose of S.N.P. (57).

Thiocyanate is excreted almost exclusively by the kidneys and has a half-life time of approximately a week in man with a normal renal function (1, 58). The plasma level of thiocyanate can be reduced rapidly by peritoneal dialysis (36).

TOXICITY

With short-term use of S.N.P. there is virtually no toxicity. One of the advantages of the drug is the absence or very low incidence of toxicity with prolonged judicious administration (1, 13, 18). Katz and Wolf, who gave it up to 32 days, reported side effects related only to a too rapid administration but no toxicity (8, 13), even with large daily doses of 100 to 140 mg S.N.P. for 10 days.

In short-term use during hypotensive anaesthesia the level of thiocyanate in plasma is very low i.e., about 0.05 mg/100 ml (8, 15). Prolonged intravenous use in hypertensive crisis had been reported to produce thiocyanate levels of 1-2.4 mg/100 ml in plasma. One case of toxicity in the form of manifest hypothyroidism was reported with plasma thiocyanate levels of 9.5 mg/100 ml after 3900 mg of S.N.P. was administered for 21 days in order to control increasing hypertension in a patient with severe renal insufficiency. Thiocyanate has an antithyroid action (59).

The main manifestations of toxicity are fatigue, nausea, and anorexia, followed by disorientation and psychotic behaviour, muscle spasm, and an 'angina-like' syndrome probably due to interference with the utilization of oxygen by cyanide and thioxyanide (36). The same mechanism applies to the extreme sensitivity of patients with vitamin B_{12} deficiency. Unduly high doses in dogs of 2 to 5 mg S.N.P. per kilogram body weight acts as a 'tetanic poison', producing trembling, laboured respiration, vomiting, rigidity, and convulsions. The smell of 'almonds' noticeable in the blood of these animals indicates that some of the toxic effects may be due to cyanide (60). Toxic symptoms begin to appear at plasma levels of 5 to 10 mg thiocyanate per 100 ml, and fatalities have been reported at levels of 20 mg per 100 ml (58).

Many authors consider plasma thiocyanate levels below 10 mg per 100 ml acceptable (1, 61).

CLINICAL USE

S.N.P. is usually prepared in the hospital pharmacy, sterilized by ultrafiltration and kept refrigerated in the dark. The stock solution remains stabile for at least 12 weeks. Any solution which has changed to a bluish colour must be discarded. It is now available commercially (NIPRIDE Roche). Immediately before use S.N.P. should be diluted in 5% dextrose or normal saline to a strength of either 0.01% or 0.005%. Bottle, syringes, and translucent plastic tubing should be protected from the light, and solutions which are several hours old should be discarded. The drug should be given by an infusion pump with precise measurement of the rate of flow. Within seconds of the start of the infusion the blood pressure drops sharply. The infusion rate must be increased gradually until the desired hypotensive effect is obtained. Because of the potent and extremely evanescent hypotensive effect of S.N.P. even small changes in the rate of infusion can cause wide fluctuations in the blood pressure. Careful continuous monitoring of the pressure in a cannulated artery is mandatory. The dose required is highly variable and the solution must be titrated against the blood pressure responses of each patient. A dose of 1 µg per kilogram per minute (0.5-1.5 µg) usually produces a prompt drop in pressure. There are reports mentioning as much as 400 µg per kilogram per minute, but only for a short period (36). With such high dosage it is mandatory to monitor thiocyanate and cyanide levels as well.

Patients completely refractory to intravenous infusion of S.N.P. have not been reported and tolerance to the drug is very rare (4, 18).

Most investigators have reported no evidence of tachyphylaxis, despite using the drug for periods of up to 21 (59) and 32 (13) days. There have been only five reports of tachyphylaxis in young previously healthy patients during hypotensive anaesthesia (14, 16, 51, 62). The total dose of S.N.P. depends on the degree and duration of hypotension required. Suggested limitation of the dose of S.N.P. varies from 1.6 mg/kg/hr (57), to 3.5 mg/kg (62). Most healthy young patients will have a constant response to a small dose of S.N.P. (< 3 mg/kg). Others, for reasons presently unknown, show metabolic disturbances on receiving doses in excess of 3 mg/kg, such as a rise in mixed venous oxygen tension ($P\bar{v}o_2$), a fall in arterial-mixed venous oxygen content difference (a-$\bar{v}Do_2$) and metabolic acidosis persisting until the administration of S.N.P. is discontinued despite buffering with sodium bicarbonate infusion (51). This represents cyanide intoxication of cellular cytochrome oxidase. S.N.P. reacts with haemoglobin to produce cyanmethaemoglobin (63) thereby reducing oxygen transport. As a potent inhibitor of carbonic anhydrase (64) red cell oxygen transport is further reduced. Tachyphylaxis gradually appearing may be treated with an infusion of 25% sodium thio-sulphate (150 mg/kg) infused during 15 minutes. This will markedly reduce the tachyphylaxis and a return to normal $P\overline{v}o_2$ and a-$\overline{v}Do_2$. The lethal dose of 10 mg/kg of S.N.P. was reported to produce 0.5 mg % of cyanide in plasma and 0.3 mg% in the urine (62).

The appearance of metabolic acidosis in the arterial blood and the cere-brospinal fluid may be an indication that the dose of S.N.P. is nearing the toxic range (57). In such a case the drug should be withdrawn promptly, sodium bicarbonate and the specific antidotes sodium nitrite, amyl nitrite, sodium thiosulphate and hydroxycobalamin should be used. Sodium, nitrite 5 mg per kg in 20 ml water given intravenously during 3 to 4 minutes or the inhalation of amyl nitrite for 30 seconds every 2 minutes will produce methaemoglobin which has a much higher affinity for cyanide than the cytochrome oxidases. Sodium thiosulphate given intravenously will supply sufficient substrate for tissue rhodanese to react with cyanide (62). Peritoneal dialysis can help rapidly (36).

Patients with maximum vasodilatation readily become hypothermic. Thiocyanate oxidase from erythrocytes acts optimally at pH 7.4 and tempe-rature 40°C. The hypothermic patient will metabolize thiocyanate to cyanide more slowly than a normothermic one. Though this may afford some protec-tion during operation, it could lead to complications due to excessive amounts of cyanide in the patient on rewarming in the recovery period (62).

An unusual and specific vasodilator, highly effective in many clinical settings, particularly during hypertensive emergencies associated with hyper-tensive encephalopathy, pheochromocytoma, intracerebral or subarachnoid haemorrhage, severe burns and drug-induced hypertension, S.N.P. is the most potent antihypertensive drug. This ideal agent is consistently effective even when other conventional antihypertensive drugs have failed to produce a satisfactory response. Once the blood pressure is under control, oral anti-hypertensive drugs are gradually substituted for the intravenous S.N.P. Surprisingly, they are then effective.

Currently, there is considerable interest in the use of S.N.P. to produce hypotension during anaesthesia for various surgical procedures, as summar-ized in table 1.

Table 1. Clinical use of sodium nitroprusside.

Hypertensive emergencies:

  Hypertensive encephalopathy
  Pheochromocytoma
  Intracerebral or subarachnoid haemorrhage
  Severe burns
  Drug induced hypertension (ergot poisoning)

Hypotensive anaesthesia for:

  Pheochromocytoma
  Dissecting aneurysms
  Neurosurgery (aneurysms)
  Head and neck surgery
  Middle ear surgery
  Orthopedic surgery
  Urology (cystectomy, prostatectomy)
  Severe responses to vasopressors

Left ventricular dilatation
Low cardiac output
After extracorporeal circulation
Cardiogenic shock
Refractory heart failure
Acute myocardial infarction
Diagnostic angiography

Control of hypertension and dysrhythmia with S.N.P. during the surgical removal of pheochromocytoma or other catecholamine-secreting tumors eliminates the need for the use of ganglion blockers and vasopressors during-operation and prevents hypoglycemia and/or hypotension occurring postoperatively. Mild controlled hypotension induced with S.N.P. reduces bleeding and produces 'dry fields' for dissecting aneurysms, neurosurgical operations, head and neck surgery, middle ear surgery, orthopedic surgery, operations in urology, and prevents severe responses to vasopressors administered during surgical procedures.

The modern pharmacological approach to the augmentation of left ventricular function is a radical reduction of the systemic vascular resistance. Among vasodilators commonly used, S.N.P. is associated with the most favourable haemodynamic responses. By reducing perioheral resistance and venous tone after-load and pre-load can be reduced to the extent appropriate to allow the maximal stroke volume for the available left ventricular contractile force (28, 32, 33). This action accounts for the beneficial effect of the drug on the cardiac function associated with, left ventricular dilatation

(28), low cardiac output, specially after extracorporeal circulation and in cardiogenic shock, refractory heart failure, acute myocardial infarction (29, 65, 66).

CONTRAINDICATIONS

The use of S.N.P. is contraindicated in Leber's optic atrophy, tobacco amblyopia, impaired liver function, malnutrition and low plasma vitamin B_{12}. Prolonged use of S.N.P. is not recommended in patients with severe renal insufficiency, pre-existing hypothyroidism and in those developing metabolic acidosis during administration of the drug. The safety of its use during pregnancy and lactation has not been established.

REFERENCES

1. Page, I. H., A. C. Corcoran, H. P. Dustan and T. Koppanyi, Cardiovascular actions of sodium nitroprusside in animals and hypertensive patients. *Circulation* 11, 188 (1955).
2. Playfair, L., On the Nitroprussides: A new class of salts. *R. J. E. Taylor*, London 1849.
3. Hermann, L., Uber die Wirkung des Nitroprussidnatriums. *Arch. ges. Physiol.*, 39, 419 (1886).
4. Johnson, C. C., Action and toxicity of sodium nitroprusside. *Arch. Int. Pharmacodyn. Therap.*, 35, 480 (1929).
5. Page, I. H., Treatment of essential and malignant hypertension. *J.A.M.A.*, 147, 1311 (1951).
6. Gifford, R. W., Jr., Current practices in general medicine. 7. Treatment of hypertensive emergencies including use of sodium nitroprusside. *Proc. Staff Meet. Mayo Clin*, 34, 387 (1959).
7. Gifford, R. W., Jr., Treatment of hypertensive emergencies associated with essential hypertension. In: Moyer, J. H., (ed.), *Hypertension.* The First Hahnemann Symposium on Hypertensive Disease. Philadelphia 1959.
8. Gifford, R. W., Jr., Hypertensive emergencies and their treatment. *Med. Clin. North Amer.*, 45, 441 (1961).
9. Gifford, R. W., Jr., The treatment of hypertensive emergencies. *Amer. J. Cardiol.*, 9, 880 (1962).
10. Loggie, J. M. H., Hypertension in children and adolescents. II. Drug therapy. *J. Pediat.*, 74, 640 (1969).
11. Mani, M. K., Nitroprusside revisited. *Brit. Med. J.*, 3, 407 (1971).
12. Nourok, D. S., G. Gwinup and G. J. Hamwi, Phentolamine-resistant pheochromocytoma treated with sodium nitroprusside *J.A.M.A.* 183, 841 (1963)
13. Katz, R L and C E Wolf, Sodium nitroprusside for controlled hypotension and hypertensive emergencies In: Mark, L C. and Ngai, S. H. (ed.), *Highlights of Clinical Anaesthesiology*, New York (1971).
14. Eppens, H., Correspondence. Sodium nitroprusside in hypotensive anaesthesia. *Brit. J. Anaesth.*, 45, 124 (1973).

194   L. STAMENKOVIĆ

15. Jones, G. O. M. and P. Cole, Sodium nitroprusside as a hypotensive agent. *Brit. J. Anaesth.*, 40, 804 (1968).
16. Lowson, J. A., Correspondence. Sodium nitroprusside in hypotensive anaesthesia. *Brit. J. Anaesth.*, 44, 908 (1972).
17. MacRae, W. R., Induced hypotension for middle ear surgery. *Proc. Roy. Soc. Med.*, 64, 1223 (1971).
18. Moraca, P. P., E. M. Bitte, D. E. Hale, C. E. Wasmuth and E. F. Poutasse, Clinical evaluation of sodium nitroprusside as a hypotensive agent. *Anesthesiology*, 23, 193 (1962).
19. Ditzler, J. W., Current status of deliberately induced hypotension. *Anesth. Analg.*, 43, 116 (1964).
20. Schiffmann, H. and P. Fuchs, Controlled hypotension effected by sodium nitroprusside. *Acta Anaesth. Scand.* (Suppl.), 23, 704 (1966).
21. Siegel, P., P. P. Moraca and J. R. Green, Sodium nitroprusside in the surgical treatment of cerebral aneūrysms and arteriovenous malformations. *Brit. J. Anaesth.*, 43, 790 (1971).
22. Taylor, T. H., M. Styles and A. J. Lamming, Sodium nitroprusside as a hypotensive agent in general anaesthesia. *Brit. J. Anaesth.*, 42, 859 (1970).
23. Styles, M., A. J. Coleman and W. P. Leary, Some hemodynamic effects of sodium nitroprusside. *Anesthesiology*, 38, 173 (1973).
24. Wildsmith, J. A., R. L. Marshall, J. L. Jenkinson, W. R. MacRae and D. B. Scott, Haemodynamic effects of sodium nitroprusside during nitrous oxide/halothane anaesthesia. *Brit. J. Anaesth.*, 45, 71 (1973).
25. Stoyka, W. W. and H. Schutz, The cerebral response to sodium nitroprusside and Trimethaphan controlled hypotension. *Canad. Anaesth. Soc. J.*, 22, 275 (1975).
26. Adams, A. P., Techniques of vascular control for deliberate hypotension during anaesthesia. *Brit. J. Anaesth.*, 47, 777 (1975).
27. Griffiths, D. P. G., B. H. Cummins, R. Greenbaum, *et al.*, Cerebral blood flow and metabolism during hypotension induced with sodium nitroprusside. *Brit. J. Anaesth.*, 46, 671 (1974).
28. Brown, D. R. and P. Starek, Sodium nitroprusside – induced improvement in cardiac function in association with left ventricular dilatation. *Anesthesiology*, 41, 521 (1974).
29. Franciosa, J. A., N. H. Guiha *et al.*, Improved left ventricular function during nitroprusside infusion in acute myocardial infarction. *Lancet*, 1, 650 (1972).
31. Guiha, N. N., C. J. Limas *et al.*, Treatment of refractory heart failure with sodium nitroprusside. *Circulation*, 46 (Suppl. II), 105 (1972).
32. Nabil, H., M. D. Guiha, J. N. Cohn *et al.*, Treatment of refractory heart failure with infusion of nitroprusside. *The New England Journal of Med.*, 12, 587 (1974).
33. Miller, R. R., L. A. Vismara, R. Zelis *et al.*, Clinical use of sodium nitroprusside in chronic ischemic heart disease. *Circulation* 51, 328 (1975).
34. Tuzel, I. T., Sodium nitroprusside, a review of its clinical effectiveness as a hypotensive agent. *The Journ. of Clinical Pharmacol.*, October, 494 (1974).
35. Carliner, N. H., D. P. Denune, C. S. Finch Jr., *et al.*, Sodium nitroprusside treatment of ergotamine-induced peripheral ischemia. *J.A.M.A.*, 22, 308 (1974).
36. Palmer, R. F. and K. C. Lasseter, Sodium nitroprusside. *The New Engl. Journ. of Med.*, February, 294 (1975).
37. Hollenberg, M., S. Carriere and A. C. Barger, Biphasic action of acetylcholine on ventricular myocardium. *Circ. Res.*, 16, 527 (1965).
38. Tountas, C. J., A. J. Georgopoulos, K. W. Kyriakou and A. A. Marselos, The effect of sodium nitroprusside on coronary circulation. *J. Cardiovasc. Surg. (Torino)*, 6, 100 (1965).
39. Adams, A. P., T. N. S. Clarke, J. Edmonds-Seal *et al.*, The effects of sodium nitrop-

russide on myocardial contractility and haemodynamics. *Brit. J. Anaesth.*, 46, 807 (1974).

40. Ross, G. and P. V. Cole, Cardiovascular action of sodium nitroprusside in dogs. *Anaesthesia*, 28, 400 (1973).

41. Goodman D. J.. R. M. Rossen E. L. Holloway, E. L. Alderman and D. C. Harrison, Effect of nitroprusside on left ventricular dynamics in mitral regurgitation. *Circulation*, 50, 1025 (1974).

42. Rowe, G. G., R. H. Henderson, Systemic and coronary hemodynamic effects of sodium nitroprusside. *Am. Heart J.*, 87, 83 (1974).

43. Adams, A. P., T. N. S. Clarke, J. Edmonds-Seal *et al.*, Effects of sodium nitroprusside on myocardial contractility and haemodynamics. *Brit. J. Anaesth.*, 45, 120 (1973).

44 Schlant, R. C., T. S. Tsagaris, R. J. Robertson Jr., Studies on the acute cardiovascular effects of intravenous sodium nitroprusside. *Am. J. Cardiol.*, 9, 51 (1962).

45. Bhatia, S. K., E. D. Frohlich, Hemodynamic comparison of agents useful in hypertensive emergencies. *Am. Heart J.*, 85, 367 (1973)

46. Bastron, R. D., G. J. Kaloyanides, Effect of sodium nitroprusside on function in the isolated intact dog kidney. *J. Pharmacol. Exp Ther.*, 181, 244 (1972).

47. Kaneko, Y, T. Ikeda, T. Takeda *et al.*, Renin release during acute reduction of arterial pressure in normotensive subjects and patients with renovascular hypertension. *J. Clin. Invest.*, 46, 705 (1967).

48. Hill, H. E., A contribution to the toxicology of sodium nitroprusside. I. The decomposition and determination of sodium nitroprusside. *Austral. Chem. Inst. J. Proc.*, 9, 89 (1942).

49. Goldstein, F. and F. Rieders, Formation of cyanide in dog and man following administration of thiocyanate. *Amer. J. Physiol.*, 167, 47 (1951).

50. Goldstein, F. and F. Rieders, Conversion of thiocyanate to cyanide by an erythrocytic enzyme. *Amer. J. Physiol.*, 173, 287 (1953).

51. Davies, D. W., L. Greiss, D. Kadar and D. J. Steward, Sodium nitroprusside in children: Observations on metabolism during normal and abnormal responses. *Canad. Anaesth. Soc. J.*, 22, 553 (1955).

52. Lang, K., Die Rhodanbildung in Tierkörper. *Biochem. Ztschr.*, 259, 243 (1933).

53. Pines, K. L. and M. M. Crymble, In vitro conversion of thiocyanate to cyanide in the presence of erythrocytes. *Proc. Soc. Exper. Biol. Med.*, 81, 160 (1952).

54. Boxer, G. E. and J. C. Rickards, Studies on the metabolism of the carbon of cyanide and thiocyanate. *Arch. Biochem.*, 39, 7 (1952).

55. Williams, R. T., *Detoxication mechanisms.* Chapman and Hall (ed.) London 1959.

56. Wilson, L., Leber's hereditary optic atrophy: a possible defect of cyanide metabolism. *Clin. Sci.*, 29, 505 (1965).

57. McDowall, D. C., N. P. Keaney, J. M. Turner and Y. Okuda, The toxicity of sodium nitroprusside. *Brit. J. Anaesth.*, 46, 327 (1974).

58. Deichmann, W. B., H. W. Gerarde, Toxicology of Drugs and Chemicals. *Academic Press*, New York (1969).

59. Nourok, D. S., R. J. Glassock, D. H. Solomon, *et al.*, Hypothyroidism following prolonged sodium nitroprusside therapy. *Am. J. Med. Sci.*, 248, 129 (1964).

60. Cromme, F., *Beitrag zur Kenntnis der Wirkung des Nitroprussidnatrium.* Dissertation, Kiel, (1891)

61. Gifford, R. W. Jr., Hypertensive emergencies and their treatment. *Med. Clin. North Am.*, 45, 441 (1961).

62. Davies, D. W., D. Kadar, D. J. Steward and I. R. Munro, A sudden death associated with hypotensive anaesthesia using sodium nitroprusside. *Canad. Anaesth. Soc. J.*, 22, 547 (1975).

63. Smith, R. P. and H. Kruszyna, Nitroprusside produces cyanide poisoning via a reaction with hemoglobin. *J. Pharmacol. Exper. Ther.*, 191, 557 (1974).
64. Vesey, C. J., P. V. Cole and J. C. Linnel, *et al.*, Some methabolic effects of sodium nitroprusside in man. *Brit. Med. J.*, 2, 140 (1974).
65. Chatterjee, K., W. W. Parmley, W. Ganz *et al.*, Hemodynamic and metabolic responses to vasodilator therapy in acute myocardial infarction. *Circulation*, 48, 1183 (1973).
66. Parmley, W. W., K. Chatterjee, Y. Charuzi *et al.*, Hemodynamic effects of noninvasive systolic unloading (nitroprusside) and diastolic augmentation (external counterpulsation) in patients with acute myocardial infarction. *Am. J. Cardiol.*, 33, 819 (1974).

PART FIVE

MUSCLE RELAXANT DRUGS

19. PHARMACOKINETICS OF THE NON-DEPOLARIZING MUSCLE RELAXANTS

S. A. FELDMAN

There have been several attempts to construct mathematical models of the behaviour of the neuromuscular blocking drugs following intravenous injection into patients (1, 2, 3). However, all of them are subject to errors due to the lack of information about some of the physical constants involved and the difficulty of predicting variable physiological changes that occur during the course of an anaesthetic.

It is useful to reflect upon the fundamental information that must be considered if we are to obtain an accurate model of the pharmacokinetics of the non-depolarizing agents.

PHARMACOKINETICS DETERMINING AMOUNT OF NEUROMUSCULAR BLOCK

In order to obtain neuromuscular blockade, sufficient cholinergic receptors must be occupied by the drug, to prevent threshold depolarization of the post synaptic membrane by acetylcholine. This requires that a critical concentration of the drug must be reached at the synapse and must remain there for a sufficient time to allow association of the drug with the receptor (the association constant for that drug).

In order to predict the amount of neuromuscular block produced the biological factors that influence the concentration of the drug that reaches the synapse after a given dose is injected intravenously must be understood. Some of these factors are predetermined and predictable, some are variable and some unknown.

The immediate distribution volume of drugs such as the non-depolarizing relaxants, which are highly ionised and therefore fat insoluble, is the extra cellular volume (E.C.F.). Assuming that for an average 70 kg adult the circulating fluid volume is 3 L and the total E.C.F. is 15 L, it follows that passage into the E.C.F. should reduce the plasma concentration of the drug to 20%. Providing that the neurolemal sheath around the end plate is

physically permeable, the synaptic cleft of the neuromuscular junction can
be regarded as a sub-division of the E.C.F. and the concentration of drug
reaching the receptors should therefore be 20% of the peak plasma level,
assuming even and equal distribution of the drug. The observation that the
plasma level of gallamine (4) and d-tubocurarine (5) falls rapidly to less than
10% of its calculated peak plasma level indicates that this simple dilution
does not fully explain the effective distribution volume of this drug.

The simple dilution effect is affected by 3 factors (fig. 1):

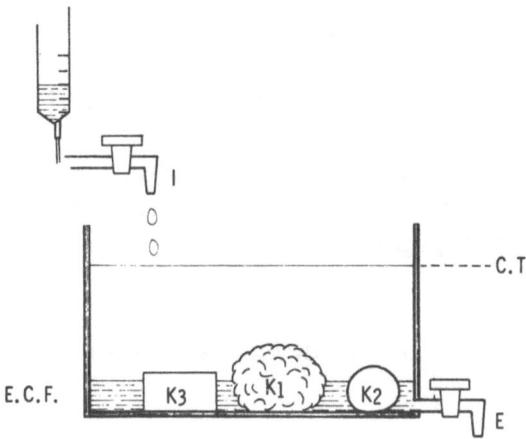

Fig. 1. Factors affecting the ability of a given dose of relaxant (I) to reach the critical value
(CT) for neuromuscular block.
E.C.F. = extracellular fluid volume. K^1 = quantity passing rapidly to non-reactive
acceptor sites. K_2 = quantity passing into cells. K^3 = quantity passing to plasma proteins.
E = excretion and/or metabolism.

1. The rate at which the relaxant is sequestrated from the circulation and
   E.C.F. to nonactive acceptor sites such as plasma protein and cell membranes.
2. The rate at which the relaxant is transported into cells.
3. The rate at which the relaxant is excreted or metabolised.

If the rate constant for any of these is greater than that for the drug entering the synaptic cleft it will affect the simple dilution concept. If this occurs
the concentration reaching the receptors will be less than 20% of the peak
plasma level. These are the factors that affect the 'apparent rapid distribution' of the drug.

Unfortunately, direct measurements of the rate at which these processes proceed in the intact patient are difficult to make and we can therefore only guess at the significance of these factors from indirect observations.

Although equilibrium dialysis shows that d-tubocurarine is bound to plasma protein and in vitro studies show its affinity for γ globulin, the quantitative significance of this action, in the three or so minutes required to affect neuromuscular block with this agent, is questionable. Indirect evidence demonstrating a relationship between γ globulin levels and d-tubocurarine requirements suggest it does play a part in the pharmacokinetics of this drug (6) but I would suggest that its role is less important than that of the redistribution of the drug into or on to the surface of cells. The amount of γ globulin is very small and in many liver diseases in which there is increased curare requirement there is only a relative increase in γ globulin due to a primary fall in plasma albumen.

The autoradiographs produced by Cohen et al. (7) (fig. 2) demonstrate

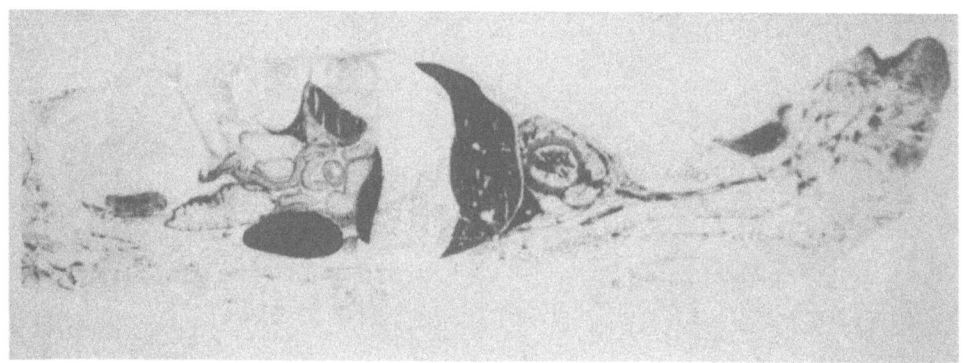

Fig. 2. Autoradiograph of rat after H^3 d-tubocurarine. This demonstrates the amount of drug sequestrated in the paranchymatous organs and salivary gland. Cohen *et al.* (1968), *Anesthesiology*, 29, 987.

the extent of the uptake of d-tubocurarine by cells of the body. They also demonstrate rapid redistribution of gallamine to the liver, kidney and mucopolysaccharide.

The work of Agoston and his co-workers (Chapter 20) has shown how rapidly the liver can scavenge the blood of some steroid relaxants. It would appear that the rate constant for cellular redistribution together with the large volume of the liver, spleen and kidneys make these more significant sequestration sites for most non-depolarizing relaxants than the plasma proteins. In the first 3 to 4 minutes following the injection of the drug into a vein meta-

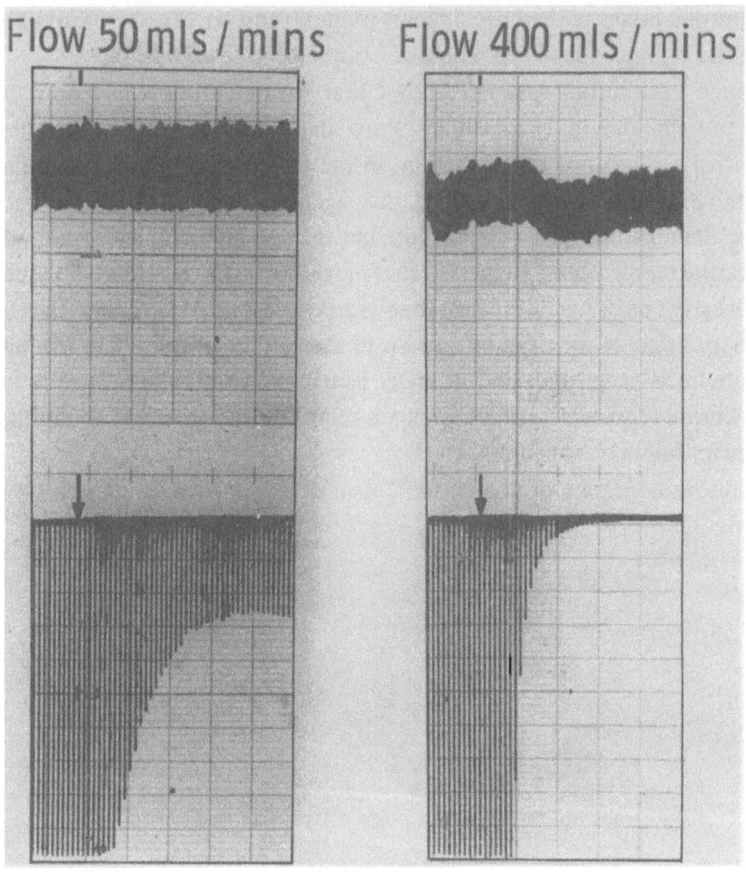

Fig. 3. The effect of alteration in blood flow upon the rate of onset and the degree of neuromuscular block induced by 0.5 mg/kg gallamine in dogs (Goat *et al*. 1976).

bolism and excretion of non-depolarizing relaxants is too slow to be of major importance, compared to the effect of sequestration of drug to non-active sites in the body.

The unknown factor in all these assertions is the relative rate at which these processes occur. The drug receptor union that determines the amount of neuromuscular block occurs within 3-4 minutes of intravenous injection provided the circulation is not abnormally slow (8). Autoradiographs taken 5 minutes and 10 minutes after the injection of d-tubocurarive and gallamine show the majority of the injected dose of drug in the liver, spleen and kidneys, and it is reasonable therefore to assume that even in the initial 3-4 minutes redistribution of the drug to those sites will be an important factor in limiting the drug available to produce neuromuscular block. The initial rate of plasma protein binding may be high, but the total quantity of drug bound to protein in the first 3-4 minutes is far less than that taken up by the parenchymatous organs.

The proportion of the injected drug that reaches the active receptors in the synaptic cleft depends to some extent upon blood flow. It is probable that patients with a low cardiac output and poor tissue perfusion will lose a higher proportion of a given dose of drug to non-active sequestration sites, especially in the parenchymatous organs, before an effective critical threshhold for neuromuscular block is reached in the synaptic cleft. The effect of a reduction in blood flow, such as may occur in elderly patients, patients with cardiac disease or during halothane anaesthesia, is to slow the rate of onset of neuromuscular block and to reduce the effectiveness of a given dose of non-depolarizing muscle relaxant (8) (fig. 3).

PHARMACOKINETICS OF RECOVERY OF NEUROMUSCULAR TRANS-MISSION

Having considered some of the variable factors determining the amount of neuromuscular block, we must consider the pharmacokenetics affecting the recovery of normal neuromuscular transmission following the administration of a non-depolarizing muscle relaxant. Recovery cannot occur unless the E.C.F. level of the drug is reduced below that required to produce critical receptor occupancy. The fall in E.C.F. concentration following establishment of neuromuscular block is the result of redistribution to the tissues. Excretion and metabolism only becomes important if large total doses are administered. Excretion in the urine is of major importance for gallamine (4), alcuronium and curare, although curare has alternative routes of excretion through the saliva, bile and gut (5). Metabolism can play a significant role in the lowering of the plasma level of steroid relaxants although the majority of pancuronium is excreted in the urine.

Recovery of neuromuscular transmission is impossible unless the E.C.F. level of drug is reduced below a critical threshhold level. However, it has been demonstrated that it is not the reduction in drug concentration that is the rate limiting process in the reversal of the neuromuscular block, it is the dissociation constant of the drug with the receptor (9). This is measured by determining the rate of recovery of the twitch response following a reduction of the plasma level of drug to as near zero as possible using the isolated arm preparation. Each drug has a different dissociation constant which depends upon its molecular affinity with the receptor. The time taken for recovery from 25% to 75% of the control twitch height is termed the Recovery Index (10). The Recovery Index for gallamine, d-tubocurarine and pancuronium, obtained in a recent series of experiments, is given in table 1. These values

Table 1. Recovery index for Gallamine, d-Tubocurarine and Pancuronium using the isolated arm technique.

Drug	Recovery index (25% – 75% recovery time)
Gallamine	9.8 ± 0.81 (n = 3)
d-Tubocurare	12.2 ± 0.52 (n = 6)
Pancuronium	10.1 ± 0.73 (n = 4)

are affected by volatile anaesthetic agents by the cumulative effect of repeated doses and by any process that interferes with acetylcholine formation release or hydrolysis. Measurement of these values must be made in carefully controlled conditions which are not always attainable in a clinical environment. However, they are remarkably constant and represent a 'finger print' of the drug.

Any mathematical model of the pharmacokinetics of the non-depolarizing relaxants that does not take account of these dissociation constants can not be valid unless the rate limiting factor in reversal of the drug activity is an artificially high E.C.F. level of drug. This very rarely occurs in clinical practice. Should it happen, reversal of the action of the muscle relaxant by anticholinesterase drugs is poor and short lived.

In predicting the duration of action of drug activity in the clinical situation it is important also to appreciate that volatile anaesthetics may appreciably affect the recovery index through their action at the myoneural junction. Blood flow changes which appreciably alter the duration of action of depolarizing muscle relaxants have little effect on the non-depolarizing drugs, as it is the dissociation constant and not the plasma-receptor concentration gradient that determines reversal of neuromuscular block with these agents (6). If the reduction in plasma level produced reversal of neuromuscular block one would expect more rapid recovery with increased blood flow as occurs with the depolarizing agents. It has been demonstrated that this does not occur (8).

CONCLUSION

Pharmacokinetics is not an esoteric abstract exercise. It is of clinical importance, as it teaches us how to use drugs to the best advantage, how to adjust doses to varying clinical circumstances, and how to deal with a prolonged activity of the drug.

The dose of non-depolarizing relaxant required to produce neuromuscular block is affected by the effective distribution volumes of the drug. These are:
1. The E.C.F. volume (related to surface area rather than body weight).
2. The parenchymatous organs, the liver, spleen and kidney – by virtue of the size and the blood flow to these organs. Enlarged organs or those with an increased blood supply necessitate a large dose of relaxant drug.
3. Plasma protein binding.

The dose requirement will also be influenced by the rate of excretion and metabolism. The duration of action of the neuromuscular block depends upon:
(i) Lowering the E.C.F. concentration below that required to produce threshold receptor occupancy – this normally occurs as a result of redistribution rather than excretion or metabolism.
(ii) The dissociation constant of the drug with the receptor and the rate of production and release of acetylcholine.

Armed with this information we can make certain generalisations about the dose requirements and usage of these drugs.

The dose requirement of a muscle relaxant will be reduced if the E.C.F. volume is small as in dehydration, or if the sequestration sites are reduced as may occur in renal shut-down or in anephric patients. More drug will be required if the cardiac output is depressed and the circulation slow. Enlargement of the liver and spleen will sequestrate a greater proportion of a given dose of relaxant. An increase in the total γ globulin content of the blood, increase the dose requirements of d-tubocurarine.

The duration of the activity of all non-depolarizing relaxants will be prolonged if the plasma and E.C.F. concentration remains abnormally high. Under these circumstances it will be impossible to completely reverse the action of the drug by an anticholinesterase. The treatment of prolonged activity from this cause is by expanding the E.C.F. and promoting a diuresis whilst maintaining artificial ventilation. Finally, any interference with acetylcholine production or release will prolong the neuromuscular block produced by non-depolarizing muscle relaxants.

REFERENCES

1. Fleischli, G. and E. N. Cohen, An analog computer simulation for the distribution of d-tubocurarine. *Anesthesiology*, 27, 64 (1966).
2. Gibaldi, M., G. Levy and W. Hayton, Kinetics of the elimination and neuromuscular blocking effects of d-tubocurarine in man. *Anesthesiology*, 36, 213 (1972).
3. Matteo, R. S., S. Spector and P. E. Horowitz, Relation of serum d-tubocurarine chloride to neuromuscular blockade in man. *Anesthesiology*, 41, 440 (1974).
4. Feldman, S. A., E. N. Cohen and R. Golling, The excretion of gallamine in the dog. *Anesthesiology*, 30, 593 (1969).
5. Cohen, E. N., W. H. Brewer and D. Smith, The metabolism and elimination of d-tubocurarine H^3. *Anesthesiology*, 28, 309 (1968).
6. Stovner, J., L. Theodorsen and E. Bjelke, Sensitivity to tubocurarine and alcuronium with special reference to plasma protein pattern. *Br. J. Anaesth.*, 43, 385 (1971).
7. Cohen, E. N., N. Hood and R. Golling, Use of whole body autoradiography for the determination of uptake and distribution of labeled muscle relaxants in the rat. *Anesthesiology*, 29, 987 (1968).
8. Goat, V., M. L. Yeung, C. Blakeney and S. A. Feldman, Effect of blood flow on the action of the non-depolarizing neuromuscular blocking agents. *Br. J. Anaesth.*, 48: 69 (1976).
9. Feldman, S. A. and M. F. Tyrrell, A new theory of the termination of action of the muscle relaxants. *Proc. Roy. Soc. Med.*, 63, 692 (1970).
10. Feldman, S. A., *Measurement of neuromuscular block – in Measurement in Anaesthesia*. Boerhaave Series, Leiden Univ. Press, Holland. Ed. S. A. Feldman, J. Leigh and J. Spierdijk I (1974).

20. THE PHARMACOKINETICS OF THE STERIOD MUSCLE RELAXANTS

S. AGOSTON AND U. V. W. KERSTEN

Metabolism, in the sence of biotransformation, of the bisquaternary steroids, is usually of minimal importance in clinical circumstances since they are usually highly polar, water soluble drugs and consequently do not need to undergo extensive metabolic conversion in order to be excreted. As a result steroid relaxants are usually excreted mostly unchanged in the urine. At present the only steroid relaxant in clinical use is pancuronium bromide (fig. 1). Therefore the fate of this agent was primarily investigated in different species.

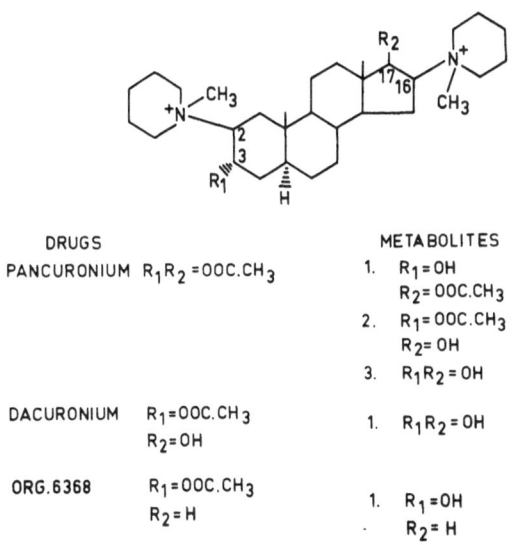

DRUGS

PANCURONIUM $R_1 R_2 = OOC.CH_3$

DACURONIUM $R_1 = OOC.CH_3$
$R_2 = OH$

ORG.6368 $R_1 = OOC.CH_3$
$R_2 = H$

METABOLITES

1. $R_1 = OH$
   $R_2 = OOC.CH_3$
2. $R_1 = OOC.CH_3$
   $R_2 = OH$
3. $R_1 R_2 = OH$

1. $R_1 R_2 = OH$

1. $R_1 = OH$
   $R_2 = H$

Fig. 1. The general structural formula of the 'pancuronium-like' agents.

Chemically the most important feature of the muscle relaxants is the presence of two quaternary ammonium groups. However, the distance between the quaternary nitrogens, the nature of radicals on the quaternary nitrogen atoms and the structure of the central part separating the cationic heads may play a very important role, not only in their activity at receptor sites, but also in determining their physicochemical properties and disposition, which in turn may change profoundly their pharmacologic effects. The only known metabolic change of the pancuronium molecule is the hydrolytic deacetylation at the 3rd, 17th or both the 3rd and the 17th carbon atoms. These are the three known metabolites: 3-hydroxy, 17-hydroxy or 3,17-dihydroxy pancuronium (fig. 1).

In addition to pancuronium and its derivatives numerous other steroid relaxants had been synthesized. A general interest in the steroid nucleus as a skeleton for non-hormonal drugs (1) and in particular as an almost rigid support for quaternary ammonium functions (2) led to the discovery of a number of mono- or bis-quaternary steroid relaxants. Some of these (table 1) were tested pharmacologically and clinically or are currently under investigation.

Table 1. The duration of action of various steroid relaxants after administration of approximately equipotent doses in different species.

Drug	Duration of action				
	Cat	Dog	Rabbit	Monkey	Man
Malouétine	–	L	L	–	–
Dipyrandium	S	–	S	L	L
NN'Dimethyl conessine	S	–	S	L	L
Stercuronium	S	S	–	L	L
HS-342	S	–	–	–	–
HS-310 (chandonium)	S	–	–	–	–
Pancuronium	L	L	–	–	L
Dacuronium	S	–	–	–	L
ORG-6368	S	S	–	L	L

S = short (< 10 min)
L = long (> 15 min)

Compounds with less than 10 min duration of action are classified in this presentation as short and those above 15 min as long acting relaxants. These arbitrary limits for the duration of action were chosen since in the last few years many research workers have been looking for ultra short acting non-depolarizing agents with time course characteristics similar to those of suxamethonium. Let me draw your attention briefly to each of these drugs:

Malouétine – the discovery (3) of the curarizing properties of this bis-quaternary alkaloid prompted the synthesis of several mono- and bisquaternary steroid compounds. *Dipyrandium* (4) showed about the same potency as d-tubocurarine in man and had approximately equal duration of action as suxamethonium in the cat and rabbit, but it was several times longer acting in the monkey than in the cat. The duration of action of this compound in man resembles that in the monkey and is far longer than in the cat and rabbit. Similarly to dipyrandium *NN-dimethylconessine* (5) showed the non-depolarizing activity of very short duration of action in the cat and rabbit. In contrast to the results in the above species, the block lasted almost 1 hour in monkeys after the administration of equipotent doses. With respect to the duration of action the results obtained in man were similar to those in monkey. *Stercuronium* is a monoquaternary conessine derivative. In the cat its potency approximated that of d-tubocurarine and its duration of action was similar to that of suxamethonium. According to Admiraal (6) and Wieriks (7) the duration of action of stercuronium in man and monkey was considerably shorter than that of tubocurarine, but it lasted several times longer in these two species than in the cat and dog. *HS-342* belongs to the novel series of the so-called aza steroids in which one or both quaternary nitrogens are incorporated in the steroid skeleton. Its pharmacological properties have been described by Singh and his associates (8) and by Marshall and co-workers (2).

Chandonium is the newest compound in this series. It is about four times more potent than d-tubocurarine and was found to very short acting in the cat. It remains to be seen whether this compound will have the same high potency, rapid onset and short duration of action in man too. *Pancuronium* (10) was found to be several times more potent than d-tubocurarine in all species, except in the rat and has, according to our definition, long duration of action. *Dacuronium* (11) is the 17-OH metabolite of pancuronium. Its duration of action is short in cat, but not in man. Since it causes tachycardia and has a longer duration of action in man than pancuronium, this drug was not studied further. *ORG. 6368* (12) is the newest analogue of pancuronium. On a weight basis it has approximately the same potency as d-tubocurarine in man. It has short duration of action in cat and dog, but not in monkey and man.

Although definite conclusions can not be drawn with regard to the exact duration of action of steroid relaxants, because of the wide variations in the experimental conditions under which they were tested the available reports indicate that all of these compounds except pancuronium and possibly malouétine have a short duration of action in the cat, but not in the monkey and man. Pancuronium is the only steroid relaxant known so far with long duration of action in all species investigated (table 1). With regard to the duration of the neuromuscular effects of most steroid relaxants the closest similarity was observed between monkey and man. Of the last three structurally similar compounds (fig. 1) listed in table 1, only pancuronium has a long duration of action in the cat, but all three were long acting in man. Pancuronium, dacuronium and ORG. 6368 differ only in their substituents on the 17th carbon atom (R_2) which is acetyl in pancuronium, hydroxyl in dacuronium and hydrogen in ORG. 6368. In spite of this very close similarity of their chemical structure they differ considerably in their pharmacologic effects in the cat. It seems that there are at least three factors which may influence the pharmacologic effects, especially the duration of action of these compounds:

1. differences in chemical structure;
2. species variation;
3. general condition of the patient and/or the type of operation.

The role that the third factor, 'general condition of the patient and/or the type of operation', may play in drug action is not obvious from the foregoing discussion, however, it is logical to assume that any drug action may be profoundly influenced by pathological conditions or by altered metabolic and/or excretory functions caused by anesthesia and surgery.

Interspecies differences in drug response may be the result of both pharmacodynamic and pharmacokinetic factors. Potency and duration of action of any drug are influenced by distribution, biotransformation and excretion and by its inherent ability to combine with receptors at the site of action and elsewhere. The study of drug disposition and metabolism is of considerable value, not only in understanding drug action, but also in defining those physicochemical properties which are important for the design of new and better neuromuscular blocking agents.

The close similarity of the chemical structures of pancuronium, dacuronium and ORG. 6368 (fig. 1) and the remarkable differences in their pharmacologic action in the cat (10), (11) and (12), prompted us to investigate and compare their pharmacokinetic behaviour in the former species. In the first experimental series the fate of these three compounds was followed for eight hours. It was observed that appreciable amounts of these compounds were excreted in the urine and bile, but striking differences were found in the hepatic accumulation of the three relaxants. By the end of the 8 hour observation period 24 percent of the injected dose of pancuronium (13), 35 percent of dacuronium and 51 percent of ORG. 6368 was found in the liver. In the second experimental series the early hepatic uptake was studied after the intravenous administration of 2 mg/kg pancuronium, dacuronium or ORG. 6368. Blood samples were obtained at 2 minutes after drug administration, the animals were sacrified at 3 minutes and the amounts of relaxants in the liver were determined. The first interesting observation in these studies was the marked differences in the rates of disappearance of the investigated drugs from the plasma. Within two minutes 48 percent of the injected pancuronium, 74 percent of dacuronium and 84 percent of ORG. 6368 disappeared from the circulation. These findings indicate that in the cat the rapid disappearance of these compounds from the plasma is probably due to their massive hepatic uptake (fig. 2).

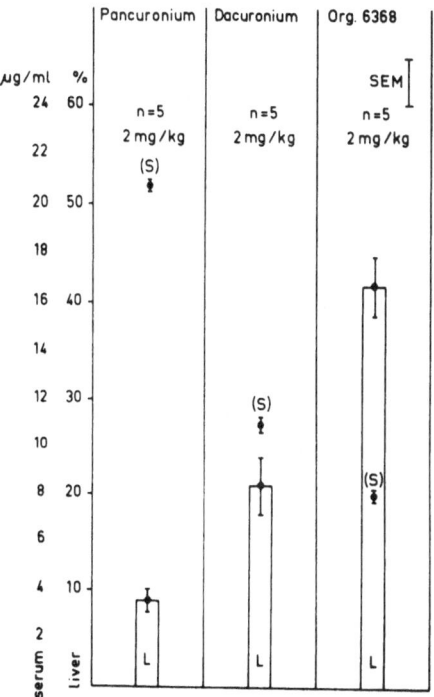

Fig. 2. The percent of the injected dose of pancuronium, dacuronium and ORG. 6368 recovered three minutes after the administration of the indicated dose from the liver of cats. The serum concentration (μg/ml) of the administered drugs two minutes after injection are indicated by dots(s) in the respective columns.

Three minutes after drug administration (fig. 2) the liver contained 41 percent of ORG. 6368, 21 percent of dacuronium and only 9 percent of pancuronium. In agreement with this, plasma concentrations were the lowest after ORG. 6368 and the highest after pancuronium. On the basis of these results it is justified to assume that the extent of early hepatic uptake has a great influence on the duration of the pharmacologic action of these compounds. Similar observations were made with stercuronium in the rat by Wieriks (7) and Hespe and his co-workers (14). However, it is probable that other factors such as binding to acid mucopolysaccharides of the connective tissue and/or differences in receptor affinity may also contribute to the observed differences in the potency and duration of action of these compounds in the cat.

In the light of the data presented it is evident that knowledge of drug distribution, biotransformation and excretion is essential for the understanding of both the pharmacologic actions and side effects of neuromuscular blocking agents.

The evidence available so far on the disposition of the steroid muscle relaxants suggest that short duration of action in the cat is most probably due to early hepatic uptake.

Now, we come to the second factor which may influence drug action, i.e. species variation.

It is highly probable that there is a considerable quantitative difference in the ability of the livers of the cat, monkey and man to accumulate bisquaternary compounds. Seemingly pancuronium is the only steroid relaxant not influenced by these differences. Further experiments with pancuronium and other relaxants in monkeys are necessary to determine whether or not this species could replace the cat as a reliable experimental model for the testing of both the pharmacologic and the pharmacokinetic properties of new neuromuscular blocking agents.

The third factor remaining to be discussed is the possible influence of the general condition of the patient on the pharmacokinetics of pancuronium. The pharmacologic effect of a drug is determined by the concentration of the drug at its cellular effector sites. Since the plasma level of a drug is in physicochemical equilibrium with its concentration at its site of action, any factor capable of affecting the plasma level of a drug is important (fig. 3).

The steep initial slope of the plasma level of pancuronium indicates a rapid distribution phase, which is followed by a more gradual decline that can be regarded as excretion phase. The half lifes of the respective phases were 4 and 32 minutes respectively (13). In man (15) the plasma disappearance exhibited three phases. The third phase in man had a half-life of 108-147 minutes and may reflect drug elimination from a large hypothetical volume

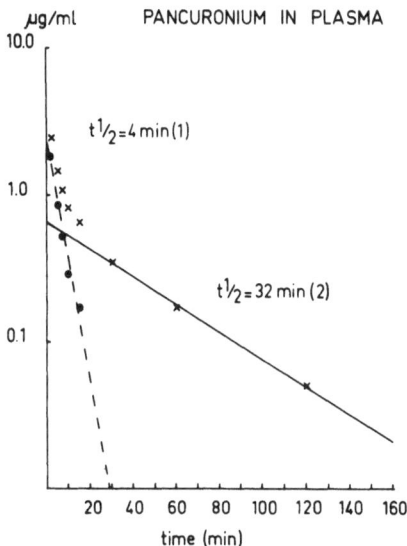

Fig. 3. The mean values in seven cats of the plasma concentration of pancuronium bromide and related compounds plotted semilogarithmically against time. (t ½ = half-life).

of distribution. It should be realised that the plasma levels in our experiments may represent both pancuronium and its deacetylated derivatives. However, the proportions of these compounds recovered in the urine indicate that the metabolites contribute only slightly to the total plasma concentration.

Since pancuronium is the only steroid relaxant in clinical use we were interested in the influence of the renal excretion on its pharmacokinetics. Therefore we investigated the fate of pancuronium in cats after bilateral ligation of the renal pedicles and compared the results (fig. 4) obtained in similar experiments (13) in cats with normal kidney function.

As expected in the animals with ligated renal pedicles the fall of the plasma level of pancuronium was slower than in the cats with intact renal function. These studies also indicated that the absence of the renal function leads to higher uptake in the liver, but no increase in biliary excretion.

It is surprising that under these circumstances the accumulation of pancuronium in the liver doubles without any concomitant increase in its biliary elimination rate. However, in spite of greater accumulation in the liver, the plasma levels also remained significantly higher. An important change was also observed in the biotransformation pattern of pancuronium. While in group with normal kidney function measurable quantities of all three known metabolites could be identified in the liver and bile, in the group without

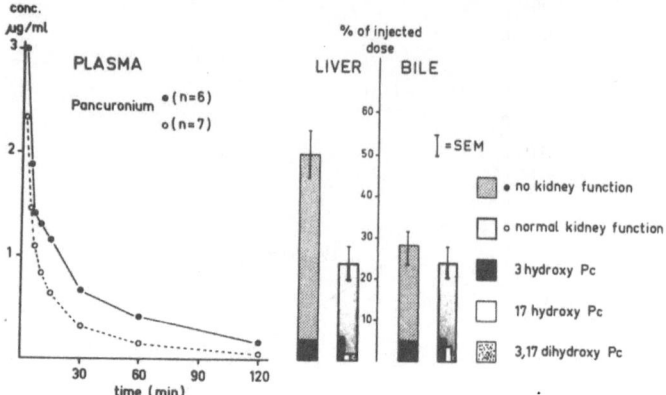

Fig. 4. The plasma levels, liver content after 8 hours and biliary excretion over 8 hours after the intravenous administration of 0.3 mg/kg pancuronium to 6 cats after bilateral ligation of the renal pedicles *c*●) and in 7 cats with normal kidney function *c*○).

renal function only 3-OH pancuronium could be identified by thin-layer chromatography. 3-OH metabolite corresponding to about 5 percent of the injected dose of pancuronium could be recovered from the liver and bile respectively. It is conceivable that under conditions of impaired or absent renal function, the liver may change its pattern of drug metabolism. It may be concluded that the absence of renal excretion, the most important route

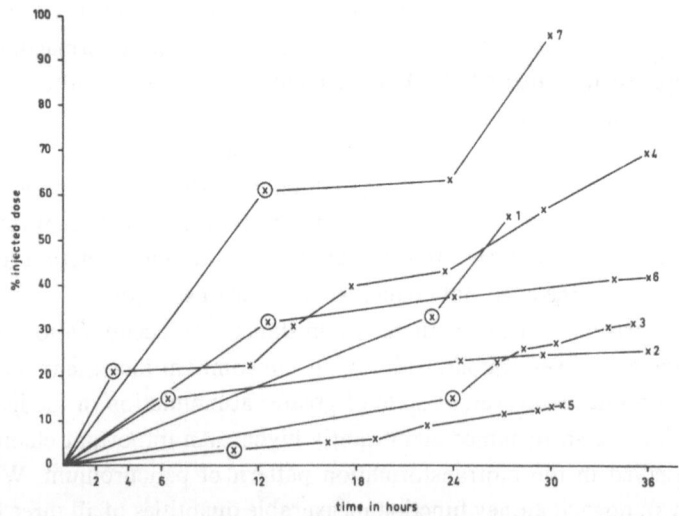

Fig. 5a.

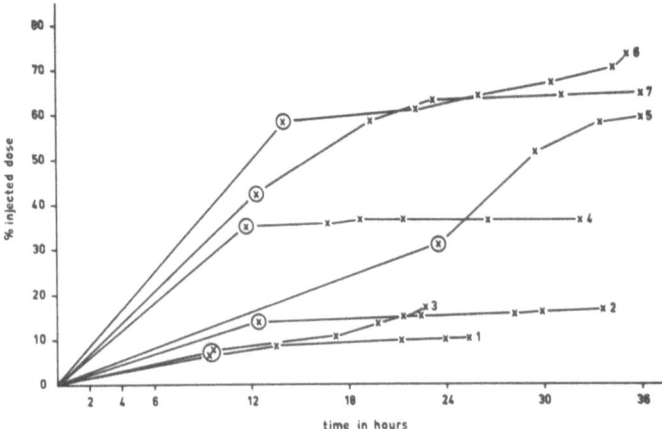

Fig.5b.

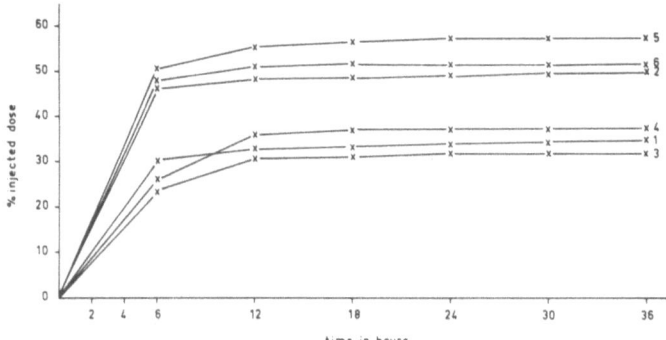

Fig. 5c.

Fig. 5. Cumulative urinary excretion (individual curves) of pancuronium after intravenous injection of a single dose of 6 mg. Urine samples were obtained separately after each
spontaneous micturition from patients in groups I and II (figs 5a and 5b). The time of the
first micturition is indicated on the curves by symbol. Patients in group III (fig. 5c) had an
indwelling urethral catheter and the samples were collected at regular 6 hour intervals.

of elimination of bisquaternary compounds, profoundly changes their pharmacokinetics. Human studies (15) have shown that much less dramatic
interventions then the ligation of the renal pedicles may also cause important
changes in the kinetics of pancuronium. In a clinical investigation of the
metabolism of pancuronium three groups of patients undergoing either
cholecystectomy and choledochostomy (group I), cholecystectomy only
(group II), or pelvic operations (group III) were studied. Urine samples were
collected for up to 36 hours after each spontaneous micturition from groups

I and II, and through indwelling urethral catheters at 6 hour intervals from group III. Bile samples were obtained through indwelling catheters inserted into the common bile duct from patients of group I.

In the first two groups (figs. 5a and 5b) pancuronium concentrations at the urine varied widely not only between the two groups, but also between successive specimens of each patient.

In contrast in group III (fig. 5c) the excretion pattern was very similar in all patients. There were considerable differences in urinary flow from patient to patient, but there was no correlation between the total volume of urine and the total amount of bisquaternary compound excreted in 36 hours. In a similar clinical experiment the same significant variation in the renal elimination of pancuronium, ranging from 28-98 percent of the injected dose in individual patients was described by Buzello (16). This irregular pattern in the urinary excretion in certain type of patients is not restricted to steroid relaxants. We have observed similar variation in the excretion of gallamine in man. Wide individual variations were also seen in the hepatic elimination of pancuronium (fig. 6).

The bile samples from the patients of group I were obtained through total bile drainage at various intervals up to 30 hours.

There was neither a positive nor a negative correlation between the rates

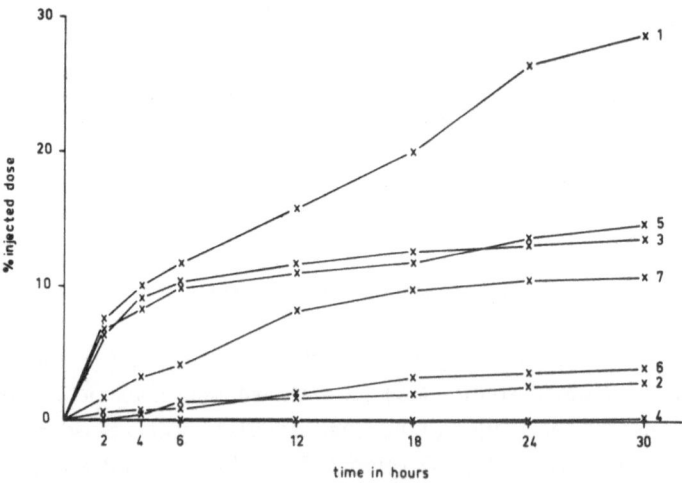

Fig. 6. Cumulative biliary excretion (individual curves) of pancuronium bromide after intravenous injection of a single 6 mg dose. The numbers of each curve correspond to the patient numbers.

of urinary and biliary excretion in the same subject. In spite of these wide variations in the urinary and biliary excretion, the total amount of pancuronium excreted in the urine was fairly consistent, approximating 43 percent of the injected dose in group I, 37 percent in group II and 43 percent in group III. The mean recovery in the bile (group I) amounted to 11 percent of the administered dose at the end of the 30 hour observation period (fig. 6).

We have no explanation for the irregularities seen in the renal and hepatic elimination of pancuronium. The fact that on one hand this phenomenon was usually seen in patients with biliary tract pathology and on the other hand in association with the altered biotransformation pattern (fig. 4) of pancuronium encountered in the absence of kidney function in cats suggest that hepatic and renal excretory functions might be interrelated.

Pancuronium bromide, at the present moment the only steroid relaxant in clinical use, belongs to the group of non-depolarizing agents which undergo partial, slow biotransformation in the body, but the major part of the administered quantity is excreted mostly unchanged in the urine. The largest part of the excreted metabolites was represented by the 3-OH derivative which in the cat possesses almost the same pharmacologic activity as pancuronium (17). Its neuromuscular activity in man, however, is unknown.

In man not more than 20 percent of the administered dose of pancuronium underwent biotransformation. From the clinical point of view it is important that the termination of the neuromuscular activity of pancuronium mainly depends on redistribution from postjunctional receptor sites to non-specific tissue acceptors after the administration of single moderate doses and on renal elimination of the unchanged drug after large or repeated doses. It is unlikely that either biotransformation or biliary excretion would significantly influence the duration of action of single, moderate doses. However, these processes might have considerable influence on the duration of action after large initial or repeated smaller doses.

GENERAL CONCLUSIONS

1. Even very closely related steroid relaxants with similar physicochemical properties may show significant differences in their pharmacokinetic behaviour. This, in turn, may profoundly change their pharmacologic effects.

2. Due to species differences animal data on pharmacokinetics are not transferable to man. It is conceivable that the differences in the pharma-

cokinetics of pancuronium between the cat and man are only quantitative and qualitative. With other words, the role of the liver in handling these compounds may be important in man too.

3. The physical condition of the patient and probably even the type of the operation may influence the pharmacokinetics of the neuromuscular blocking agents in man.

REFERENCES

1. Davis, N., The chemotherapy of Schistosomiasis. Part V[1]. Chlorestelyl and hocloy derivatives of 4-amino-2-methoxyphenyl ethers. *J. chem. Soc.* 178 (1962).
2. Marshall, I. G., D. Paul and H. Singh, The neuromuscular and other blocking actions of 4,17a-dimethyl-4,17a-diaza-d-homo-5 alfaandrostane dimethiodide (HS-342) in the anesthetized cat. *Eur. J. Pharmacol.* 22, 129 (1973).
3. Quevauviller, M. A. and M. F. Lainé, Sur la toxicité et le pouvoir curarisant du chlorure de melouétine. *Ann. pharm. franc.* 18, 678 (1960).
4. Biggs, R. S., M. Davis and R. Wien, Muscle-relaxant properties of a steroid bisquaternary ammonium salt. *Experientia* 20, 119 (1964).
5. Busfield, D., K. J. Child, A. J. Clarke, B. Davis and M. G. Dodds, Neuromuscular blocking activities of some steroidal mono and bisquaternary ammonium compounds with special reference to NN'-dimethyl-conessine. *Br. J. Pharmac. Chemother.* 33, 609 (1968).
6. Admiraal, P. V., *Klinisch onderzoek van stercuronium (Myc 1080), een kortwerkend niet-depolariserend spierrelaxans.* Acad. Proefschr. Rotterdam (1972).
7. Wieriks, J., *Farmacologisch onderzoek van Myc 1080 (stercuronium), een nieuwe kortwerkende motorisch eindplaatremmer.* Acad. Proefschr. Rotterdam (1972).
8. Singh, H., D. Paul and V. V. Parashar, Steroid skeleton modification to 4,17a-dimethyl-4,17a-diaza-D-homo-5 alfa-androstane dimethiodide-a potential neuromuscular blocking agent. In: *Abstr. IUPAC Symp. Chem. Natural Prod.* New Delhi, p. 274 (1972).
9. Gandiha, A., I. G. Marshall, D. Paul, I. W. Rodger, W. Scott and H. Singh, Some actions of chandonium iodide, a new short acting muscle relaxant, in anesthetized cats and on isolated muscle preparations. *Clin. Exp. Pharmacol. Physiol.* 2, 159 (1975).
10. Bonta, I. L., W. R. Buckett, J. J. Lewis *et al.*, 2-beta-16-beta-dipiperidino-5 alfa, androstane- 3 alfa, 17 beta-diol- diacetate-dimethbromide (NA 97) a potent neuromuscular blocking steroid. In: *Abstr. ICS no. 111*, Excerpta Medica (1966).
11. Feldman, S. A. and M. F. Tyrrell, A new steroid muscle relaxant. *Anaesthesia* 25, 349 (1970).
12. Sugrue, M. F. and N. Duff, ORG. 6368: A competitive steroidal muscle relaxant with a rapid onset and a short duration of action. *Naunyn Schmiedeberg's Archives Pharmacology*, Suppl., 279, 1230 (1973).
13. Agoston, S., U. W. Kersten and D. K. F. Meijer, The fate of pancuronium in the cat. *Acta anaesth. scand.* 17, 129 (1973).
14. Hespe, W. and J. Wieriks, Metabolic fate of short acting peripheral neuromuscular blocking agent stercuronium in the rat as related to its action. *Biochem. Pharmacol.* 20, 1213 (1971).
15. Agoston, S., G. A. Vermeer, U. W. Kersten and D. K. F. Meijer, The fate of pancuronium bromide in man. *Acta anaesth., scand.* 17, 267 (1973).
16. Buzello, W., Der Stoffwechsel von Pancuronium beim Menschen. *Anaesthesist* 24, 13 (1975).
17. Sim, A., Personal communication. Organon Laboratories (Newhouse) (1972).

21. NEW MUSCLE RELAXANTS

J. F. CRUL

Since the introduction of pancuronium some six years ago many clinicians felt that the search for new relaxants could be stopped. The predictable degree of block caused by this drug, the apparent lack of circulatory side effects and the good reversibility made it useless to try to find a drug which was clearly different and superior. Investigators, however, were not content and looked for drugs with the same specific, nondepolarizing action on the motor end plate, but with a faster onset and shorter duration of action.

This can be achieved in two ways, either by making the binding or the affinity of the drug molecule to the receptor less strong and/or by causing a rapid fall in the plasma concentration by metabolic breakdown; rapid excretion or by binding to non-specific receptor sites. If a large enough quantity of drug could be bound to non-specific receptor sites, it could contribute to a rapid decline of the plasma concentration of the drug. Developments in both these directions have been followed over the last years.

To maintain a pure nondepolarizing block the 2 quaternary-onium groups of the molecules should be shielded off from the receptor sites by large alkylradicals, diminishing in this way the intrinsic stimulating activity of the onium groups. The steroid configuration, and particularly the andostren, was seemingly a good skeleton to build upon for powerful muscle relaxants with little autonomic blocking or stimulating action.

Two derivatives of pancuronium have therefore been investigated more extensively over the last years (fig. 1). They differ from pancuronium only by the radicals on the seventeen carbon atom and are called dacuronium and Org. 6368.

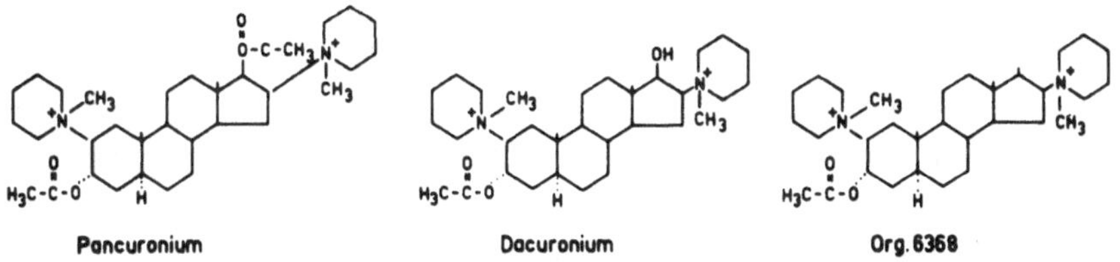

Pancuronium   Dacuronium   Org. 6368

Fig. 1.

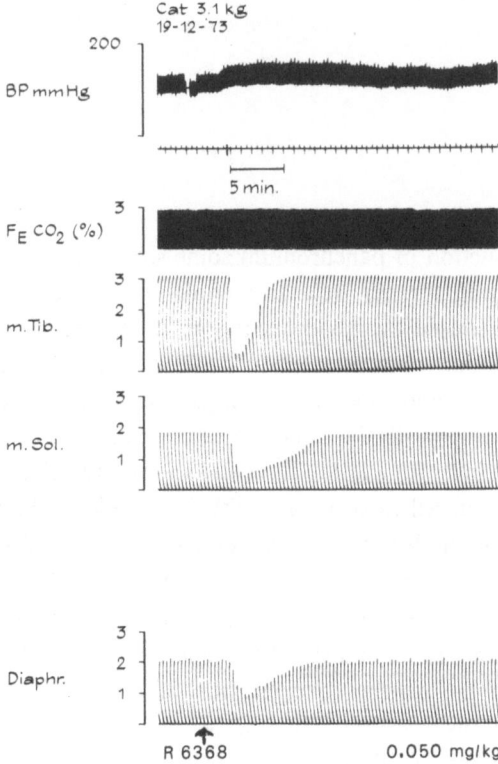

Fig. 2. Relaxation of a fast (m. tibialis anterior) and a slow (m. soleus) muscle as well as the diaphragm of the cat on a single intravenous dose of 0.05 mg/kg R 6368.
Note the stronger paralysis in the tibialis and the sparing effect of the diaphragm (see text). The upper trace is the intra-arterial blood pressure, the second trace the endtidal CO_2 curve. In between the time marking.

Dacuronium, first investigated by Buckett (1973) and Feldman (1970), has a hydroxyl group on the C 17 atom instead of the carboxyl group of pancuronium. Dose response curves in the cat showed a considerable weaker action than pancuronium and a flatter response curve. Duration of action was as short as that of succinylcholine. In the isolated arm preparation in awake volunteers and in clinical trials it was slightly weaker than gallamine and also had a somewhat shorter action in milligr. per kg body weight basis. Onset of the action of a full paralysing dose was not shorter than with equipotent doses of gallamine. Intubation was not speeded up with this drug, neither was there a pronounced respiratory muscle 'sparing' effect.

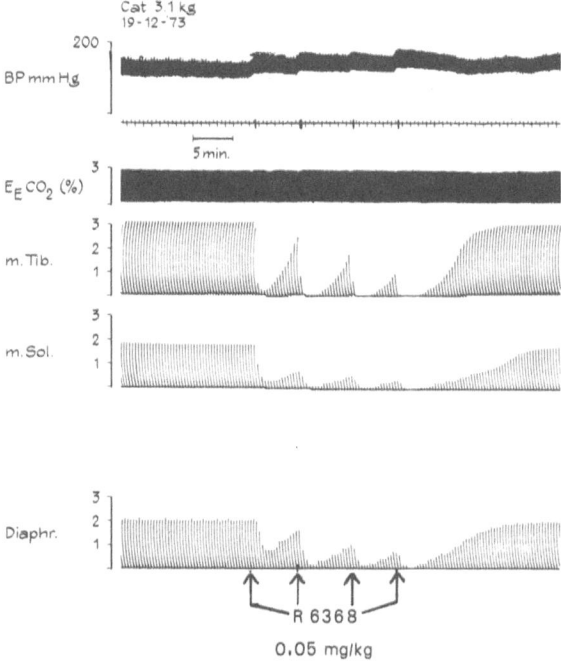

Fig. 3. Cumulative action of repeated doses of 0.05 mg/kg R 6368 on the tibialis, soleus and diaphragm muscles of the cat. Note the decrease in slope of the return of contractions after each following dose and the longer duration of the total block.

Good reversibility with esterase inhibitors was achieved. The usual cumulative effect was seen after repeated dose. Unfortunately Norman and Katz showed in many patients a marked tachycardia indicating a strong vagolytic action. This, together with its strong antichonilesterase activity, precluded this drug from further clinical studies.

The second derivative, studied more extensively, is Org. 6368, which lacks even the hydroxyl group at the C 17 position. Single injections of 0.05 mg/kg R 6368 showed short relaxation of the tibialis, soleus and diaphragm of the cat (fig. 2). Dose reponse curves in cats showed a sensitivity of $\frac{1}{5}-\frac{1}{6}$ of pancuronium with a parallel shift of the curve to the right. Cumulative effects in these species were only seen when higher doses were repeated within 30 minutes after the previous injection (fig. 3). Only mild changes in sensitivity were seen in respiratory or metabolic acidosis (fig. 4). Reversibility by esterase inhibitors was prompt and long lasting.

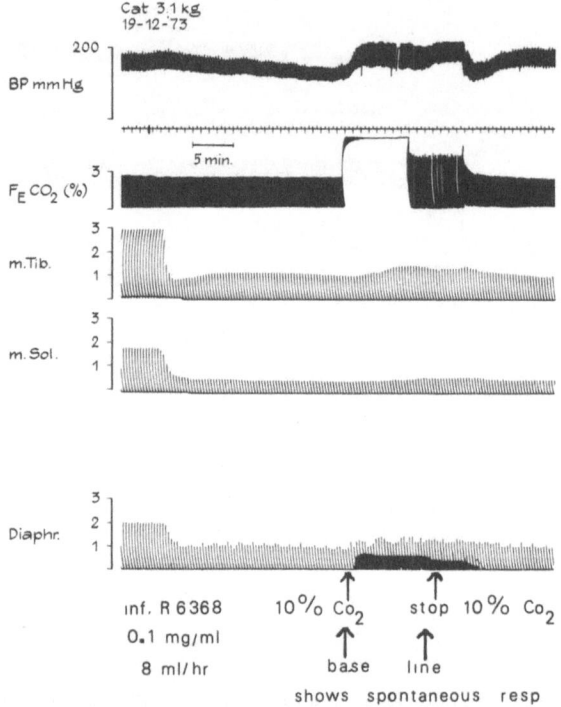

Fig. 4. Change in steady state in muscle relaxation by infusion of 0.042 mg/kg/min of R 6368 on three muscles of the cat. Only a slight increase in the blockade was seen.

In comparing the effect upon the slow and fast muscles of the leg with the diaphragm, higher dose ranges showed a slightly larger respiratory muscle sparing effect of 6368 in comparison with pancuronium in equipotent doses for the other muscles (fig. 5). Both the degree and duration of block in the diaphragm were smaller. The promising short action of this compound in rats and cats – full paralysing doses lasted only 4-7 minutes – could not be substantiated in monkeys and in man. Agoston has suggested that this short action in cats could be explained by the rapid and strong selective absorption of the drug by the liver of the cat.

In clinical experiments doses of 0.5 mg/kg body weight just caused a 100% paralysing of the adductor pollius muscle. It did show a slightly faster onset of action (2 min for a 100% block) than equipotent doses of pancuronium. Doses of 0.75 mg/kg were needed for smooth intubation. This prolonged the block considerably. Duration of action of R 6368 for a dose of 0.5 mg/kg

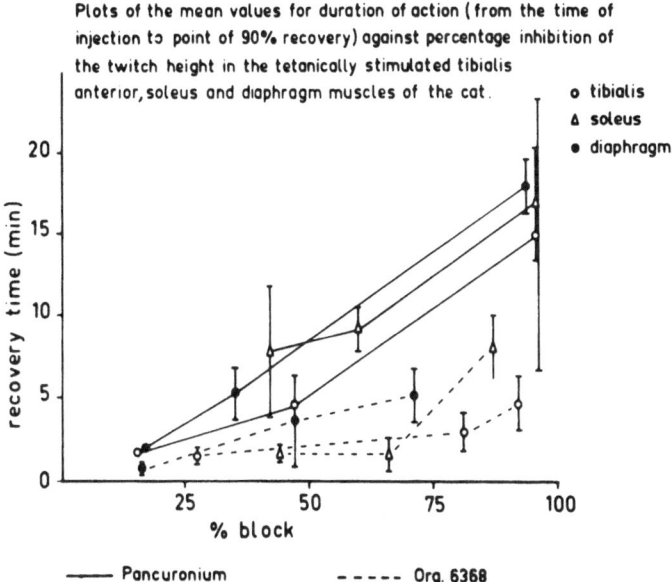

Plots of the mean values for duration of action (from the time of injection to point of 90% recovery) against percentage inhibition of the twitch height in the tetanically stimulated tibialis anterior, soleus and diaphragm muscles of the cat.

o tibialis
Δ soleus
● diaphragm

———— Pancuronium   - - - - Org. 6368

Fig. 5. Recovery time versus % block for three different muscles of the cat for pancuronium and Org. 6368. (After Hiser et al., *Anesthesiol.* 1975, 42, p. 251).

from onset of 100% block till 90% recovery was 62 minutes. Reversibility with pyridostigmine once the contractions re-appeared, was good. Dose response curves in man showed its potency to be *11* of pancuronium. In these experiments no preliminary suxamethonium was given and neurolept anesthesia without halothane was used during the operation. Patients were intubated before the drug was given and operation started. All 15 patients showed a tachycardia within 1 minute of the injection, well before the onset of the neuromuscular block. Maximal effect was reached after 5 minutes and lasted for 15-20 minutes. An average increase of 28% in pulse rate occurred with a concomitant and equivalent rise in blood pressure. No clinical signs of histamine release were noted. The relatively larger respiratory sparing effect, seen in cats in higher dose ranges, has not yet been investigated in these clinical trials.

Vagolytic action therefore seems to be stronger with this relaxant than with pancuronium. This is not outweighed by any clear advantages in onset time and duration of action. The strong plasma cholinesterase inhibiting effect of this new steroid relaxant is interesting. This could explain the threefold increase in duration of action of suxamethonium after preliminary small dose of ORG 6368 (0.1 mg/kg) (Hutschenreuter, 1974). This may even be used as an alternative to a pure, short acting, nondepolarizing type of block. It also prevents fasciculations and muscle pains if administered before suxamethonium.

Of the large series of other steroid relaxants studied, one should be mentioned brifly, namely chandonium iodide, which also is an androsten derivative (Gandiha, 1975). It has a structural formula as shown in figure 6.

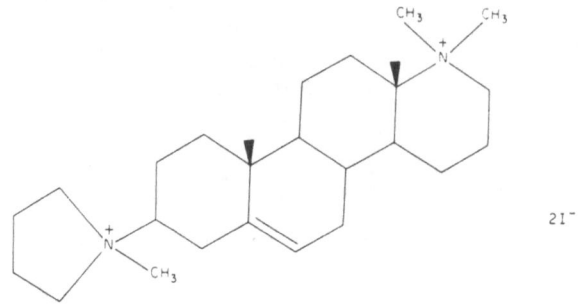

Fig. 6. Chandonium iodide.

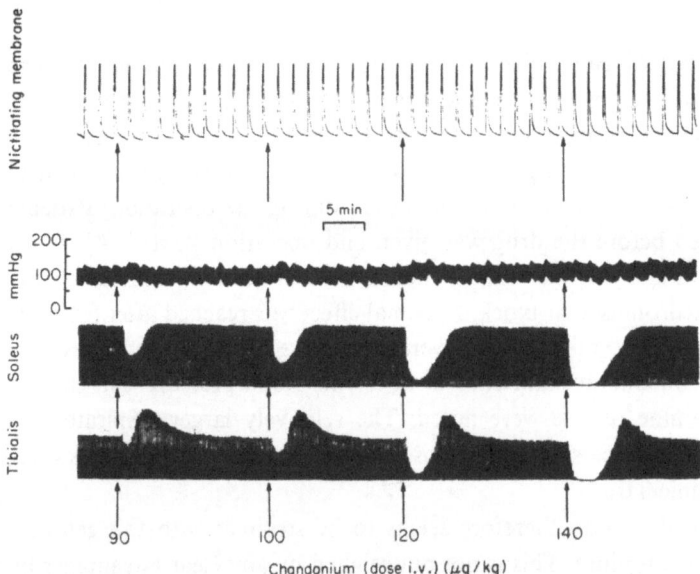

Fig. 7. Chloralose-anesthetized cat. Effects of increasing doses of chandonium on responses of the nictitating membrene to preganglionic stimulation, blood pressure and responses of the soleus and tibialis anterior to direct stimulation at 0.1 Hz. (After A. Ghandiha et al., Clinical en Experimental Pharmacology and Physiology 1975, 2, p. 159-170).

It is as potent a relaxant in cats as ORG 6368 it with a rapid onset and short duration of action. However, at low dose levels it showed an augmentation of the twitch response of the tibialis muscle in the cat and at higher dose levels a marked post-block twitch augmentation, probably caused by its weak anticholinesterase effect (fig. 7).

In the avian muscle it did not show any contracture, indicating that it is a pure nondepolarizing blocker. This was also substantiated by the tetanic fade and post tetanic facilitation. No effect was seen on either sympathic or parasympathic gangliq, but it had a lytic action on the cardiac vagus neuro effector junction, causing a mild tachycardia. No reactions were seen on either airway resistance or transpulmonary pressure, indicating a lack of histamine liberation.

No further studies on monkeys or men have been reported.

Another group of new drugs that warrants the attention of the anesthesiologists are the tetrazine dyes with nondepolarizing relaxant action. AH 8165, yet without tradename, is the best known of these and has the following structure formula (fig. 8). It is proposed as a pure nondepolarizer, but

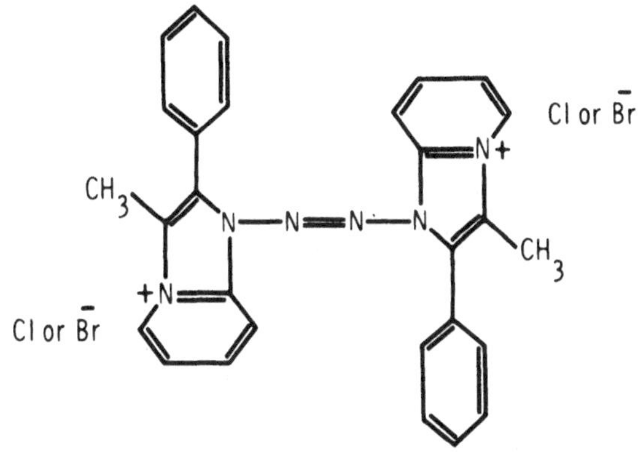

Fig. 8.

AH 8165

studies by Hiser (1975) with chick biventer vervicis muscle clearly indicated that it causes muscle contracture at low dose levels (fig. 9), indicating a depolarizing activity. At higher doses the nondepolarizing effect predominates. In the in vitro rat diaphragm preperation its onset of action turned out to be much faster than d-tubocurarine, but slower than succinylcholine. The dose response curve is parallel to that of d-tubocurarine, but shifted to the right with a 10 times weaker potency (fig. 10). The washout from the muscle preparation, indicating its affinity to the end-plates, was faster than

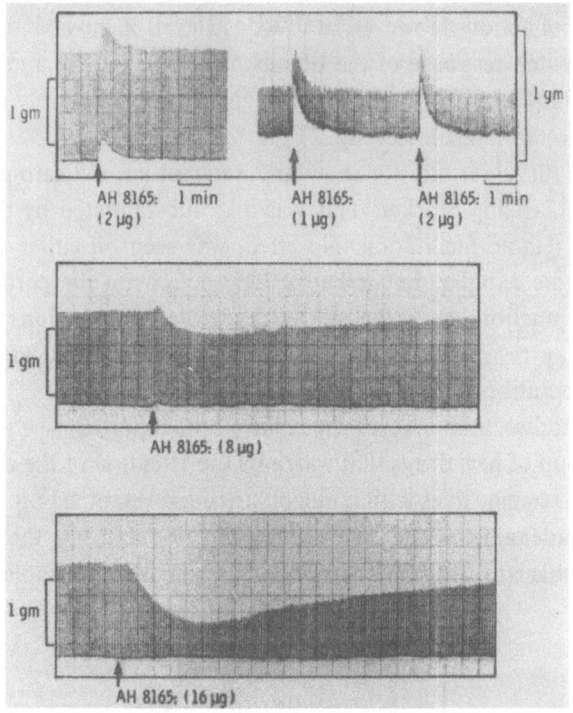

Fig. 9. Typical records of the effect of AH 8165 on the chick biventer cervicis nerve-muscle preparation. Upper left trace: effect of 1 μg AH 8165. The arrow represents the point of drug administration. Middle trace: effect of 8 μg AH 8165 on the same preparation. Lower trace: effect of 16 μg AH 8165 on the same preparation. Upper right trace: effects of 1 μg and 2 μg AH 8165 on another preparation in which the tonic component appeared to predominate. (After Hiser *et al.*, *Anesthesiol.* 1975, 42, p. 251).

of d-tubocurarine and slower than succinylcholine. Esterase inhibitors like neostigmine could only partially reverse the block by AH 8165. This also could indicate that this drug is not a pure nondepolarizing blocker. A direct effect on the muscle fibres has not been detected. Post (1974) showed that at low doses AH 8165 increased the miniature end-plate potentials in the in vitro frog sartorius muscle.

In vivo in cats and rats AH 8165 showed rapid onset and a short duration of action, with the same variation in species sensitivity as has been demonstrated with other nondepolarizing drugs. Prolonged infusions did not cause a prolongation of recovery.

Studies in man shows that AH 8165 is about 10 times weaker than pancuronium. The rapid onset of action seems to be the main advantage of this

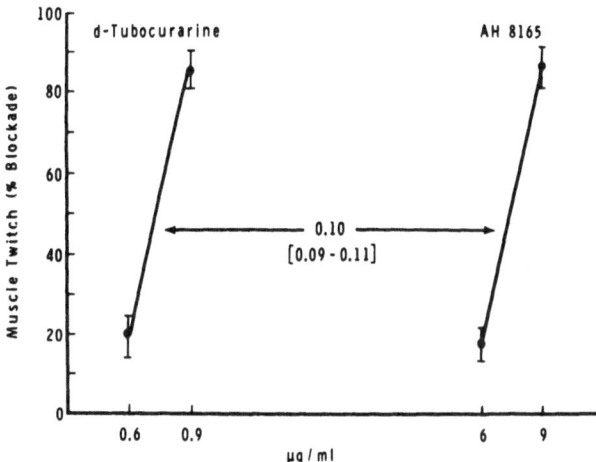

Fig. 10. Comparative effects of AH 8165 and d-tubocurarine on muscle twitch of the rat phrenic nerve-diaphragm preparation. Points represent actual data points. Values are means ± SE, n = 10. The four-point bioassay was performed and the resultant potency ratio of AH 8165 to d-tubocurarine was calculated to be 0.1. The 95 per cent confidence interval was 0.09 to 0,11. (After Hiser et al., *Anesthesiol.* 1975, 42, p. 249).

drug (Kean, 1975). Time to 100% paralysis of the adductor pollicis muscle with a dose of 0.25 mg/kg is 30-40 sec. Intubating conditions are reasonably good (Young, 1975), when a dose 3 to 5 times as high as this is used, but less perfect than with 1 mg/kg succinylcholine. The time taken to achieve a 90% recovery of twitch contraction was 49 min. with the dose of 0.75 mg/kg (Kean, 1975). Cardiovascular actions were very extensively studied by Patschke (1974) and Coleman (1975) and showed a persistant increase in cardiac rate. A tachycardia of 10-12% is usually compensated for by lowering of the peripheral vascular resistance, as a result the arterial pressure usually remains constant. When the tachycardia is larger (Coleman even reported increases of 40-60%), a concomitant blood pressure rise is seen. These circulatory effects were very persistent and tasted longer than the neuromuscular block. A vagolytic action of this drug on the cardiac vagus effector neuron has been suggested as a probable explanation of his effect.

When AH 8165 was used for relaxation in cardiac surgery (Lyons, 1975) the tachycardia was much more troublesome than with pancuronium and in high doses was even accompanied by a drop in blood pressure.

Histamine release was measured by Blogg (1973) and not found in an appreciable amount. Placental transfer was proven by Blogg (1975) in man, but not in clinically important amounts. The insensitive bio assay technique of the determintation, however, made the data rather dubious.

The only indication for the use of this drug therefore seems to be as a replacement for succinylcholine in crash induction in acute patients, when succinylcholine is contra-indicated. The mixed depolarizing and nonde-polarizing effects seen in in vitro experiments as well as the overt cardio-vascular effects, combined with the long duration of action in clinical use does not provide any advantages for this drug over pancuronium.

Lastly I want to mention the studies undertaken by Savarese (1973) and his group to synthetize a group of diesterdiquaternary ammonium com-pounds which are sensitive to plasmacholinesterase hydrolysis and break-down like succinylcholine, but lack an intrinsic receptor stimulating activity because the methylgroups have been substituted by long chain alkyl groups (fig. 11). One of these compounds, DD 188, was a very promising drug in

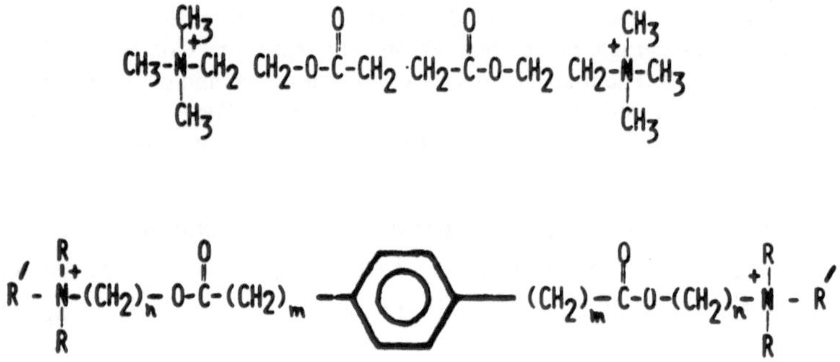

$$CH_3-\overset{\overset{\displaystyle CH_3}{+}}{\underset{\displaystyle CH_3}{N}}-CH_2 \; CH_2-O-\overset{\overset{\displaystyle O}{\|}}{C}-CH_2 \; CH_2-\overset{\overset{\displaystyle O}{\|}}{C}-O-CH_2 \; CH_2-\overset{\overset{\displaystyle CH_3}{+}}{\underset{\displaystyle CH_3}{N}}-CH_3$$

$$R'-\overset{\overset{\displaystyle R}{+}}{\underset{\displaystyle R}{N}}-(CH_2)_{\overline{n}} \; O-\overset{\overset{\displaystyle O}{\|}}{C}-(CH_2)_m -\bigcirc - (CH_2)_{\overline{m}}-\overset{\overset{\displaystyle O}{\|}}{C}-O-(CH_2)_{\overline{n}}-\overset{\overset{\displaystyle R}{+}}{\underset{\displaystyle R}{N}}-R'$$

Fig. 11. Chemical formula of succinylcholine (top) contrasted with general formula for current series of compounds (bottom). Note that both formulae contain two ester linkages, making the compounds potential substrates for hydrolysis by plasma cholines-terase. The methyl groups of succinylcholine, which confer depolarising neuromuscular blocking action, have been replaced by ethyl and larger groups, thereby producing nondepolarising agents.

animal experiments even in primates. Its action is purely nondepolarizing in all species studied. Its duration of action is shorter than succinylcholine in cats and somewhat longer in monkeys (8-12 min). Muscle fasciculations are not seen. The neuromuscular block produced by this drug can be fully antagonised by anti-cholinesterase agents. As the plasma cholinesterase activity in this species is slightly less than in human plasma (Drabkova, 1973), this fast breakdown and short action could also be expected in man. However, the affinity to the receptor site could be stronger and contra-act such a rapid decline in the plasma.

When administered as an infusion for 1 hour to primates, recovery was complete within 5 to 15 minutes after the end of an infusion and this could even be accelerated by anti-cholinesterase agents.

The inhibitory action of this drug on the vagus is equal to that of gallamine in equipotential doses, the sympathetic ganglionic blockade is about $\frac{1}{4}$ to $\frac{1}{10}$ of that of d-tubocurarine. These effects are usually of short duration. Most of these compounds, however, caused a sharp rise in blood pressure of 1-2 min. in the cat, followed by a hypotensive period of 5-8 min. Nicotinic stimulation followed by inhibition at the peak of the block is the most probable cause of these effects. In the monkey this nicotinic hyperactivity and block is absent. Only a moderate rise in pulse frequency and blood pressure was seen here regularly.

It is worthwhile to note that in vitro experiments showed that this drug is hydrolysed by human plasma slightly slower than succinylcholine. In spite of the light vagolytic action of these compounds their short action may justify clinical trial. Patients with atypical variants of plasma cholinesterase may show a prolonged effect, but in these cases anticholinesterase drugs should accelerate spontaneous recovery.

It would be interesting to try to synthetize steroid relaxants with an ester linkage, sensitive to esterase hydrolysis in human plasma and where the metabolites of this hydrolysis loose their muscle relaxant properties. For the time being none of the drugs presented offers sufficient advantages over pancuronium that it should replace it.

It seems as if the shorter action of these drugs is inevitably combined with a weaker potency and a more pronounced stimulation of acetylcholine receptor in the autonomic nerve system, thereby causing more circulatory side effects.

REFERENCES

1. Buckett, W. R., C. L. Hewett and D. S. Savage, Pancuronium bromide and other steroidal neuromuscular blocking agents containing acetylcholine fragments. *J. Med. Chem.* 16, 1116 (1973).
2. Feldman, S. A. and M. F. Tyrell, A new steroid relaxant – dacuronium NB-68 (Organon). *Anaesthesia* 25, 349 (1970).
3. Norman, J. and R. L. Katz, Some effects of the steroidal muscle relaxant dacuronium bromide in anesthestized patients. *Brit. J. Anaesth.* 43, 313 (1971).
4. Agoston, S., Personal communication.
5. Hutschenreuter, K., Erste klinische Erfahrungen mit einem Pavulon Derivat. Abstr. no. 280 in: *International Congress Series no. 330*, Excerpta Medica, Amsterdam (1974).
6. Gandiha, A., I. G. Marshall, D. Paul, I. W. Rodger, W. Scott and H. Singh, Some actions of chandonium iodide, a new short-acting muscle relaxant, in anaesthetized cats and on isolated muscle preparations. *Clin. Exp. Pharmacol. Physiol.* 2, 159 (1975).

7. Hiser, P. Th., K. L. Dretchen and G. O. Kruger, In-vitro investigation of a new neuromuscular relaxant, AH 8165. *Anesthesiology* 42, 245 (1975).
8. Post, E. L., M. D. Sokoll, K. L. Dretchen, Effects of a new blocking agent AH 8165 on neuromuscular transmission. *Fed. Proc.*, 33, 579 (1974).
9. Kean, H. M. C., The neuromuscular blocking properties of AH 8165 during halothane anaesthesia. *Anaesthesia* 30, 333 (1975).
10. Young, H. S. A., R. S. J. Clarke and J. W. Dundee, Intubating conditions with AH 8165 and suxamethonium. *Anaesthesia* 30, 30 (1975).
11. Patschke, D., J. B. Brückner, J. Tarnow und A. Weymar, Einfluss von AH 8165 – eines neuen, nicht depolarisierenden Muskelrelaxans – auf die Hämodynamik des Menschen. *Anaesthesist* 23, 430 (1974).
12. Coleman, A. J., P. T. Walling, J. W. Downing and L. T. Bees, The effect of carbon dioxide on the neuromuscular and haemodynamic effects of AH 8165, a new non-depolarizing muscle relaxant. *Br. J. Anaesth.* 47, 365 (1975).
13. Lyons, S. M., R. S. J. Clarke and H. S. A. Young, A clinical comparison of AH 8165 and pancuronium as muscle relaxants in patients undergoing cardiac surgery. *Br. J. Anaesth.* 47, 725 (1975).
14. Blogg, C. E., T. M. Savege, J. C. Simpson, L. A. Ross and B. R. Simpson, A new muscle relaxant – AH 8165. *Proc. R. Soc. Med.* 66, 1023 (1973).
15. Blogg, C. E., B. R. Simpson, M. B. Tyers, L. E. Martin and J. A. Bell, Human placental transfer of AH 8165. *Anaesthesia*, 30, 23 (1975).
16. Savarese, J. J., S. Ginsburg, C. Lee and R. J. Kitz, The pharmacology of new short-acting nondepolarizing ester neuromuscular blocking agents: clinical implications. *Anesth. Analg. Curr. Res.* 52, 982 (1973).
17. Drábková, J., J. F. Crul and E. Van der Kleijn, Placental transfer of ^{14}C labelled succinylcholine in near-term Macaca Mulatta monkeys. *Br. J. Anaesth.* 45, 1087 (1973).

22. THE IDEAL MUSCLE RELAXANT

S. A. FELDMAN

An ideal muscle relaxant drug would provide complete neuromuscular blockade in every patient and, provided artificial ventilation were maintained, it would have no other pharmacological effects. Its activity would be capable of complete reversal, in all patients, without any residual effects at any time within a few minutes of its administration.

I would suggest that it is unlikely that a drug with all these desirable properties will ever be synthesised. It is therefore more profitable to consider where our present neuromuscular blocking drugs are inadequate, in the expectation that drugs will be synthesised that will avoid some or all of these disadvantages. Indeed, Galindo (1) asserted with much justification that we already possess excellent safe muscle relaxants, provided they are used with due attention and care. Certainly all the non-depolarizing relaxants have a far higher therapeutic index than virtually any other drug used in anaesthetic practice. Some of them, however, have specific side effects that make them less suited to patients with certain physiological abnormalities.

There are two possible starting points for considering likely improvements in the muscle relaxants – the first is safety, the second is convenience. I will discuss the ideal relaxant by considering firstly the side effects that must be avoided and then the factors necessary to make it convenient as well as safe when used.

HAZARDS OF NEUROMUSCULAR BLOCKING AGENTS

Cardiovascular system
The ideal of a muscle relaxant, free of any effect upon the cardiovascular system irrespective of dose, has yet to be achieved. However, in spite of this it is doubtful whether the cardiovascular effects of any non-depolarizing muscle relaxant have ever resulted in the death of a patient with a normal cardiovascular system. When considering the safety record of the three commonly used non-depolarizing drugs – alcuronium, pancuronium and d-tubocurarine – against the occasional death from suxamethonium, it is

apparent that suxamethonium is a *relatively* dangerous drug due to its effect on the cardiovascular system, yet even suxamethonium would hardly figure in a statistical analysis of the causes of anaesthetic mortality. The ideal muscle relaxant would not have any chronotropic effect on the heart, even in doses up to 5 times those required to produce neuromuscular block. I use a safety factor of 5 as experience on both sides of the Atlantic has demonstrated that what constitutes a therapeutic dose varies by 5 fold according to the anaesthetic department involved and whether one is referring to common American or European practice.

Hypotension due to ganglion blockade is an undesirable side effect, although a moderate fall in peripheral resistance at high dose levels would not necessarily be a disadvantage.

Certainly it is less harmful than the depression of myocardial performance and increase in oxygen utilisation by the heart that appears to occur in dogs when d-tubocurarine is administered (2). Similarly, a slight fall in peripheral resistance is probably preferable to any increase in this parameter. The occurrence of hypertension due to a rise in peripheral resistance not only increases the work load of left ventricle but may also cause bloody operating conditions.

In a study of various muscle relaxants by Hughes (3) he found tachycardia to be a disadvantage of gallamine and AH 8165 at 80% paralytic doses, whilst pancuronium and dimethyl curare only produced vagolysis at high doses. We have found that vagolysis occurs with pancuronium at about twice the therapeutic dose level (4). Sympathetic blockade was a major disadvantage of d-tubocurarine and occurred at high doses with AH 8165 Hughes (1974) concluded that dimethylcurine had the best cardiovascular profile.

Histamine release
Until one experiences acute bronchospasm in a patient oneself, one is apt to discount the significance of histamine release by muscle relaxant drugs. Certainly its effects are rare but when they do occur they can be alarming due to bronchospasm or allergic manifestations. An ideal relaxant must not only not release histamine but it must also be free of the possibility of producing true sensitisation and anaphyllactic response in patients.

Passage across vital barriers
The ideal muscle relaxant would not only not pass into brain but also would not cross the placental barrier. However, when one considers the evidence

that plasma protein and red blood cells can cross the placental membrane during the third trimester one realises that the placenta is far from a true physical barrier. It is other factors such as the concentration gradient and the blood flow rather than the characteristics of the drug that ultimately determine the passage across the membrane.

Convenience factors

1. Rapidity of onset
The ideal relaxant would produce a rapid onset of paralysis. The rate of onset is largely a function of the concentration gradient between the plasma and receptor site and this depends upon the dose of drug given. The ideal drug would produce a rapid onset of action even in a dose that just produced 100% neuromuscular block. This would indicate an ability to penetrate rapidly to the receptor site.

2. Lack of cumulative effect
Most muscle relaxants have a cumulative effect. A second dose administered many hours after apparent recovery of neuromuscular transmission produces a more profound effect. This is especially true of gallamine. The presence of a cumulative effect indicates that neuromuscular transmission, with its normal large margin of safety, has not been restored to normal in spite of apparent recovery of twitch response at the end of the operation. I consider this to be a potentially dangerous side effect of many non-depolarizing muscle relaxants. The ideal relaxant should be capable of complete reversal leaving the receptor site free of any depression of cholinergic response.

3. Ability to terminate the action at any time
It has been held that the ideal relaxant is a short acting non-depolarizing drug. Certainly such a drug would have an activity that could be terminated soon after the drug was discontinued. However, the shorter the duration of action the more likely is the drug to have autonomic or other acetylcholine-like properties. I would like to suggest that it is more practicable to seek a drug which would be long acting, that is one with a high affinity constant for the receptor, but one whose activity was at any time completely and absolutely reversible by a small dose of a short acting anticholinesterase such as edrophonium. This drug would combine all the virtues of the 3 drugs suggested as being desirable by Savarese and Kitz (5). I believe that reversibility is a more valuable and realistic virtue than brevity of action. It

could be achieved by a drug whose plasma level fell rapidly following the fixing of the drug at the receptor site. This might be achieved by enzymatic hydrolysis or by renal or hepatic clearance. Such a drug should be readily reversible and would be equally suited for long and short procedures.

SUMMARY

I look forward to improvements in the muscle relaxant drugs resulting from an increase in their safety resulting from avoiding any deleterious cardio-vascular effects and histamine release together with an increase in their convenience in use associated with rapid onset and to a more ready and complete reversibility.

REFERENCES

1. Galindo, A., Discussion on the Ideal Muscle Relaxant. 4th European Congress of Anaesthesiology – Symposium on Muscle Relaxant Drugs, Madrid (1974).
2. Blackburn, J., Personal communication (1974).
3. Hughes, R., Pharmacological concepts. Presented at 4th European Congress of Anaesthesiology – Symposium on Muscle Relaxant Drugs (Madrid (1974).
4. Goat, V. A. and S. A. Feldman, The effect of non-depolarizing muscle relaxants on cholinergic mechanisms in the isolated rabbit heart. *Anaesthesia* 27, 143 (1972).
5. Savarese, J. J., and R. J. Kitz, Does clinical anaesthesia need new neuromuscular blocking agents: *Anesthesiol.* 42, 236 (1975).

PART SIX

PROFESSIONAL HAZARDS TO ANAESTHETISTS OF VOLATILE ANAESTHETIC AGENTS

23. PROFESSIONAL HAZARDS TO ANAESTHETISTS OF VOLATILE ANAESTHETIC AGENTS

JOH. SPIERDIJK

INTRODUCTION

In 1929, Julius Hirsch and Adolf L. Kappers (1) – who were then working under Professor Geheimrat M. Hahn at the Institute for Hygiene in Berlin – published a paper on air pollution in operating rooms. The following quotation is taken from the summary: 'The inhalation anaesthetic agents present in the air of operating rooms has an injurious effect on the health of the surgeons and those who assist them'. Several factors are mentioned, among which two groups can be distinguished:

a. active factors, such as headache and fatigue, and
b. factors whose influence only becomes noticeable in the long term, for instance heart complaints.

In addition other causes of complaints were considered, including prolonged standing, often in awkward positions, a warm and humid atmosphere, and poor illumination.

The authors drew the following conclusions:

1. The question of whether possibly injurious anaesthetic gases have an acute effect cannot be answered.
2. Acute toxicity is unlikely, because:
   a. it has not been reported, and
   b. it is not to be expected in view of the low observed concentrations.
3. Chronic toxicity cannot, however, be excluded. The measured ether concentrations were considered sufficiently strong to have an effect, and must be characterized as toxic in over a prolonged period. The almost daily inhalation of small quantities of toxic substances must, according to the authors, lead to changes, even though evidence had not been obtained in animal experiments.

The industrial hygienist were of the opinion that conclusive evidence did not have to be available before steps were taken to provide for the removal of ether vapours. Since 1918, a number of systems were designed for the removal of anaesthetic gases from the operating room (fig. 1, fig. 2).

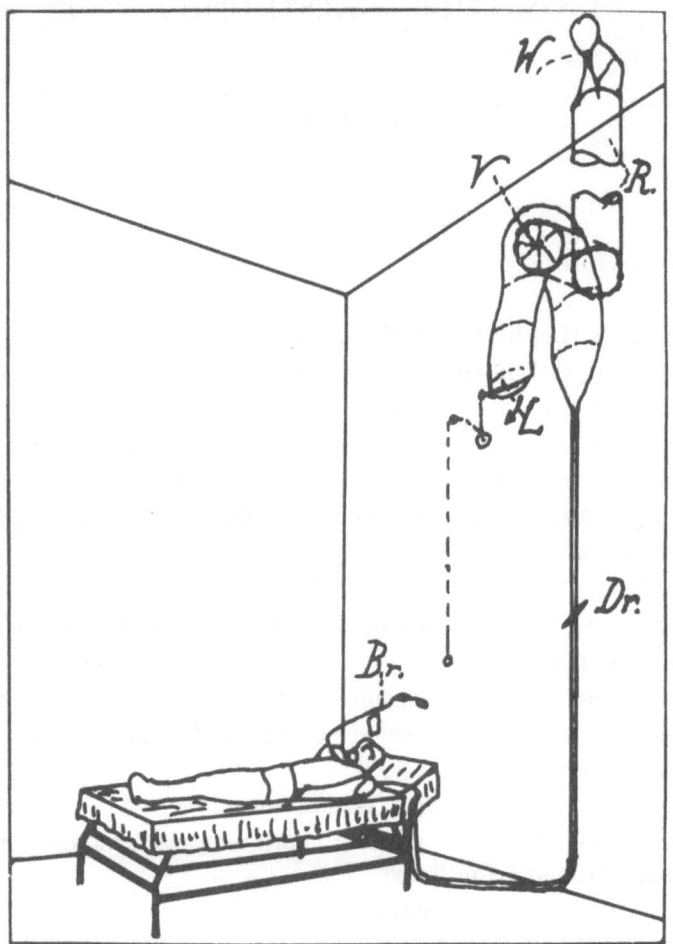

Fig. 1. From: G. Kelling, Uber die Beseitigung der Narkosedämpfe aus dem Operations-saale. *Zbl. Chir.*, p. 602 1918.

Today, almost fifty-sixty years later, the situation is very much the same as it was then. We now have new apparatus for anaesthesia, we have new anaesthetic agents, and in many places we also have air-conditioning. But in spite of all this, the complaints have increased. However, conclusive evidence that there is a relationship between the presence of anaesthetic agents in the air of the operating room and these complaints is still lacking.

Little by little, milieu specialists have begun to take an interest in the problems encountered in operating rooms. Their opinion is unequivocal:

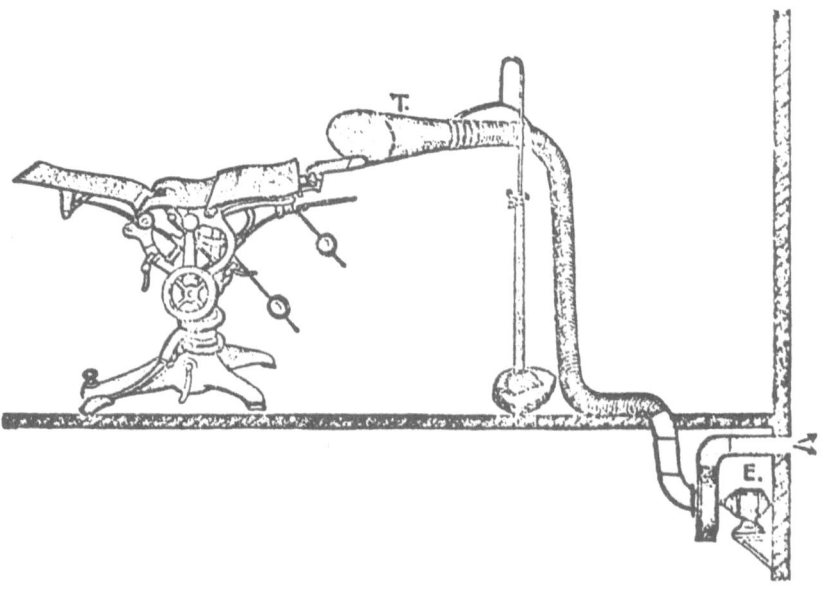

Fig. 2. From: G. Perthes, Schutz der am Operationstisch Beschäftigten vor Schädigung durch die Narkosegase. *Zbl. Chir.*, p. 852, 1925.

'Conclusive evidence can wait; injurious gases should be removed from the operating room'. In this respect, certain criteria are imperative:

1. The removal must be as safe as possible, i.e.:

   a. the exhaust system must not impose an undesirable pressure on the patients ventilation, and
   b. the exhaust system must not distract the anaesthetist's attention from the patient.

2. The presence of an air-conditioning system should be made compulsory by law.

3. The efficiency of the scavenging system should be regularly evaluated by an independent service. Simple methods should be developed for these measurements.

   Nevertheless, a number of questions remain unanswered:

   a. Does the chronic inhalation of anaesthetic gases have a toxic effect on the health of those who work in operating rooms?
   b. If so, does this toxic action extend to the offspring of male or female anaesthetists?

c. Is there an acute effect, that is, is the performance of the anaesthetist directly affected by low concentrations of anaesthetic gases?

d. Are there other factors involved that could influence the health and performance of the anaesthetist and his staff, for instance stress situations, long working hours and a heavy load.

If we are to clarify this situation it will be necessary, in my opinion, to have problems investigated by specialists in other disciplines besides anaesthesiology. The contributions of those who work in the fields of labour hygiene and toxicology, technicians in the field of anaesthetic apparatus, and specialists in the field of air-conditioning are indispensable. As you will hear from Professor Whitcher, a study group has been formed in the U.S.A. In Germany, the *Berufgenossenschaft für Gesundheitsdienst und Wohlfahrspflege* is dealing with the problem. In The Netherlands an advisory committee is being set up to advise the Ministry of Health and Environmental Hygiene on such matters, and a specialized engineering committee will attempt to solve the mainly technical problems. In Sweden legislation has been passed to control air-pollution in operating rooms; some of the provisions went into force on 1 April 1975 and the rest are to do so on 1 January 1976. The stipulations of the law concern twelve points, of which I shall mention only three:

a. Employers are held responsible for informing those in charge and other employees about the dangers involved in working with anaesthetic gases and how the risks can be avoided.

b. Anaesthesia must be performed in a way that protects the personnel from exposure to the gases used for this purpose. This must be taken into account in the choice of the method to be applied.

c. A number of standards are given for the ventilation of operating rooms, recovery rooms, and induction rooms. Stipulations are also made with respect to scavenging systems. Supervision is assigned to the labour inspectorate (an independent body that reports on compliance with industrial safety regulations).

In approaching the problem of pollution it is well to keep in mind that halothane is not the only agent to be considered: other fluorinated hydrocarbons are suspect, and nitrous oxide has not yet been exonerated.

Wood, O'Malley and Stevenson (4) investigated the question of whether there is a change in the 'drug metabolizing ability in operating theatre personnel', and then found indications which led them to conclude that 'it would seem that halothane brings about some induction of liver microsomal metabolizing enzymes in man. However, the extent of induction is much less than that produced by hypnotic doses of an inducer like amylbarbitone or brought by occupational exposure to insecticides'. This drug-metabolizing ability requires further study.

At the end of this session we should have a much clearer idea of the problems involved:

1. Are good scavenging systems available that satisfy the two requirements: a. no danger to the patient, and b. simple to regulate?
2. What steps should personnel be advised to take in the absence of scavenging, particularly women who are or wish to become pregnant?
3. Is it necessary to perform further studies on the chronic toxicity of anaesthetic gases?
4. Is further analysis of the work and performance of the anaesthetist necessary?
5. Should there be international approved standards? Is it therefore necessary to issue recommandations for:
   a. health authorities
   b. hospital designers.

It is my hope that the combined contribution of the speakers and their audience will make it possible to reach a common standpoint.

REFERENCES

1. Hirsch, J. G., A. L. Kappers, Uber die Mengen des Narkoseäthers in der Luft van Operationssälen. *Hyg. Infekt.* 110, 391 (1929).
2. Kelling, G., Uber die Beseitigung der Narkosedämpfe aus dem Operationssaale. *Zbl. Chir.* pg. 602 (1918).
3. Perthes, G., Schutz der am Operationstisch Beschäftigten vor Schädigung durch die Narkosegase. *Zbl. Chir.* p. 852 (1925).
4. Wood, M., K. G. O'Malley, I. H. Stevenson, Drug metabolizing ability in operating theatre personnel. *Br. J. Anaesth.* 46, 726 (1974).

24. INHALATION ANAESTHETICS AS CAUSE FOR OCCUPATIONAL DISEASE IN ANAESTHESIOLOGISTS

R. FREY, E. HERRMANN, E. G. STAR

Toxicity of anaesthetic agents has been known for a long time. But until recently very little attention was paid to it. Already in 1883 Hewitt (1) noted that decomposition products of chloroform inhaled by anaesthesiologists could lead to cough, throat irritation and headache. Reports about possible toxic effects of minute concentrations of halothane, methoxyflurane, trichlorethylene in the operating room and enflurane followed more than half a century later (5, 8, 9, 22, 34, 42).

But not only halogenated agents were incriminated of causing toxic symptoms on chronic exposure to small quantities. Diethyl ether was also found to have adverse effects. Typical are the symptoms of an operating team in which surgeon, nurse and anaesthesiologist experienced symptoms of depression, fatigue, headache, anorexia and loss of memory. All these symptoms disappeared during vacation and did not recur after ventilation equipment had been installed into the operating room (Werthmann, 1949) (43). Even nitrous oxide, generally claimed as being 'inert', was found to cause bone marrow depression and aplastic anemia in man after long term inhalation of subanaesthetic concentrations (24, 30). To the rat it is embryotoxic and teratogenic (21).

Impurities of halothane, once believed to be hepatotoxic, have now been removed (14, 15). Commercially available nitrous oxide is about 99% pure. The remainder contains potentially toxic substances as nitric oxide, nitrogen dioxide, carbonmonoxide and others (1). According to the manufacturer our nitrous oxide presently contains less than 5 ppm nitric oxide, less than 5 ppm nitrogen oxide and less than 10 ppm of carbonmonoxide. Because of their low concentration these substances have probably no effect on operating room personnel.

Radiation probably is no hazard to operating room personnel either. It was found that the doses received are usually well below acceptable limits (32). The incidence of leukemia is not higher in anaesthesiologists than in the rest of the population (6). However, an additive effect to potentially toxic anaesthesia gases is a possibility.

In 1967 Vaisman (40) reported about subjective complaints of Russian anaesthesiologists and a significantly higher rate of spontaneous abortions in 18 out of 31 pregnancies. Furthermore he observed an increased frequency of toxicosis among those pregnancies which were carried to term. It is interesting to note that in this report ether as well as halothane and nitrous oxide were listed and that the operating rooms were poorly ventilated.

This publication initiated a number of epidemiological studies in the USA and Europe. These studies showed that a number of diseases are particularly frequent among operating room personnel:
1. Malignancies
2. Spontaneous abortions
3. Malformation of offspring
4. Damage to parenchymal organs, particularly liver and kidneys
5. Central nervous system disturbances
Bruce et al. (6) found a significantly higher rate of malignancies of the lymphatic and reticuloendothelial system among the members of the American Society of Anaesthesiologists in comparison with statistics of the general population furnished by the Metropolitan Life Insurance Company.

Corbett et al. (20) evaluated in 1973 the data of 621 nurse anaesthetists. The incidence of neoplastic disease was three times as high as expected. A study of the American Society of Anaesthesiologists in 1974 (2) demonstrated a statistically higher rate of malignancies of anesthesiologists in comparison to pediatricians.

It is of interest that chemists chronically exposed to low concentrations of volatile liquids and gases were also found to have a significantly higher proportion of deaths from malignant lymphomas and cancer of the pancreas than professional men in general (31).

Askog 1970 in Denmark (3), Cohen in California (16) and Knill-Jones in England (29) reported an increased number of spontaneous abortions in female anaesthesiologists and nurse anaesthetists.

Concentrations of halothane in the operating room were measured as about 10 ppm in the vicinity of the anaesthesiologist (32, 44). It was found that the concentration of halothane in the operating room was practically zero in the morning and increased steadily during the day (44). High concentrations were measured in the vicinity of the anaesthesiologist, especially when drapes partially covered the anaesthesia machine as it is customary during certain operations.

Determinations of halothane levels in the blood demonstrated that anaesthesiologists within a relatively short time of 3-4 hours incorporate quantities of halothane which cannot be completely eliminated until the next morning. Anaesthesiologists and the remaining operating room personnel are under a constant halothane level during the whole week (25). The reason is a slow elimination of the lipoid soluble vapor from the fatty tissues.

Similar observations were made when methoxyflurane was used as anesthetic. Methoxyflurane is detectable in the end-expired air of patients for 10 to 18 days after anaesthesia and in anaesthesiologists for as long as 30 hours (18). Samples of air collected in the area of the operating room from which the anaesthesiologist inspired air contained 1,3 to 9,9 ppm methoxyflurane (18).

Nitrous oxide was present in concentrations ranging from 350 to 9700 ppm (21) in the inhalational zone of the anaesthesiologist during routine conditions (21). Concentrations ranged from 310 to 550 ppm in the inhalational zone of the surgeons (21). Nitrous oxide was demonstrated in the exhaled air of anaesthesiologists for 6-7 hours, and in patients for 56 hours (19).

In animal experiments it was found that a chronic exposure to 10 ppm halothane causes a decrease of cerebral functions (35). Bruce et al. (7, 8) demonstrated that already minimal concentrations of nitrous oxide, methoxyflurane and enflurane effect perceptual, cognitive and motor skills in volunteers.

All these data do not only have toxicological implications but raise a lot of other questions too. Is an anaesthesiologist still fully capable of performing his work after the exposure to small concentrations of anaesthetics for more than 24 hours (for instance when taking night calls)? Secondly, when is a patient again in the possession of his full will power after an anaesthetic? When and after what time would he be able to give legal consent to a second operation, if necessary? As data show these intervals certainly would vary from case to case and depend upon the type of anaesthetic agent used.

In the United States Study of 1974 Cascorbi (2) reported a significant increase of malformations in children of female anaesthesiologists and nurse anaesthetists in comparison to female pediatricians. There was also an increase of 25% in the incidence of congenital abnormalities for the babies of wives of exposed male anaesthesiologists. Knill-Jones et al. (29) found that the babies of female anaesthesiologists working during pregnancy had a significantly higher frequency of congenital abnormalities (6,5%) than those not at work (2,5%).

The rate of hepatitis is significantly higher in anaesthesiologists than in pediatricians. The chronic inhalation of anaesthetic agents might be one cause. Undoubtedly the daily exposure to blood carries a risk also (2). Already minute amounts of blood as 0,00004 ml are sufficient for the transmission of the hepatitis virus. The incidence of posttransfusion hepatitis in the United States is listed as about 0,5%, with the number of anicteric and subclinical cases more than ten times greater (38). Kidney diseases in the United States Study, excluding pyelonephritis and cystitis, showed a slightly higher frequency in female anaesthesiologists. No increase was noted among male anaesthesiologists (2).

Bruce et al. (6) reported a two fold increase in chronic renal disease as a cause of death among anaesthesiologists in the period from 1957-1966.

Several possibilities are available in order to improve the working conditions for anaesthesiologists:

1. Technical facilities to decrease pollution with anaesthetic agents
   a. Air conditioning of operating rooms with circulation of fresh air
   b. Scavenging of excess anaesthetic gases and vapors
   c. Filters with activated charcoal
   d. Use of closed circuits, resp. minimal gas flows
   e. Preference for regional anaesthesia if no venting of the operating room is available
2. Adequate Staffing of Anaesthesia Personnel
   a. To eliminate excess working hours
   b. Relief of anaesthesiologists during long lasting cases
   c. Minimizing the working hours in the operating room and by this exposure to anaesthetic gases
   d. Restrictions for pregnant anaesthesiologists and nurses in operating rooms where no scavenging system for anaesthetic gases is present.

The venting of anaesthetic gases and vapors to the operating room floor is ineffective. Although anaesthetics generally are heavier than air, turbulence created by air conditioning systems, the opening of doors and the like will stir up these agents with the result of an almost equal distribution throughout the operating room (2).

A simple and effective method of decreasing the concentration of anaesthetic agents in the operating room is the attachment of a scavenging system to the pop-off valve of the gas machine and to conduct the excess gases and vapors through a hose and a hole in the wall to the outside. A more efficient way is to connect the scavenging system to the wall suction, provided no flammable anaesthetic agents are being used and a pressure-balancing system is integrated. Non-rebreathing systems for pediatric anaesthesia and ventilators create some problems. Ventilators discharge at least 1-2 liters of anaesthetic gas flow plus about 10 liters of driving gas per minute which all have to be scavenged away.

The use of charcoal filters is insufficient. They are capable of absorbing halothane quite effectively. But after about 3 hours they become exhausted. Nitrous oxide passes through these filters unchanged (37).

The use of regional anaesthesia does not eliminate the necessity for scavenging. In long cases or if the block does not provide satisfactory pain relief, general anesthesia might become a necessity.

Non-recirculating air conditioning systems with a disposal of waste anaesthetic agents into the exhaust duct are an effective method. Many air conditioning systems use partial recirculation of air. Recirculating air-conditioning systems may be used, provided that the waste gases are introduced into the exhaust duct downstream from the point of recirculation (2).

The Department of Safety of the State of Rhineland-Pfalz has recently ordered that every newly built operating room within the state must have a scavenging system directly from the pop-off valve of the anaesthesia machine and to the outside. In the older hospitals similar systems will be added (26).

Scavenging systems are about 85 to 90% successful in removing waste anaesthetic gases (44). Approximately half of the remaining anaesthetics can be removed by an effective air conditioning system. The rate of removal depends upon the rate at which fresh air enters and the air turbulence inside the operating room. The combined effect of scavenging, air-conditioning and low-flow anaesthetic techniques can reduce halothane concentrations to less than 0,05 ppm and nitrous oxide concentrations to less than 1 ppm (2). It is fortunate that safety departments begin to realize the importance of these facts. The establishment of threshhold limit values (TLV's) for all anaesthetic agents is needed. At the moment in most countries only TLV's for chloroform and diethyl ether are available (17). However, efforts are being made to define TLV's for other anaesthetics as well.

New threshhold limit values will eventually have to take into account recent information about possible teratogenicity, anaesthetic metabolism and enzyme induction.

It has been suggested that it might not necessarily be the anaesthetic agents which cause organ toxicity. Breakdown products of the biotransformation of volatile anaesthetic agents have been incriminated as well (13). The metabolism of these substances continues for days and weeks or even longer, as long as they remain in the body. The rate of metabolic breakdown is steered by enzymes. These are influenced by many substances again, some of them being anesthetic agents themselves (4). How much these enzyme inducers can influence the breakdown of anaesthetics was demonstrated by the fact that anaesthesiologists have a considerable higher rate of halothane metabolism than pharmacists who are not exposed to anaesthetic drugs (11). The amount of each enzyme in an individual is controlled genetically, but the synthesis of certain enzymes can be altered by long term administration of a variety of chemicals. An increase in metabolites or their intermediates may then produce toxic effects (4, 10, 12, 13, 33, 41).

Elimination of anaesthetic gases and vapors from the operating room solves only part of the problem. An optimal number of anaesthesiologists has to be recruited also. Otherwise the result is chronic overwork, excessive working hours, undue stress and strain among anaesthesiologists and nurse anaesthetists.

Rosenberg (36) in his report about the high incidence of spontaneous abortions of Finnish anaesthesia nurses mentioned besides anaesthetic agents the long working hours, shift work, night calls and chronic stress as causes. Knill-Jones (29) in England came to similar conclusions in his evaluation of the high abortion rate in female anaesthesiologists. The higher rate of irregular menstrual cycles in anaesthesia- and intensive care nurses is probably an indicator for the exposure to stress also. Premature uterine contractions and increased edema during pregnancies in anaesthesia nurses may likewise be a reflection of excessive work load.

Besides the toxicological hazard there is also a gap between demand and supply of physician and nurse anaesthetists. We share our concern for optimal working conditions in the operating room with our colleagues throughout the world. However, among all our emotions, don't let us forget the patient.

After all what has been said before, we must also question the safety of administering anaesthesia to the pregnant patient who might need surgery during the first trimester. Will our anesthetics induce abortion or cause deformity of the fetus? There are no conclusive surveys to date which have explored this possibility. Noticable concentrations of halothane, methoxyflurane, ether and nitrous oxide have been found in the expired air of patients for days after surgery (18). Embryotoxicity has been demonstrated in animals at concentrations of 1000 ppm nitrous oxide (21). To investigate these possibilities and to establish firm guidelines seems to be a great challenge.

Especially in this field we should do more than ever in order to finally end the 'immense uncontrolled human experiment' as it was demanded by Settergren (39) already several years ago.

CONCLUSION

In conclusion we can say that anaesthesiologists and operating room personnel have a higher incidence of occupational disease and shorter life expectancy than the average population. We should strive for complete elimination of anesthetic pollution in our operating rooms. This is technically easy to accomplish. We should, however, also try to end chronic overwork due to a shortage of manpower. Breaking this vicious circle would help to make the field of anesthesia more attractive to younger physicians again. Only combined efforts will be successful and eventually accomplish optimal working conditions for all of us.

REFERENCES

1. Adriani, J., *The Chemistry and Physics of Anesthesia*, p. 197-198 Charles C. Thomas, Springfield, Illinois, U.S.A. (1962).
2. American Society of Anesthesiologists, A National Study Occupational Disease among Operating Room Personnel: Report of an Ad Hoc Committee on the Effect of Trace Anesthetics on the Health of Operating Room Personnel. *Anesthesiology* 41, 321-340 (1974).
3. Askog, V., B. Harvald, Teratogen effect of inhalations-anesthetika. Saertyk Fra. *Nordisk. Medicin.* 3, 490 (1970).
4. Berman, M. L., J. F. Bochantin, Nonspecific stimulation of drug metabolism in rats by methoxyflurane. *Anesthesiology* 32, 500-506 (1970).
5. Brody, G. L., R. B. Sweet, Halothane anesthesia as a possible cause of massive hepatic necrosis. *Anesthesiology* 24, 29-37 (1963).
6. Bruce, D. L., K. A. Eide, H. W. Linde, J. E. Eckenhoff, Causes of Death among Anesthesiologists: A 20 Year Study. *Anesthesiology* 29, 565-569 (1968).
7. Bruce, D. L., M. J. Bach, J. Arbit, Trace Anesthetic Effects on Perceptual, Cognitive and Motor Skills. *Anesthesiology* 40, 453-458 (1974).
8. Bruce, D. L., M. J. Bach, Psychological Studies of Human Performances as Affected by Traces of Enflurane and Nitrous Oxide. *Anesthesiology* 42, 194-196 (1975).
9. Bunker, J. P., C. M. Blumenfeld, Liver necrosis after halothane anesthesia: Cause or coincidence? *N. Engl. J. Med.* 268, 531-534 (1963).
10. Carney, F. M., R. A. Van Dyke, Halothane Hepatitis: A Critical Review. *Anesth. and Analg., Curr. Res.* 51, 135-160 (1972).
11. Cascorbi, H. F., D. A. Blake, M. Helrich, Difference in the biotransformation of halothane in man. *Anesthesiology* 32, 923-926 (1968).
12. Cascorbi, H. F., E. S. Vesell, D. A. Blake, Genetic and environmental influence on halothane metabolism in twins. *Clin. Pharmacol. Ther.* 12, 50-55 (1971).
13. Cascorbi, H. F., Biotransformation of drugs used in anesthesia. *Anesthesiology* 39, 115 (1973).
14. Cohen, E. N., J. W. Bellville, H. Budzikiwicz, D. H. Williams, Impurity in halothane anaesthetic. *Science* 141, 899 (1963).
15. Cohen, E. N., H. W. Brewer, J. W. Bellville, R. Sher, The chemistry and toxicology of dichlorohexa-fluorobutene. *Anesthesiology* 26, 140-153 (1965).

16. Cohen, E. N., J. W. Belville, R. W. Brown, Anesthesia, pregnancy and misearriage: A study of operating room nurses and anesthetists. *Anesthesiology* 35, 345 (1971).
17. Conney, A. H., Pharmacological implications of microsomal enzyme induction. *Pharmacol. Rev.* 19, 317-366 (1967).
18. Corbett, T. H., G. L. Ball, A Possible Occupational Hazard to Anesthesiologists. *Anesthesiology* 34, 532-537 (1971).
19. Corbett, T. H., Anesthetics as a Cause of Abortion. *Fertility and Sterility* 23, 866-869 (1972).
20. Corbett, T. H., R. G. Cornell, K. Lieding, J. L. Endres, Incidence of Cancer among Michigan Nurse-Anesthetists. *Anesthesiology* 38, 260-263 (1973).
21. Corbett, T. H., R. G. Cornell, J. L. Endres, R. I. Millard, Effects of Low Concentrations of Nitrous Oxide on Rat Pregnancy *Anesthesiology* 39, 299-301 (1973).
22. Corbett, R. H., G. C. Hamilton, M. K. Yoon, Occupational exposure of operating room personnel to trichlorethylene. *Canad. Anaesth. Soc. J.* 29, 675-678 (1973).
23. Corbett, T. H., R. G. Cornell, K. Lieding, J. L. Endres, Birth defects of children among Michigan nurse anesthetists. *Anesthesiology* 41, 341 (1974).
24. Eastwood, D. W., C. D. Green, M. A. Lambdin, R. Gadner, Effect of Nitrous Oxide on the White-Cell Count in Leukemia. *N. Engl. J. Med.* 268, 297-299 (1963).
25. Gostomzyk, J. G., G. Eisele, F. W. Ahnefeld, Chronische Narkosegasbelastung des Anaesthesiepersonals im Operationssaal. *Anaesthesist* 22, 469-474 (1973).
26. Hagedorn, F., Personal communication.
27. Hallén, B., H. Ehrner-Samual, M. Thomason, Measurements of Halothane in the atmosphere of an Operating Theatre and in Expired Air and Blood of the Personnel During Routine Anaesthetic Work. *Acta anaesth. scand.* 14, 17-27 (1970).
28. Hewitt, F. W., *Anaesthetics and Their Administration*. Charles Griffin and Co., London (1883).
29. Knill-Jones, R. P., D. D. Moir, L. V. Rodrigues, A. A. Spence, Anaesthetic Practice and Pregnancy: Controlled Survey of Women Anaesthetists in the United Kingdom. *The Lancet* 1326-1328 (1972).
30. Lassen, H. C. A., Treatment of Tetanus Severe Bone-Marrow Depression after Prolonged Nitrous-Oxide Anaesthesia. *The Lancet* 270, 1, 527-530 (1956).
31. Li, F. P., J. F. Fraumeni, M. A. Mantel, R. W. Miller, Cancer mortality among chemists. *US Nat. Cancer Inst. J.* 43, 1159 (1969).
32. Linde, H. W., D. L. Bruce, Occupational Exposure of Anesthetists to Halothane, Nitrous Oxide and Radiation. *Anesthesiology* 30, 363-368 (1969).
33. Linde. H. W., M. L. Berman, Nonspecific Stimulation of Drug Metabolizing Enzymes by Inhalation Anesthetic Agents. *Anesth. and Analg., Curr. Res.* 50, 656-667 (1971).
34. Lindenbaum, J., E. Leifer, Hepatic necrosis associated with halothane anesthesia. *N. Engl. J. Med.* 268, 525-530 (1963).
35. Quimby, K. L. et al., Enduring learning deficits and cerebral synaptic malformation from exposure to 10 parts of halothane per million. *Science* 185, 625 (1974).
36. Rosenberg, P., A. Kirves, Miscarriages Among Operating Room Theatre Staff. *Acta anaesth. scand. Suppl.* 53, 37-42 (1973).
37. Schulze, H. H., D. Kästner, P. Lange, Zur Frage der chronischen Toxicität von Halothankonzentrationen in der Operationsluft. *Anaesthesist* 18, 378-381 (1969).
38. Senior, J. R., Post-transfusion hepatitis. *Gastroenterology* 49, 315-320 (1965).
39. Settergren, G., Long-term toxicity of volatile anaesthetic agents. Swed. Soc. Anaesth. Ann. Meet. Stockholm, Nov. 1967, *Opusc. Med.* 13, 251 (1968).
40. Vaisman, A. I., Working conditions in surgery and their effect on health of anesthesiologists. *Eksp. Khir. Anes.* 3, 44 (1967).
41. Van Dyke, R. A., M. B. Chenoweth, A. Van Poznak, Metabolism of Volatile Anesthetics. *Biochem. Pharmacol.* 13, 1239-1247 (1964).

42. Virtue, R. W., K. W. Payne, Postoperative death after Fluothane. *Anesthesiology* 19, 562-563 (1958).
43. Werthmann, H., Beitrag zur chronischen Ätherintoxikation der Chirurgen. *Beitr. klin. Chir.* 178, 149-156 (1949).
44. Whitcher, C. E., E. N. Cohen, J. R. Trudell, Chronic Exposure to Anesthetic Cases in the Operating Room. *Anesthesiology* 35, 348-353 (1971).

25. THE WORK AND WORKING CONDITIONS OF THE ANAESTHETIST IN DUTCH HOSPITALS

J. J. SCHWARZ AND V. REJGER

PREFACE

In this study the work and working conditions of the anaesthetist is equated to that of a control and regulating system.

This task is not analysed from a medical point of view, but the anaesthetist is seen as a worker who controls and regulates a biological system until that system can again resume independent performance of its own functions.

INTRODUCTION

Interest in the work of the anaesthetist has been increasing rapidly due to recurring reports in the news media of mistakes in anaesthesia leading to patient injury and death. The most recent publications in the Netherlands on this subject put the main emphasis on the problems connected with the supervision of the patient during the operation (1) and the prolonged exposure of the anaesthetist to low concentrations of volatile anaesthetics (2). The view that the work and working conditions of the anaesthetist can cause problems that can result in sub-optimal anaesthesia during operations and in the long run adversely affect the anaesthetist's health, has led to investigations in which an attempt is made to analyse the influence of the various factors involved. Ultimately, the interrelationship between the work and the working conditions will have to be investigated as well, in order to arrive at conclusions concerning the consequences of these factors.

The two most important factors recognized by the analysis of the work and working conditions of the anaesthetist are, respectively: the work load and the stress, here defined as the effect of all the surrounding influences which can lead to physiological changes. Both of these factors can be further subdivided into a mental and physical component:

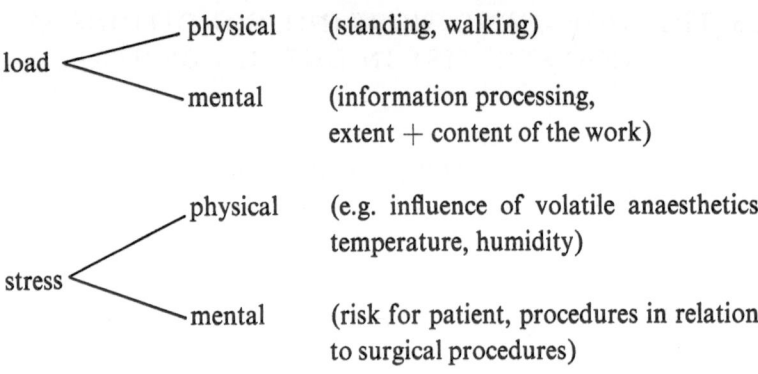

THE ANAESTHETISTS'S WORK

The work performed by the anaesthetist can be divided into two parts, one of them surgical and the other non-surgical. The surgical part consists of the preparations for and administration of anaesthetics to patients undergoing operation. The non-surgical part consists of the care of the patient before and after surgical treatment and a number of associated activities such as the administration of blood transfusions, ventilation, relief of pain, and intensive care. Because the operations are usually done in rapid succession during an average "operating day" and advances in the field of anaesthesia and surgery have led to an increase in the complexity of surgical treatment, there is usually relatively little time left for the non-surgical part of the anaesthetist's work. The estimates of anaesthetists in three provincial hospitals indicate that on the average operating day (excluding weekends), 8 to 10 anaesthesias* are administered by one anaesthetist. In addition, depending on the number of anaesthetists on the staff of a given hospital and upon other factors, regular weekend duties must be performed.

As a result of all this, it is often difficult to properly organize the anaesthetist's work so that optimal division of his tasks can be achieved. Furthermore, both the schedules and the duration of the operation are usually determined by the surgeon. In interviews with anaesthetists attached to three hospitals, the following problems were mentioned:

– Varying work tempo, which complicates division of the work.
– The need to give attention to several cases simultaneously (working in

---

* This estimate agrees reasonably well with the results of a questionnaire applied in hospitals (see reports of the *Commissie voor Anesthesiologie van de Gezondheidsraad*) (3), i.e., about 2,000 per anaesthetist per year.

more than one operating theatre and with different types of operations at the same time).
- Irregular working hours (weekend and night duty, substituting for a colleague).
- Long working hours.
- Tension (emergency cases, poor risk patients, complicated and long operations).
- Relationship with surgeon.
- Relationship with assistents (supervision of monitoring, correction).
- Inhalation of volatile anaesthetics.
- Much standing and walking.

Thus, as seen by the just mentioned interviews, the surgical part of the work gave the most problems. Consequently the rest of this paper will be devoted to this task.

THE SURGICAL TASK OF THE ANAESTHETIST

This part of the work can be seen as a control and regulation task. On the basis of available information and with the use of technical facilities and pharmacological substances, a biological system (the patient) is brought into and kept in a state that is desirable for surgical treatment. In this process of control and regulation, the following phases can be distinguished: induction, maintenance, and termination of anaesthesia plus transfer to the recovery room.

In the first of these phases the patient (regarded here as a biological system) is brought into a state such that an operation can be performed with the least possible difficulty for the patient and the surgeon. Here, the anaesthetist's work is mainly concerned with a form of interference in an existing state, i.e., *"controlling and regulating" a biological system until the desired "stable"* state is reached.* During the period of "stabilization" an attempt is made to maintain the biological system (the patient) in the desired state. The control and regulation are now performed by the anaesthetist, monitoring and supervision being left to auxiliary personnel, in this case specially trained assistants.

The termination period consists of the restoration of the "original" state of the biological system as rapidly as possible so that it can perform its own

---

* This phase concerns stabilization of the system's state. The operation itself will of course make a truly stable state impossible.

functions again independently (i.e., control and regulate itself). The final phase starts when the anaesthetist is satisfied that the biological system is able to perform its own functions adequately. To this end the patient is kept for a while under supervision in a recovery room or, if necessary, in the intensive care department.

In this four-phase process the anaesthesiological work is seen, as already mentioned, as controlling and regulatory, in other words as work by which a biological system is brought into a state making it possible to perform surgical treatment without causing the system to stop functioning, i.e., the patient to die.

For the sake of clarity it should be mentioned that the concept of the patient as a biological system is only applied to obtain a better understanding of the anaesthetist's work. This does not mean that we are not concerned with a person with whose condition and progress both the surgeon and the anaesthetist are emotionally involved. It may also be noted that the concept that the anaesthetist's work consists of control and regulation is also adopted in an informative brochure given in some Dutch hospitals to patients admitted for surgical treatment (4).

THE OBJECTIVES OF THE SURGICAL PART OF THE ANAESTHETIST'S WORK

The objectives of the surgical part of the anaesthetist's work is in fact determined by the overall objective of the surgical treatment. The latter objective is to attain the best possible surgical results without undermining the condition of the patient. The degree to which this objective can be achieved depends primarily on the degree to which the operation is successful and upon the patient's condition during the period of admission for surgery. In the long run, therefore, the surgical and anaesthesiological objectives more or less coincide. However, shortly before, during, and just after the operation, this agreement between objectives is less distinct. Especially in those cases where the patient's physical condition is not very satisfactory, problems can be encountered in attempting to achieve both objectives. Strong concern for the condition of the patient often complicates the surgeon's work. On the other hand giving more emphasis to the surgical procedure can complicate the anaesthetist's task. This conflict of interests arises from the fact that both the surgical and the anaesthesiological procedures carry short-term risks for the adequate functioning of the biological system. The surgical risks are associated with the traumatic effect of the operation. The anaesthesia entails risks because pharmacologically active substances are introduced into the biological system whereby, among other actions, one of their effects is to reduce the patient's resistance. Consequently, this means that during the operation the patient's condition can only be maintained at sub-optimal levels. This may in turn affect the long-term objectives of both the surgical and the anaesthesiological procedures. During the short-term period, however, maintenance of the patient's condition is the responsibility of the anaesthetist.

Although the anaesthetist cannot be held responsible for surgical errors (5), he is primarily responsible for the health and well-being of the patient. As a result, a conflict can easily arise between the surgeon and the anaesthetist with respect to the borderline between the responsibility borne by the two disciplines. When such conflicts arise during an operation, they are virtually insoluble. If the anaesthetist gives way he in fact can no longer bear the responsibility for the patient's condition, and if the surgeon gives way the results of this operation will be less satisfactory.

CONTROL AND REGULATION ASPECTS OF THE SURGICAL TASK

If it is accepted that the immediate responsibility for the anaesthetized patient is to be borne by the anaesthetist, it is then imperative to determine what means he has at his disposal to discharge this responsibility. Here again we shall interpret the anaesthetist's work along control and regulation lines whereby the system is controlled and regulated on the basis of certain available information. This control is mainly done by means of pharmacological agents. To do so it is necessary to estimate beforehand what dosage will be required in order to obtain a given state.

Furthermore, a large part of the control and regulation must be performed during a period of more or less severe disturbance, i.e. during an operation. As already mentioned, the anaesthetist's work consists of short-term and long-term objectives. The short-term objective for control and regulation can be defined as the direct goal achievement of the system in question, which is here the patient's condition during and immediately after the operation. The long-term objective can be seen as the preservation of the system, in other words the maintenance of its future effectiveness (6). This can be shown in the next figure.

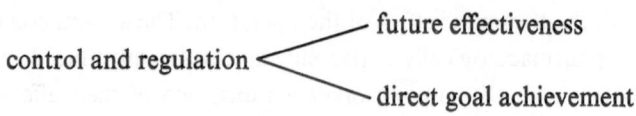

In general, it may be said that if the system develops a disturbance, the control and regulation will be directed mainly towards the future effectiveness of the system. This requires making a compromize between direct goal achievement and future effectiveness. This can be clearly observed by control and regulation of a biological system during an operation. The output, i.e. the direct goal achievement or more simply put, the patient's activity is mainly limited by means of the anaesthetic given in order to make the surgical procedure possible. The abnormal element in this is that it is done with agents which themselves endanger the future effectiveness of the system. The crux of the problem here is that when dealing with a biological system its functions cannot be suspended without making its future effectiveness impossible (death). Whereas a technical system can be completely stopped when it develops a severe defect, the activity of a biological system can only be reduced to a given degree and for a given amount of time. And even then the biological system must be controlled under conditions which may endanger its future effectiveness. This means that the available information about the system and its functioning must permit clear-cut decisions with respect to the control and regulation of that system. The necessary information concerning the patient's condition before, during, and after the operation can be classified as follows:

a. Pre-operative investigation respecting the patient's condition and any relevant anomalies.
b. Control of the vital functions during the first three phases of the anaesthesia.
c. Control of the vital functions after the operation (in the recovery room).
d. Post-operative investigation respecting possible detrimental results of the anaesthesia and/or the surgical treatment.

This is the kind of information with which the anaesthetist is usually concerned, although he does not always make the observations himself. This is an important point, because it may be necessary for him to have followed the surgical procedure, in order to better assess and more rapidly correct the failure of one or more of the vital functions.

The information indicated under point a. provides a basis upon which the selection of an anaesthetic is possible so that the surgical requirements are met without endangering the patient's general condition. This information has the disadvantage of only giving a picture which reflects the situation at the time when the data was collected. Changes occurring there-after may well go unobserved, even though they could lead to undesirable situations during the operation.

With respect to point b. the following may be said. The information obtained during the operation, is either collected continuously or at intervals depending upon the parameter. When compared to a technical system the number of parameters utilized here is restricted, making it more difficult to notice small, relatively slow changes arising in the biological system. The parameters monitored during an operation can be summarized as follows:

Patient parameters: A number of these can be called standard parameters, and only some of these are applied in 'special' cases according to the judgement of the anaesthetist. Those applied in the three hospitals investigated are:

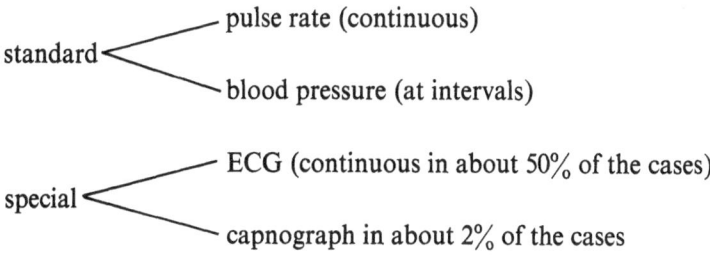

standard — pulse rate (continuous)
          — blood pressure (at intervals)

special — ECG (continuous in about 50% of the cases)
        — capnograph in about 2% of the cases

In addition to the mechanical and electronic collection of information, subjective information is also gathered. This is done directly for example by feeling the patient's face (clamminess) and pulpating the pulse (at intervals), in order to obtain an impression of its strength rather than its frequency. Attention is also given to facial colour and so on.

Other circumjacent parameters: These include factors outside the patient himself:
the operation (progress, complications, etc.)
the infusion or possibly blood transfusion
the loss of blood
the functioning of the apparatus (checking of exhaled carbon dioxide, respiratory volume, ventilation pressure and leakage, disconnection, level in gas cylinders).

This latter group of parameters also plays an important role in the evaluation of the condition of the biological system. The character of the parameters providing information about the state of the biological system often makes it difficult to rapidly determine the cause of a serious disturbance. In situations of this kind the anaesthetist's work will in the first instance be directed towards the treatment of symptoms mainly because the time in which potentially fatal processes can be reversed is very short. Consequently, it is imperative that constant and strict supervision of the biological system be provided for not only during the operation, but also going into and during the post-operative period.

In provincial hospitals this supervision is often transferred into the hands of auxiliary personnel, because the anaesthetist must attend to several operations simultaneously. Under these conditions it is relatively difficult to obtain sufficient information to find the cause of complications very quickly, especially when the problem is acute. An additional problem is created here by the fact that the anaesthetist cannot follow the process continuously and is therefore not in a position to observe slow changes in the parameters as they occur.

It is even considered imperative to keep the patient under supervision in the recovery room for some time after the operation. This period is characterized by the more or less continuous monitoring of a number of vital functions. This too is performed by specially trained personnel. Nevertheless, the responsibility for the patient is still borne by the anaesthetist, which means that the same objection as during surgery applies here: namely that the anaesthetist does not continuously follow the process and is therefore not always in a position to identify the cause of problems rapidly.

After the operation it may sometimes be necessary to examine the patient for possible harmful effects of the anaesthesia and/or the operation. This constitutes the final phase of the period of hospitalization, and is not expected to require any additional effort on the part of the anaesthetist. It follows from all this that the surgical part of the anaesthetist's work is characterized by an intermittent supply and processing of information. The content of this (control) task may change relatively fast because operations are performed in rapid succession. The controlling and regulatory work is also typified by the expenditure of a relatively large amount of time on procedures related to the future effectiveness of the system, i.e. in dealing with parameters which provide information concerning the state of the biological system.

The necessity to attend more than one operation at a time as well as maintaining supervision of the recovery room can result in a tendency to transfer a great deal of the responsibility to the auxiliary personnel.

The anaesthetists questioned in the present study were all in agreement that there are actually no routine situations during the administration of anaesthetics. Consequently, the anaesthetist must be unceasingly prepared to cope with (difficult) problems and to make rapid decisions about how to deal with them.

STRESS

Two forms of stress should be considered when dealing with an anaesthetist's work. The first is that due to physical influences and the other that due to psychosocial influences. With respect to the physical influences, it is generally accepted that those who work in operating theatres are exposed to stress resulting from the inhalation of low concentrations of volatile anaesthetics over appreciable periods of time. Experiments done by Bruce, Bach and Arbit (7) on the performance of audiovisual work, reaction time, and the like, have shown that traces of volatile anaesthetics have an effect on a subject's performance. In most of the cases the subject's achievement was significantly reduced under conditions in which small amounts of anaesthetics were inhaled. It has yet to be determined as to whether this holds as well for those procedures usually performed as part of the anaesthetist's work.

With respect to the psychological influences it is more difficult to determine whether there are elements in the work and work conditions of the anaesthetist which in themselves indicate the presence of this form of stress. In terms of the concept of psycho-social stress as applied by such authors as Dirken (8), stress can occur when an individual is in a situation in which his attention is shifted from the work to the Ego. This can take place both consciously and unconsciously. The warning sometimes heard by anaesthetists: 'Take care if you don't want to be on the front page tomorrow', could be interpreted as an expression of psychological stress.

The following aspects of the work can give rise to stress reactions in anaesthetists (or their assistants):

a. the operating room atmosphere (leakage of volatile anaesthetics, temperature, ventilation);
b. the relationship with the patient and the condition of the patient (reference is not made here to the biological system, because what is involved here is the realization that a human being is concerned);
c. the relationship with the surgeon and the surgical team (which also includes the degree of difficulty of the operation concerned); and

d. delegation of authority to auxiliary personnel (with respect to supervision of the patient).

The stress undergone by the anaesthetist as the result of inhalation of anaesthetics must be evaluated by further research. Since this also applies to the supervision of the patient by auxiliary personnel, the anaesthetist must pay extra attention to the supervision of these auxiliaries.

In addition to the reduction of vigilance due to the influence of volatile anaesthetics in the air of the operating theatre, the reduction of attention related to the patient and the patient's condition is of importance. All of the interviewed anaesthetists agreed that a patient in a weak condition requires extra attention during the anaesthesia, but they were also of the opinion that good supervision is equally necessary for young patients in good condition undergoing less serious operations. Playing a role in this last formulation was the fact that the death of the low-risk patient during or shortly after the operation would make the question of blame loom larger (psychosocial stress). In the discussion on the controlling and regulating work of the anaesthetist reference has already been made to the relatively small amount of information available concerning the state of the biological system, during the operation. This factor undoubtedly plays a role in the occurrence of stress with respect to the evaluation of the patient as a human being.

The potential stress which can result from a less than optimal relationship between the anaesthetist and the surgeon can find its origin in the problem of the divergence in their objectives over the short term. This has already been discussed with respect to the objectives of the surgical part of the anaesthetist's work, and it will suffice here to mention that the risk factor in both the anaesthesiological and surgical procedures can give rise to conflicts between the anaesthetist and the surgeon. These conflicts can be both latent and manifest.

Finally, the delegation of the supervision of the patient to auxiliary personnel during the operation can also involve stress for both the auxiliaries and the anaesthetist. The heart rate of auxiliary personnel measured during research in the mentioned hospitals sometimes gave high mean values* during surgery.

The supervision of a patient during an operation has a strong resemblance to the work performed by the operator of a highly automated technical system (e.g. an electrical power plant). Sudden disturbances can change the nature and intensity of the work drastically and can therefore give rise to stress.

* These values were measured over half hour periods during surgery (9).

CONCLUSIONS

It is evident from the foregoing that the work and working conditions of anaesthetists in provincial hospitals in the Netherlands comprise a number of elements which can give rise to problems. Some of these problems were mentioned by interviewed anaesthetists attached to three hospitals and others were observed during the collection of data in the operating theatres of these hospitals. The most important factors as far as the work load is concerned include: lack of information about the state of the biological system, the many facets of the work, the objectives of the work, and the necessity to assign supervision of the patient to auxiliary personnel. Stress can arise not only from a physical factor such as exposure to volatile ana-esthetics but also from a number of psycho-social factors such as the reac-tion to the patient's condition, the relationship with the surgeon, the evalua-tion of the surgical procedure, and the supervision of the patient by auxiliary personnel. All this must be seen against the background of a less than optimal division of the anaesthetist's work as well as the limitations of his influence on the scheduling of operations and the steadily increasing tendency to perform more complicated operations.

Although anaesthetists and surgeons often think of themselves as working in a single team, it is clear – for instance from the division of responsibility, the division of the work, and the autonomous organization of the work – that there are actually two separate teams working together, a surgical and an anaesthesiological team. It would be worthwhile to explore the possibi-lities for the formation of one team to find ways to gather more information about the patient's condition and to improve the work conditions to obtain an optimal anaesthesia and health of the anaesthetist.

REFERENCES

1. Smalhout, B., Anesthesie, het kan gewoon anders, het kan beter. *Elsevier* 30 maart 1974.
2. Spierdijk, J., Hoe gevaarlijk is het beroep van anesthesist? *Elsevier* 29 juli 1972.
3. Rapporten van de *Commissie voor Anesthesiologie van de Gezondheidsraad*, Volks-gezondheid, 5 verslagen en rapporten, Ministerie van Volksgezondheid en Milieuhy-giëne, 55-56.
4. Van Hegelsom, J. A., Onder Narcose, Informatie over anesthesie voor patienten die binnenkort geopereerd worden. *Exerpta Medica* 1974.
5. Crul, J. F., L. N. Marlet, A. E. D. v/d Vijver, *De beroepsverantwoordelijkheid en aan-sprakelijkheid van de anesthesist*, rapport: Nederlandse Anesthesistenvereniging, mei 1974.
6. Schwarz, J. J., De mens in moeilijke arbeidssituaties. Menselijke stuur en regeltaken, *Mens en Onderneming* 27, 1973, 373-87.

7. Bruce, L. D., M. J. Bach and J. Arbit, Trace Anesthetic Effects on Perceptual Cognitive and Motor Skills, *Anesthesiology* 5, mei 1974 453-58.
8. Dirken, J. M., *Arbeid en Stress* dissertatie Wolters-Noordhof, Groningen 1967.
9. Ekkers, C. L., W. T. M. Ooijendijk en J. J. Schwarz, *Menselijke Stuur- en regeltaken, verslag van een onderzoek bij vier stuur- en regeltaken* rapport NIPG/TNO Leiden 1975.

26. CONCENTRATIONS OF ANAESTHETIC AGENTS IN THE AIR IN OPERATING ROOMS*

A. G. L. BURM, JOH. SPIERDIJK AND V. REJGER

The first reports on air pollution in operating rooms and its possible unto-ward effects on those who work there appeared many years ago (1-3). After a number of studies showed that certain complaints might occur relatively frequently among anaesthetists and the nurses assisting them (Frey and Herrmann, this volume) there was renewed interest in this form of air pollution. At present studies are being done in this field in many institutes.

One question to arise concerns the degree to which the air in operating rooms is polluted. In order to answer this question the concentrations of two commonly used agents, nitrous oxide and halothane, have been measured in several operating rooms.

THE SOURCE OF POLLUTION

Anaesthetic gases enter the atmosphere because the circuit between the apparatus and the patient is not completely closed. In all cases more of the gas(es) is supplied than the patient takes up. Most of the remaining gas leaves the system via an outlet which may or may not be provided with a valve. A smaller amount excapes via leaks in the supply system or around a poorly fitting tube or mask. For the sake of completeness, it may be men-tioned that a small – probably negligible – amount of anaesthetic gases reaches the air via the patient's skin and the wound.

From the points at which they escape, the anaesthetic gases are spread over the room. The pattern of the distribution is determined mainly by the air currents in the room, which in their turn are dependent on several factors (Bossers, this volume). In most cases all of the air in the room is polluted, the concentration of the gases usually varying from place to place. The con-centration of a given agent at a given place is mainly dependent on the amount of that agent released, the level of ventilation of the room, the pat-

* These investigations were possible by a grant from the Preventiefonds Nederland.

tern of the air currents, and the location of the given place in relation to the places at which the gas is escaping. The precise influence of each of these factors is difficult to predict. Exact determination of the degree of pollution requires measurement of the concentrations.

MEASUREMENT OF ANAESTHETIC GASES IN OPERATING-ROOM AIR

Methods
Various techniques are available for the determination of the concentration of anaesthetic gases in the air. The literature indicates that such analyses are

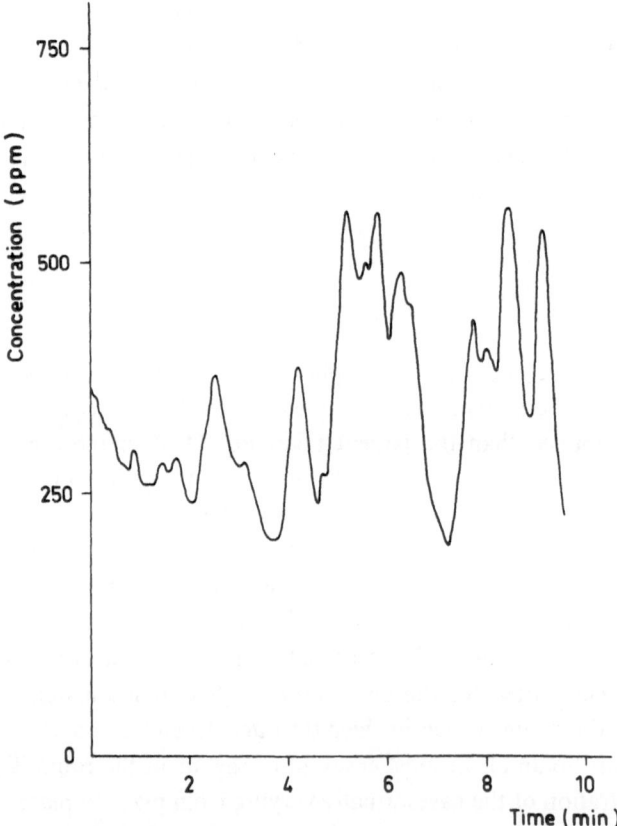

Fig. 1. Variation in time of the nitrous oxide concentration in the 'breathing zone' of the anaesthetist in one of the operating rooms, as registered by a Miran I portable gas analyzer (time constant analyzer: ± 12 sec).

usually done by gas chromatography. When this method is applied, special attention must be given to the sampling technique, because the concentration can fluctuate rather strongly and rapidly at some points (fig. 1), the size and frequency of the fluctuations being dependent on the place in the room and the mixing of the gases with the air. In general, the use of a rapid sampling method means that a rather large number of samples must be taken. The number of samples to be taken per site can be derived from the differences in the concentration of the gas in a successive series of samples. If a slow sampling technique is used, a smaller number of samples will suffice. In all cases it is necessary to make certain in advance that the flask, syringe, or bag in which the sample is collected is adequately gas-tight and that no adorption or absorption of the anaesthetic agent can occur in it.

The collection of samples can be avoided by the use of a continuous method of measurement. Whitcher et al. (4) and Knights et al. (5) have described the use of a mass spectrometer and a halogen leak detector respectively. For the present study, use was made of a Miran portable gas analyser. A pump mounted on the analyser draws in air through a dust filter. The air then passes through a gas sample cell crossed by infared rays of a certain adjustable wavelength. If the air contains a component which absorbs radiation of this wavelength, the intensity of the rays falling on the detector is lower than when this component is absent, the difference in intensity being dependent on the specific extinction coefficient and the concentration of the component in question, and the distance travelled by the rays in the cell (pathlength). The values chosen for the wavelength and the pathlength were as follows:

Anaesthetic agent	wavelength	pathlength
	(μ)	(m)
Nitrous oxide	7.78	0.75
Halothane	12.38	20.25

Under these conditions, the interference between nitrous oxide and halothane as well as disturbances by other components of the air are negligible.

Sampling sites
The best picture of the amount of anaesthetic gas taken up during work in

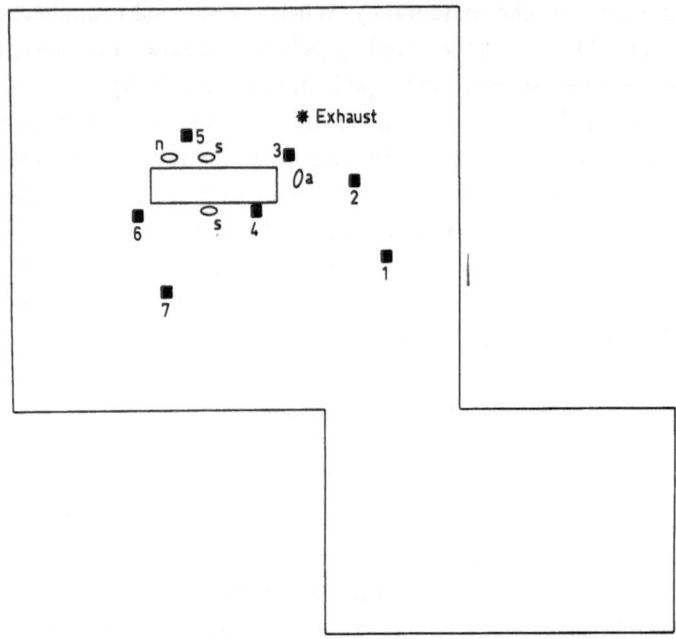

Fig. 2. Location of the measuring sites in one of the operating rooms (viewed from above); operating room not separated from the adjacent scrubbing room. scale 1:120.

■   measuring site (1.5 m above the floor).

○   'stationary persons', s = surgeon, n = scrub nurse; a = anaesthetist.

✳   exhaust valve of the anaesthetic apparatus (± 90 cm above the floor).

the operating room is obtained by analysing the air inhaled and exhaled by the personnel. This requires repeated sampling; a single sample taken at the end of the period of exposure does not supply sufficient information. It is also important to take the samples at the places where the persons involved perform their work. In practice, however, this method is not feasible, and the air in the room must be analysed. Since enough is known about the pharmacokinetics of the commonly used anaesthetic agents, the amount taken up can be calculated from such measurements with adequate accuracy.

For this latter method, the choice of the places at which the measurements are made is important. Enough must be known about the air-current pattern, for one thing. As Bossers' findings show, this pattern largely determines the distribution of the gas in question. The distribution is always inhomogeneous to a varying degree, and the greater the inhomogeneity the more measuring sites are required.

Furthermore, the area in which each of the individuals works must be taken into account. The concentrations just under the ceiling or just above the floor may be of interest in a study of the distribution of the gas but do not provide any information about the quantity taken up by personnel.

The choice of measuring sites is limited by the limited accessibility of the sterile zone. Even the use of a sterilized tube for distant sampling would impede the surgical team. Consequently, the final choice of sites is always a compromise between the desirable and the feasible.

For our study, a minimum of six measuring sites was applied. An example of the locations is given in figure 2. The air to be analysed was collected 1.5 m above the floor (nose level). The positions of the 'stationary' personnel are also shown in figure 2. Concentrations were measured alternately at the various sites over a period of 5 to 15 minutes per point depending on the fluctuation of the signal. The total measuring period amounted on average to about five hours per operating room per day.

The use of a continuous method means that the concentrations of nitrous oxide and halothane in one operating room are measured on different days. It should also be kept in mind that it has been shown that nitrous oxide and halothane, which are released as a homogeneous mixture, are also distributed as a homogeneous mixture, and therefore the concentration of one of them can be calculated from that of the other if the ratio of the agents in the escaping mixture is known (6).

OPERATING ROOMS AND ANAESTHESIA EQUIPMENT

Nitrous oxide concentrations were measured in eight operating rooms. In five of them, where halothane is used regularly, the concentrations of this agent were also measured.

Five of the eight operating rooms are equipped with a mechanical ventilation system in which the removed air is not recirculated. The amount of fresh air introduced is shown in table 1. Two of the operating rooms are not provided with a ventilation system, and the last has an aircooling installation designed for complete recirculation.

Nitrous oxide and halothane were almost always administered to the patient via the so-called semi-closed circle system in which use is made of a mechanical ventilator (Spiromat 650, Bird 4 N 8). Intubation was applied in all cases.

Table 1. Concentrations of anaesthetics in mechanically ventilated operating rooms.

Room	Anaesthetic	Mean conc. in ppm (v/v)		Air supply in the room (m³/h.)	Supply anaesthetic (l/min)	Calculated conc. (ppm (v/v))**
		Working zone anaesthetist	Other sites			
1	Nitrous oxide	300	130–260	2200	4	110
2*	Nitrous oxide	290	60–230	2025	4	120
2*	Nitrous oxide	320	80–130	2025	4	120
3	Nitrous oxide	270	200–420	1800	4	130
4	Nitrous oxide	370	290–440	1700	5	180
5	Nitrous oxide	490	80–250	1550	4	155
4	Halothane	4.1	2.1–4.4	1700	0.035	1.2
5	Halothane	5.3	0.8–2.4	1550	0.03	1.2

* Anaesthetic apparatus on different places in the same room.
** See Bossers, this volume.

RESULTS

From the signal tracings the mean concentration for each 5-15 minute
period was determined. This gave, for each measuring site, a series of values
C_{p_i} representing the mean concentration at that site at various times.
The concentrations are expressed in ppm:

$$1 \text{ ppm} = 1 \frac{cm^3}{m^3} = 0.0001 \text{ vol}\%$$

The nitrous oxide concentration as a function of time at the various sites in
one of the operating rooms lacking an air-conditioning system is demonstrated in figure 3.
The location of the sites and the position of the stationary personnel
are shown in figure 2.

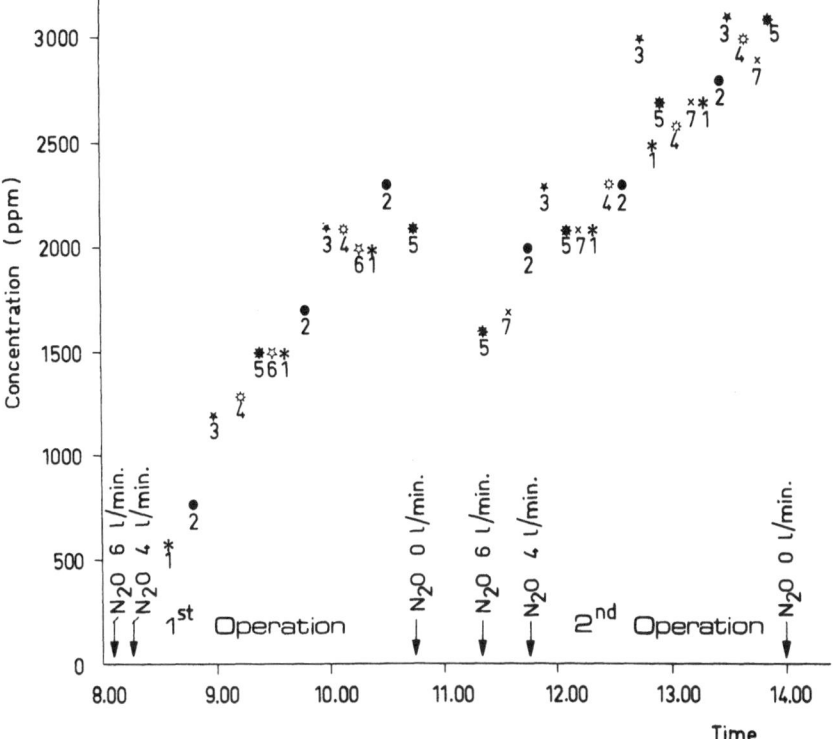

Fig. 3. Concentration of nitrous oxide at several measuring sites in a naturally ventilated
operating room given as a function of time. Location of the measuring sites: see fig. 2.
Volume of the operating room + scrubbing room: 200 m³.

As can be seen from figure 3 the concentrations increase steadily during the operations and there is a decrease between operations. A similar pattern was found for the other two 'unventilated' operating rooms. The measured concentrations almost always lie between 1500 and 3000 ppm for nitrous oxide (rate of supply 4-6 1/min) and between 15 and 35 ppm for halothane (supply rate 0.02-0.07 1/min, mean supply 0.03-0.04 1/min).

It is noteworthy that no distinct relationship was found between the degree of pollution and the size (volume) of the operating rooms (200, 100 and 110 m³). This can only be explained by differences in the natural ventilation rate in these operating rooms (Bossers, this volume). In general the concentrations measured shortly after one another at different places differ little. This means that the anaesthetic gases are ultimately distributed rather homogeneously over the room.

The nitrous oxide concentrations at the various sites in one of the operating rooms with mechanical ventilation is shown in figures 4 and 5. The location of the sites and the positions of the stationary personnel are shown in figure 6. In these operating rooms the concentration at each site rises

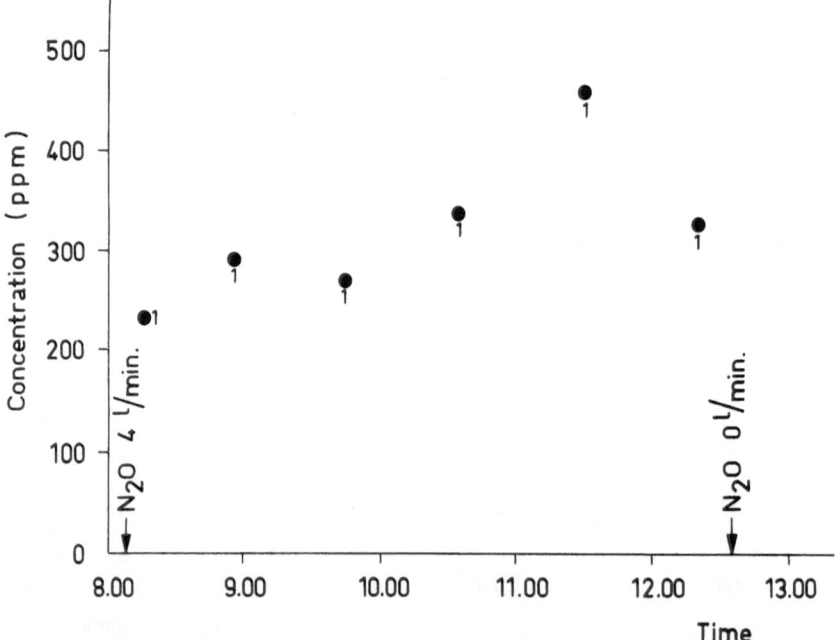

Fig. 4. Concentration of nitrous oxide in the 'breathing zone' of the anaesthetist in a mechanically ventilated operating room given as a function of time. Location of the measuring site: see fig. 6.

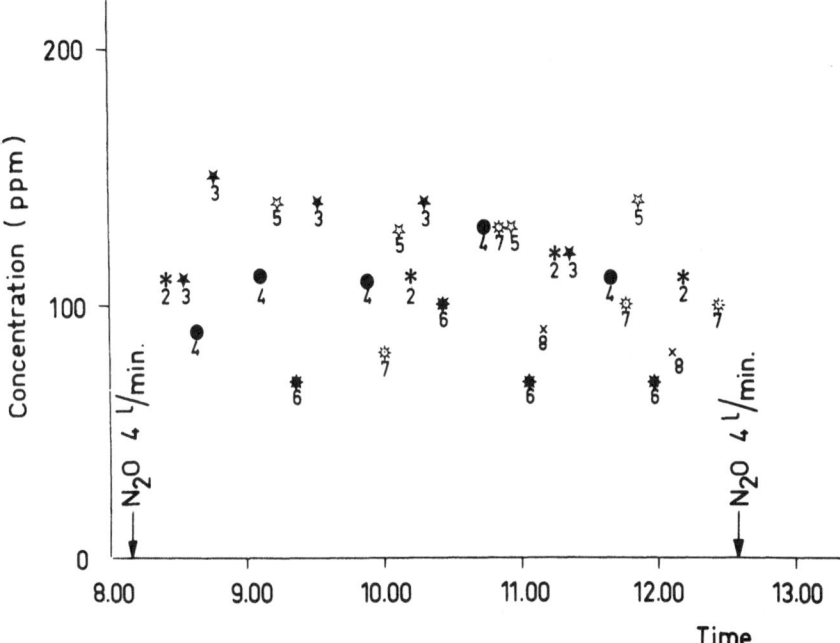

Fig. 5. Concentration of nitrous oxide at several measuring sites in a mechanically venti-lated operating room given as a function of time. Location of the measuring sites: see fig. 6.

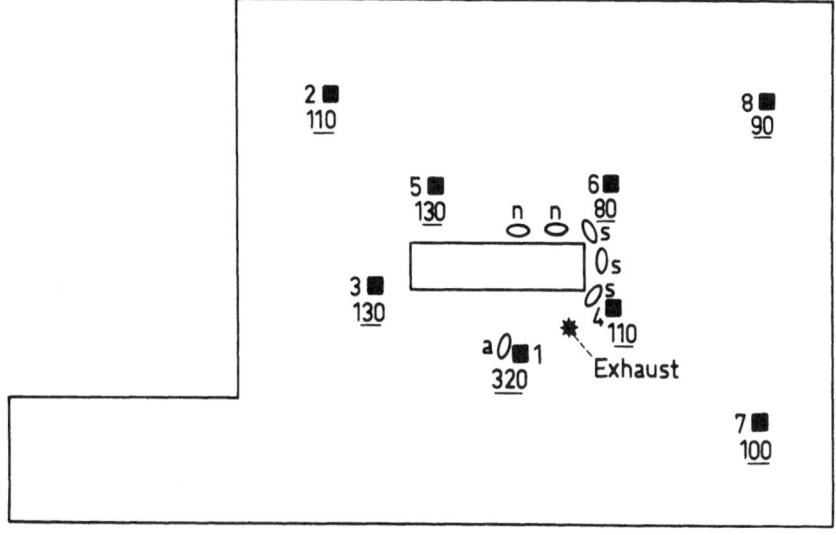

Fig. 6. Mean concentrations of nitrous oxide in ppm (v/v) found at several measuring sites in a mechanically ventilated operating room (underlined numbers). Measuring sites 1.5 m above the floor, exhaust valve 90 cm above the floor. Supply rate N_2O: 4 l/min; supply fresh air: 2025 m^3/h. scale 1:85

rather rapidly initially and after some time reaches a more or less constant level. Here, too, there is a decrease between two operations.

From the concentrations $\overline{C}_{pi}$ measured during operations at various times the mean $\overline{C}_p$ was determined for each site P:

$$\overline{C}_p = \frac{\sum\limits_{i=1}^{n} C_{pi}}{n},$$

in which n is the number of measuring periods at point P. The difference between $\overline{C}_p$ and C_{pi} was in general less than 30%.

The values obtained for $\overline{C}_p$ are summarized in table 1, where, to permit comparison with data in the literature, a distinction is made between the concentrations in the 'breathing zone' of the anaesthetist and the other sites. Table 1 also shows the amount of the anaesthetic gases supplied and data concerning the ventilation in the room, as well as the mean concentrations calculated from them for the imaginary case in which there is a complete mixing of the anaesthetic gases with the air in the operating room occuring immediately.

An example of the distribution over the various measuring sites is given in figure 6. It can be seen from figure 6 and table 1 that in operating rooms with mechanical ventilation the distribution is always more or less inhomogeneous. This inhomogeneity is related to the air-flow pattern.

DISCUSSION

The measurements made in the present study indicate that the degree of pollution in operating rooms can differ widely. The concentrations depend upon the amount of anaesthetic gases released, the ventilation applied, and the air-current pattern. The concentrations found for nitrous oxide and halothane differ by a factor of roughly 100, which is consistent with the ratio of the two gases in the escaping mixture.

In operating rooms not provided with a mechanical ventilation system a constant level of the polluting gases is not reached. The mean concentration is therefore irrelevant, because the degree of exposure is dependent on the course of the concentration. In mechanically ventilated operating rooms a mean can usually be determined for each site.

Comparison of our results with the values reported in the literature is difficult because most authors do not give the necessary information about ventilation and/or the amount of escaping anaesthetic gases. Furthermore, there is little uniformity in the choice of measuring sites. The concentrations reported for the 'breathing zone' of the anaesthetist range from a few ppm (vol/vol) to more than 1,000 ppm for halothane and from about 100 to 10,000 ppm for nitrous oxide (4, 7-18).

The degree to which the personnel is exposed to anaesthetic gases is dependent not only on the degree of pollution but also on the amount of time spent in an operating room or other space polluted with such agents. The duration of the period between exposures is also important, since a role is played by the elimination of the anaesthetic agents from the body. All of these factors, which can vary widely, complicate the problem to such an extent that it is impossible to reach a general conclusion about the exposure to anaesthetic gases in the operating room.

REFERENCES

1. Hewitt, F. W., *Anaesthetics and their administration*, p. 33, Charles Griffin London (1893).
2. Hirsch, J. and A. L. Kappus, Uber die Mengen des Narkoseäthers in der Luft von Operationssälen. *Zeitschrift für Hygiene und Infektionskrankheiten* 110, 391 (1929).
3. Werthmann, H., Beitrag zur chronischen Ätherintoxikation der Chirurgen. *Beitrage zur Klinischen Chirurgie* 178, 149 (1949).
4. Whitcher, C. E., E. N. Cohen and J. R. Trudell, Chronic exposure to anaesthetic gases in the operating room. *Anesthesiology* 35, 348 (1971).
5. Knights, K. M., J. M. Strunin and L. Strunin, Measurement of low concentrations of halothane in the atmosphere using a portable detector. *Br. J. Anaesth.* 47, 635 (1975).
6. Spierdijk, J., A. G. L. Burm, P. A. Bossers, F. C. van Beukering and E. van Gunst, *Distribution of anaesthetic gases in an operating room*. München 1974. (In press)
7. Askrog, V. and R. Petersen, Forurening af operationsstuer med luftformige anaesthetika og røntgenbestråling. *Nordisk Medicin* 83, 501 (1970).
8. Hallén, B., H. Ehrner-Samuel and M. Thomason, Measurement of halothane in the atmosphere of an operating theatre and in expired air and blood of the personnel during routine anaesthetic work. *Acta anaesth. Scandinav.* 14, 17 (1970).
9. Jenkins, L. C., Chronic exposure to anaesthetics: a toxicity problem? *Canad. Anaesth. Soc. J.* 20, 104 (1973).
10. Langley, D. R. and A. Steward, The effect of ventilation system design on air contamination with halothane in operating theatres. *Br. J. Anaesth.* 46, 736 (1974).
11. Linde, H. W. and D. L. Bruce, Occupational exposure of anaesthetists to halothane and nitrous oxide. *Anesthesiology* 30, 363 (1969).
12. Mehta, S., W. J. Cole, J. Chari and K. Lewin, Operating room air pollution: influence of anaesthetic circuit, vapour concentration, gas flow and ventilation. *Canad. Anaesth. Soc. J.* 22, 265 (1975).
13. Murrin, K. R., Atmospheric pollution with halothane in operating theatres. *Anaesthesia* 30, 12 (1975).

14. Nikki, P., P. Pfäffli, K. Ahlman and R. Ralli, Chronic exposure to anaesthetic gases in the operating theatre and recovery room. *Annals of Clinical Research* 4, 266 (1972).
15. Strunin, L., J. M. Strunin and C. C. Mallios, Atmospheric pollution with halothane during outpatient dental anaesthesia. *Brit. Med. J.* 4, 459 (1973).
16. Schulze, H. H., D. Kästner and P. Lange, Zur Frage der chronischen Toxicität von Halothankonzentrationen in der Operationssaalluft, *Der Anaesthesist* 18, 378 (1969).
17. Usubiaga, L., J. A. Aldrete and V. Fiserova-Bergerova, Influence of gas flows and operating room ventilation on the daily exposure of anaesthetists to halothane. *Anaesthesia and Analgesia . . . Current Researches* 51, 968 (1972).
18. Yanagida, H., C. Kemi, K. Suwa and H. Yamamura, Nitrous oxide content in the operating suite. *Anaesthesia and Analgesia . . . Current Researches* 53, 347 (1974).

27. AIR-CONDITIONING IN OPERATING ROOMS*

P. A. BOSSERS

1. INTRODUCTION

Air-conditioning is designed to control the environment of humans within an enclosed room such that the factors determining the climate, i.e. the temperature, the velocity and the relative humidity of the air, remain within certain limits. These limits are chosen such that a percentage as high as possible of the people experience the climate thus offered as comfortable. The temperature and relative humidity are chosen in dependence on metabolism, clothing and other factors. We might call this: the thermal climate control.

Besides, air-conditioning is meant to control the climate in a hygienic sense. For that purpose an amount of fresh air is fed to a room so that human smells or odours, carbon dioxide from the air resulting from expiration and solid or gaseous impurities that are released into the room, all remain below the limit at which they are inconvenient or noxious. The way in which the air is fed to a room has an effect on the local concentration of these admixtures. Furthermore, heat sources play a role as to the distribution of such impurities in the room. In the following chapters we shall mainly deal with airconditioning in the hygienic sense.

2. SOURCES OF AIR POLLUTION IN OPERATING ROOMS

Two types of air pollution prevail in operating theatres: solid particles (dust), and gaseous impurities. The first type especially affects their bacteriological purity because germs adhere to the dust. This type of pollution will not be discussed in further detail here. We shall now focus on gaseous impurities; they originate in particular from the anaesthesia facilities and from the very persons in the operating room. The most important 'human' impurities are water vapour via exhaled air and via evaporation at the skin, carbon

* Publ. no. 551 of the TNO Research Institute for Environmental Hygiene, Delft.

dioxide and smells exuded along with perspiration. Long before any carbon dioxide concentration can be noxious to human health, the concentration of water vapour and those smells will have become a nuisance. In particular the latter group of admixtures causes a sultry and stuffy atmosphere. A relatively small amount of fresh air (minimum approximately 30 m³/h a head) is sufficient to maintain an adequately hygienic atmosphere.

Anaesthetic gases are odourless, in the concentrations that normally occur in operating rooms, and as a result they are not directly objectionable. As there are indications, however, that they may have noxious side effects for humans on prolonged exposition, it is useful to ascertain what levels of concentration may be expected, if exhaust of these gases is effected into, and not away from, the operating room. Moreover, also at low concentrations they tend to cause headaches.

It is assumed that the anaesthetic gases are mixed with air to such an extent that they have no rate of fall of their own, and that they do not unmix either. Measurements have shown that these assumptions are justified.

3. TRANSPORT OF GASES IN A ROOM

If exhaust of anaesthetic apparatus is into the operating room, the highest concentration of gases will occur close to the apparatus. This concentration is equal to that administered to the patient.

When the air is perfectly stationary (an imaginary situation), spreading of anaesthetic exhaust can only occur because the gas discharged is 'pushed up' by a new supply, and by diffusion. Then, finally, a cloud with a high concentration of anaesthetic gases would occur, which, at its edges, has a somewhat lower concentration than in its core, just because of diffusion. The air movements that occur in a room are so intense, however, that the occurrence of such an exhaust cloud is prevented. Incidentally, the causes of air movements will be discussed in the next chapter. The distribution of anaesthetic gases by diffusion can, in fact, be neglected. Even hydrogen, which has a relatively high diffusion rate, does not attain any more than some cm/sec at great differences in concentration (1).

Movement of anaesthetic gases of their own accord can be observed in very quiet air, at rather high concentrations. Because of their greater specific mass, the anaesthetic gases will tend to drop.

From measurements it has been found that, if these gases are mixed with air, such movements because of differences in mass are negligible. As a result, there is no unmixing.

4. THE GENESIS OF AIR MOVEMENTS IN ROOMS

For transport of impurities in a room, it is mainly the movements and flows of air that are responsible. Such a pattern of movements can only result from the influence of some driving force. The generating forces that play a role here may be divided as follows:
1. the impulse of the air which, at a certain speed, flows into the room;
2. differences in temperature;
3. the 'stirring effect' of moving objects, and that of human beings.

4.1. Movement of air as a result of ventilation
Practically always an amount of air will enter a certain room and an equal amount will leave that room, even if there is no mechanical ventilation. Under the influence of wind pressure upon the façades of a building, and the differences in temperature of the air that are usually present in the building,

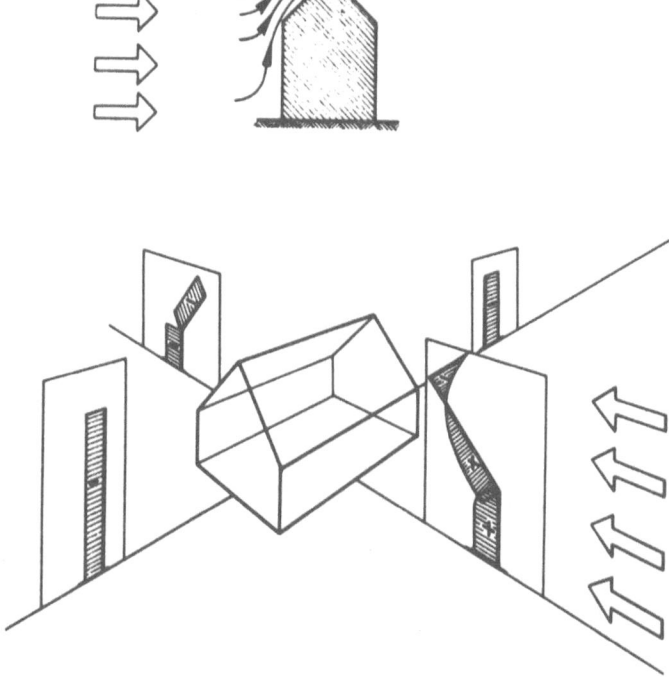

Fig. 1. Air pressures on a building subjected to wind.

and also outside it, differences in pressure will arise. These differences in pressure cause a transport of air. For instance, via cracks of windows and doors, open windows and the like. In this way, 'natural' ventilation takes place (fig. 1). Operating rooms are generally provided with a mechanical ventilation system, so that the pressure ratios are better controlled and undesirable air transports, e.g. from the nursing departments or patients' rooms to the operating theatre, can thus be avoided. The supply of air, whether by perforated panels, grills, ceiling outlets or the like, is practically always implemented in the form of one or more 'jets' of air. Whether such a jet is great or small does not essentially affect its composition. Basically it is always composed of a core zone, in which the quality and speed of the air are equal to those of the air in the inlet opening, and a mixing zone in which mix the air fed to and that present in the room (fig. 2). The entering air jet mostly has a higher speed than that of the air in the room. The circumference of the air jet then entrains particles of air and, in the eddies thus created, the mixing process takes place. This mixing relates to speed, differences in temperature and to impurities present in the room.

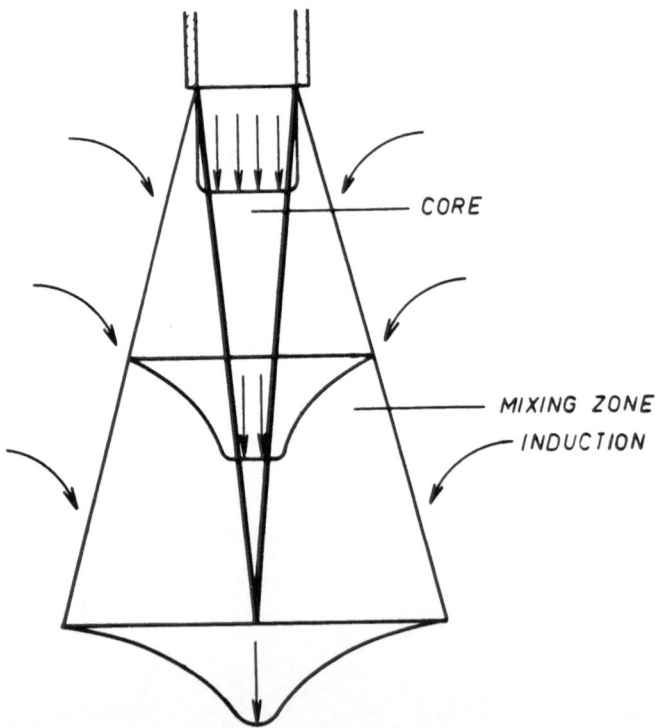

Fig. 2. Sketch of an air jet

AIR SUPPLY

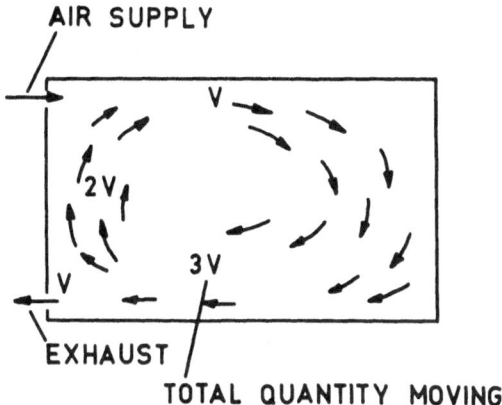

TOTAL QUANTITY MOVING

Fig. 3. Quantities of air moving in a ventilated room.

In its course through the room, an air jet puts an amount of air into motion that is approximately two times its own volume. Since as much air is exhausted as is supplied, the amount of air that is moving will be about three times as large as the amount fed, though at relatively low speeds (fig. 3).

The mixing process, as much as it relates to speed and temperature, benefits the degree of comfort experienced in the room. If the air jet would not be subject to this process, then persons present in the route followed by the jet would feel a draught. With regard to the impurities carried, mixing is often less desirable; particularly so in view of bacteriological impurities. In proportion as mixing intensifies, the impurities are better divided over the entire room.

The difference in temperature between the air in the jet and that in the room also has an effect on the course of the jet. If the air in the jet is warmer than that in the room, the jet will tend to rise and if the air in the jet is colder, the jet will decline. This influence of differences in temperature on the course of a jet also highly depends on the way it is blown in (fig. 4). For instance:

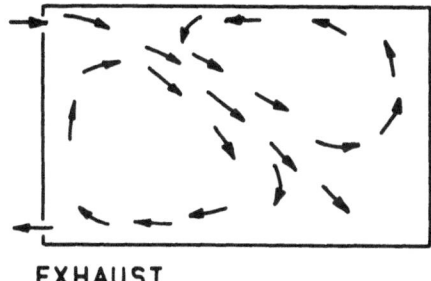

EXHAUST

Fig. 4. Air-flow pattern when cold air is supplied.

the course of a jet of air that has been blown in horizontally and has a temperature lower than the air in the room, will decline and a jet directed vertically downwarhs will gain some extra speed.

Some examples of flow patterns resulting from ventilation are shown in figures 5-8.

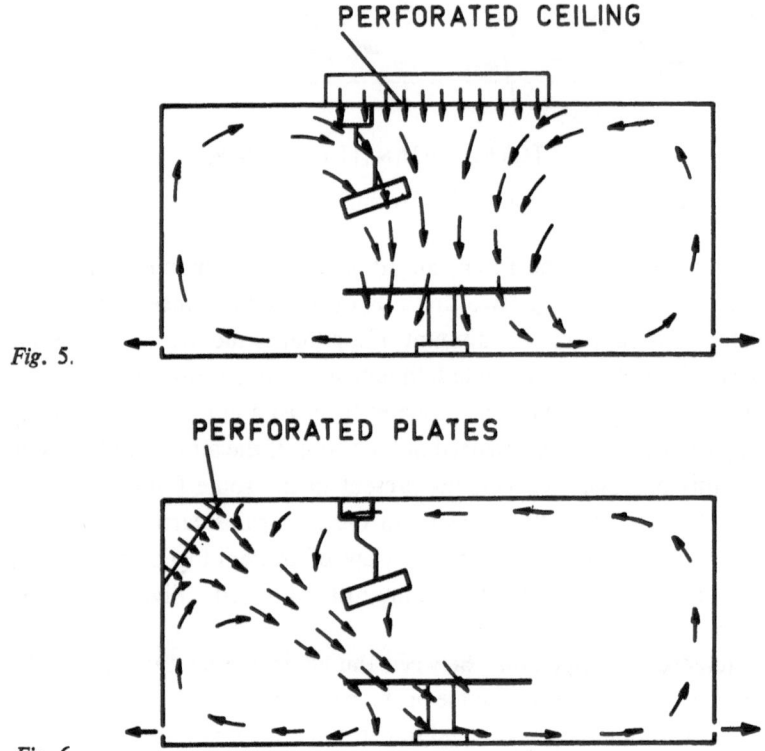

Fig. 5.

Fig. 6.

It will be clear from the above that the way of supply has much influence on the shape of the flow pattern. For an operating theatre that is not in use, the very way in which the air is fed to it is determinative for its air-flow pattern.

In contrast to our remarks about ways of feeding air to operating rooms, the place where exhaust takes place, and even the speed in the exhaust device, have hardly any influence on the total air-flow pattern. As appears from figure 9, the speed rapidly decreases with the distance to the exhaust opening. With a circular opening, of a diameter d, at a distance of 1 d the speed is only approximately 10% of the speed in that exhaust opening.

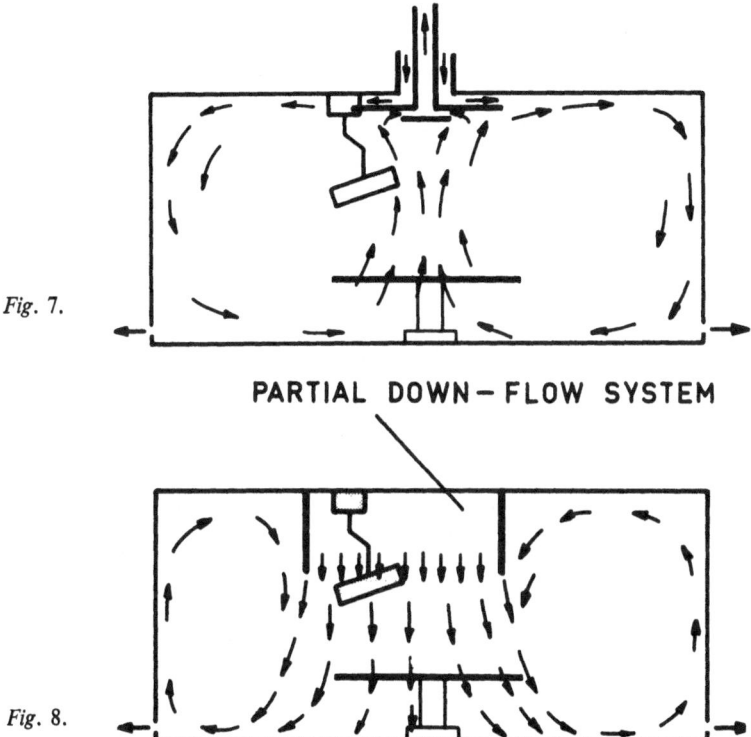

Fig. 7.

PARTIAL DOWN-FLOW SYSTEM

Fig. 8.

Figs. 5-8. Air-flow patterns in rooms with different systems of air-supply; without heat load in the rooms.

4.2. *Air movement caused by differences in temperature*

A second important factor in the genesis of air movement in a room, and accordingly for the transport of impurities, is that of air movements resulting from differences in temperature.

The specific mass of air highly depends on temperature; if air in a room is heated locally, then the heated part will rise in respect of the rest of the room's air. This heating may take place simply because there are persons present in a room and, also, it may be caused by equipment that is mounted in it and that produces heat; think of monitors, lamps, and the like.

At the surface of these heat sources heat is transferred to the air, which therefore rises and is replaced by cooler air. Let us consider, by way of example, a person standing in quiet air. The surface temperature of his/her clothing is higher than the environmental temperature because internal heat production is partially discharged via clothing. As a result a layer of warm air flows upwards past the body. Over the head, this flow of air reaches a speed

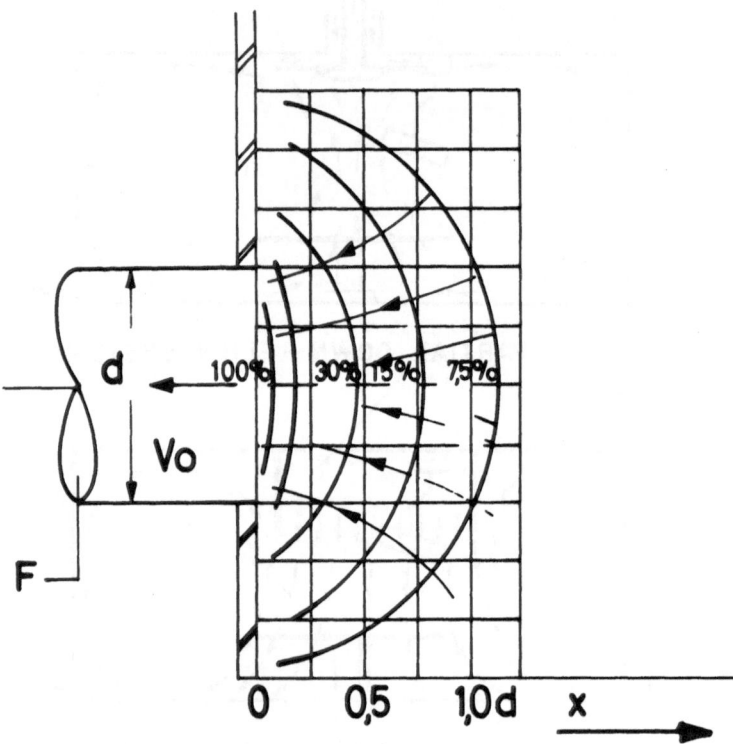

Fig. 9. Velocities near an exhaust opening.

of 0.2-0.3 m/s (fig. 10) (2). Largely determinative for the final speed of this convectional flow are two things: the magnitude of the difference in temperature, and the height over which this temperature difference prevails. It will be clear that the air-flow pattern in a room, as a result of the supply of air for ventilation, is also influenced by these convectional flows. In particular when the human and other heat sources are rather near, one to another, as is the case with a team of operating surgeons around a patient, the convectional flows are of some considerable intensity. For the same ventilation systems as shown in figures 5-8, the influence of convection on flow patterns is presented in figures 11-14. In this way, the temperature of the air blown in has also an influence on the air-flow pattern, as has already been elucidated. The movements as a result of the differences in temperature in the jet have been pinpointed by a number of investigators, and can be largely predicted via calculations (4).

An important source of air movement as a result of differences in tem-

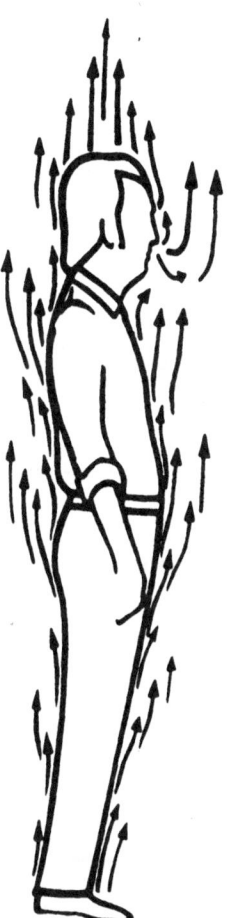

Fig. 10. Convection along a stationary person.

perature is that via the door opening between two adjacent rooms. If there is a difference in temperature between rooms, then in the door opening, or in the cracks when the door is closed, two opposite flows of air will occur. In the lower half, air flows from the cooler room to the warmer one, and in the upper half from the warmer to the cooler. To give an impression about the size of these flows, the following example may serve: at a difference in temperature between the rooms of only 1 °C, at least 350 m³/h flows from one room into an other (4). Even when the door is closed, and without particular measures to seal the cracks, still approx. 30 m³/h flows under these conditions from one room into an other (5).

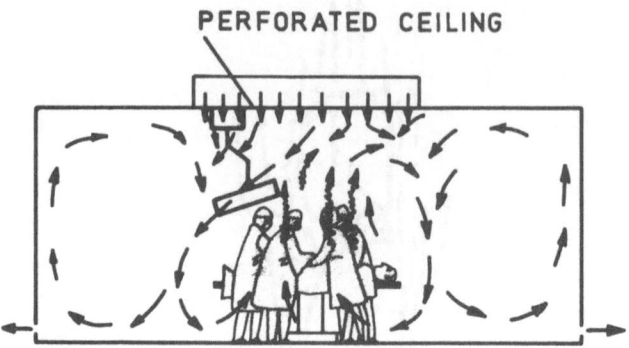

Fig. 11. Air-flow pattern in rooms with different systems of air-supply: with heat load in the rooms.

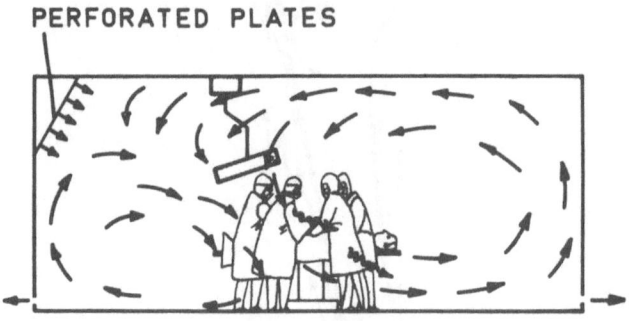

Fig. 12. Air-flow pattern in rooms with different systems of air-supply: with heat load in the rooms.

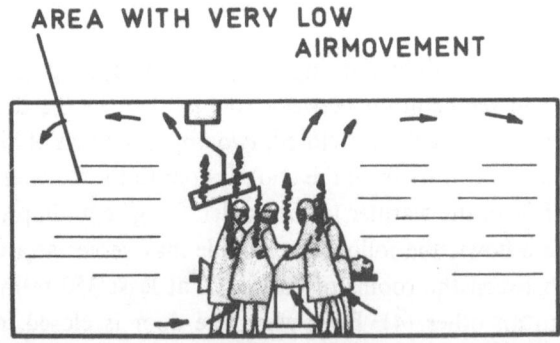

Fig. 13. Air flow pattern caused by natural convection of the operating team in the absence of mechanical ventilation.

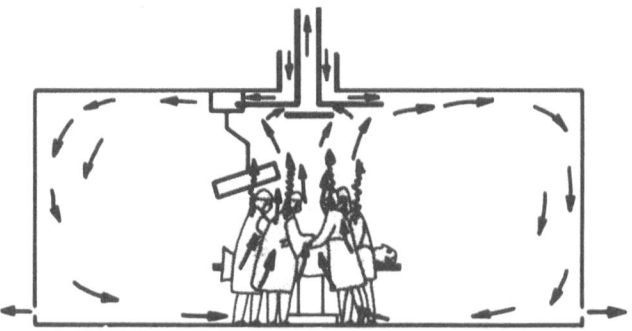

Fig. 14. Air-flow pattern in rooms with different systems of air-supply: with heat load in the rooms.

4.3. Movement of persons or objects

The third cause of air movement is that which results from movement of persons or objects. When people are walking, a vortex area is produced behind them and air is brought from one spot to an other. Naturally, this likewise applies to all objects that are moved. If, locally, there are differences in concentration of impurities, these will be smoothed down by this 'stirring' effect.

5. CONCENTRATION OF IMPURITIES

If, in a restricted space, a known amount of impurities is released, how great is then the concentration to be expected? This question can only then be answered exactly, if mixing of the impurities takes place immediately and completely. Though in practice this will never happen, investigation of the pertinent phenomena will give an insight in the process.

How the concentration will proceed from a point of time $t = 0$, in which concentration $C_0 = 0$, can be shown by the formula:

$$C_t = \frac{q}{aV} (1\text{-}e^{-at})$$

Where C_t = concentration at point of time t

     q = amount of anaesthetic gas that is supplied (in $1/h$)

     a = air change rate (h^{-1})

     V = volume of the room in m^3.

Product aV represents the amount of ventilation air that per hour is fed into the room. From the formula it can be seen that the final concentration only depends on the amount of air that is fed, for after a sufficiently long period of time term e^{-at} has approached zero. The size of the room has no influence on the final concentration. There is a relationship, though, between the size of the room and the period of time in which the final concentration is reached. In figure 15 this has been pictured for rooms of 50 m³, 75 m³ and

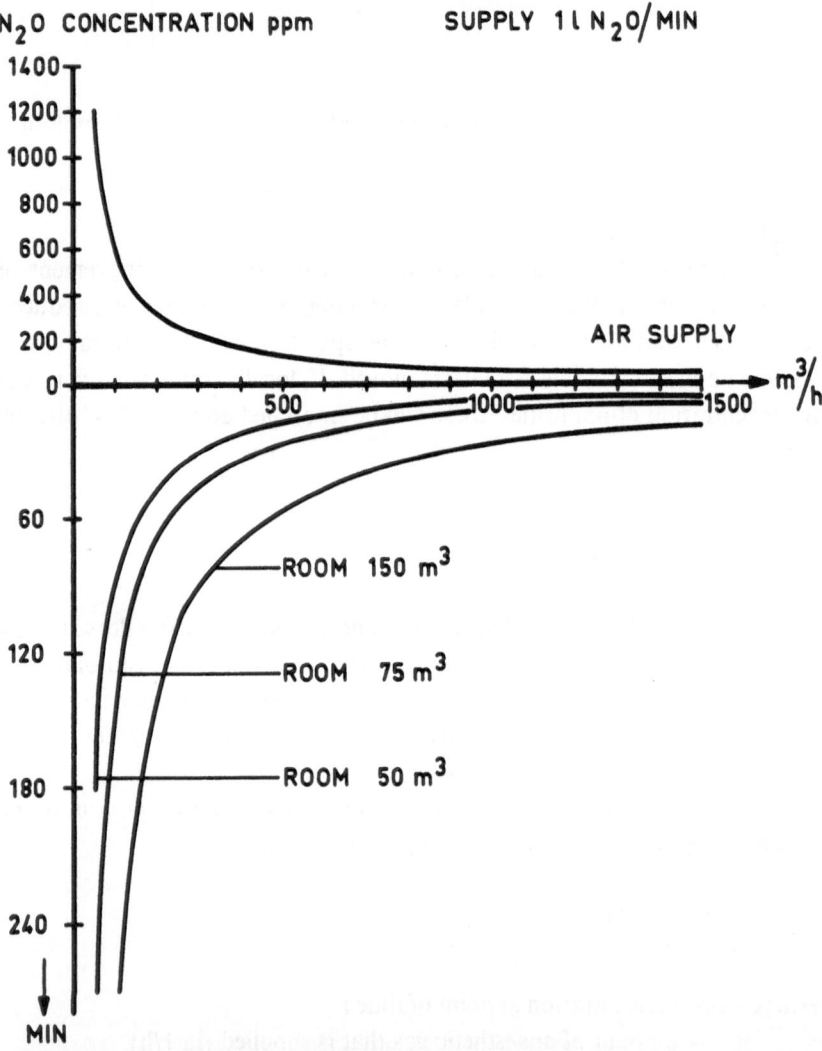

Fig. 15. N₂O concentration depending on the amount of air supplied. The time to reach 95% of the end concentration for rooms with different volumes.

150 m³. The horizontal axis plots the amount of air supplied that is responsible for the concentration plotted on the upper vertical axis. A supply of nitrous oxide of 60 1/h (1 1/min) has been assumed. For other amounts, the concentrations can be multiplified with the real amount of nitrous oxide supplied. On the lower vertical axis is plotted the period of time in which 95% of the final concentration is reached. From this can be concluded that human beings in a large room, with one and the same amount of air for ventilation, receive a dose (i.e. concentration x period of time of exposure) that is smaller than the dose in a smaller room. This will especially be of importance for rooms that are fed with a small amount of clean air, such as is the case when ventilation is natural.

Immediate and complete mixing is a purely theoretical case; it suitably serves as a base of comparison for conditions found in practice. In practice, if clean air is supplied to a room, it will take some time before mixing has taken place. As a result, in a surgery there will be locations of highly different concentrations. The distribution of anaesthetic gases very much depends on the flow pattern that is: on the way in which the air is supplied to the operating theatre, and on the nature and the positions of its heat sources. If we consider the outlet of the anaesthetic equipment as a point-source, it will make a great difference for the anaesthesist or the operating team, in respect of the concentration of anaesthetic gases, whether the air movements carries those gases directly in their direction or whether they first pass through the entire room. The longer path thus covered gives more opportunity for mixing, the concentration level meanwhile dropping.

If a flow with a high concentration goes past exhaust opening, the average concentration in the room will be lower than follows from the above theoretical approach; effectively, fewer impurities have then been introduced. The extreme case, which in respect of the persons present would have to be aimed at, is that exhaust for the room air is being implemented at the very location of exhaust of the anaesthetic equipment. Then the effective source of pollution approaches zero and, of course, so do the concentrations in the room. The concentration that is measured at a certain point in the room varies rather considerably with time. Apparently the mixing process takes place in such great eddies that, as it were, waves with alternate high and low concentrations pass the measuring point. If the surgeons and nurses walk much in the room, the amplitude of the 'waves' is smaller and then the differences in concentration from place to place are also smaller (see also Burm, this volume).

6. FINAL REMARKS

Restriction of the concentration of the anaesthetic gases to which persons
working in a operating room are exposed, can be warranted in different
ways. The most obvious way is: directly discharging the gases to outside the
room. This has practically the same effect, both with naturally and mechanically ventilated rooms. Leakages, if any, in the anaesthetic system result in a
greater concentration in case of rooms that are not ventilated mechanically.
Mechanical ventilation achieves a reduction in the concentration in respect
of rooms that are ventilated naturally. The differences in concentration,
from place to place, then depend on the air-flow pattern. If that pattern is
not known, measured concentrations may show a distribution over the
operating theatre that seems inexplicable. Furthermore it may be expected
that a greater distance from the exhaust of the anaesthetic equipment to the
persons concerned results in a lower concentration near those persons. The
longer path then covered creates more opportunity for mixing. This measure
would generally be most beneficial to the anaesthesist, as he stands closest to
the path of gases being discharged.

The best method for restricting exposition to anaesthetic gases remains, of
course, their direct discharge from the operating room. In many places, the
construction of systems suitable for this purpose, and perfectioning of
existing solutions, are in progress. In particular for operating theatres that
are not ventilated mechanically, the use of this method is necessary in view
of the high concentration that may be expected in them.

REFERENCES

1. Crommelin, R. D., P. A. Bossers, De Beoordeling van reinheid en comfort in operatie-
   kamers (The evaluation of cleanness and comfort in operating theatres) Publ. no. 434,
   IG-TNO (= TNO Research Institute for Environmental Hygiene), pp. C 519-C 21
   (only available in Dutch).
2. Clark, R. P., R. N. Cox, *Dispersal of bacteria from the human body surface, Airborne
   transmission and airborne infection,* Oosthoek p. 413-426.
3. Regenscheit, B., The air movement in air-conditioned rooms, *Kältetechnik* Jahrgang 11,
   1959 Heft 1 pp. 3-11 (= Refrigeration engineering, volume 11, 1959 No. 1 pp. 3-11).
4. Bouwman, H. B., Mogen deuren in ziekenhuizen open blijven staan? (Is it allowed to
   leave doors in hospitals open? Publ. no. 437 *IG-TNO*, pp. F2-F15.
5. Whyte, W. and B. H. Shaw, *Air-flow through doorways, Airborne transmission and
   airborne infection,* Oosthoek 513-516.

28. CONTROLLING OCCUPATIONAL EXPOSURE TO INHALATION ANAESTHETICS

CH. WHITCHER

The anaesthetist has always concerned himself primarily with the homeostasis of the patient. In the 1970's he has assumed an additional concern, the health of the operating room team with respect to its possible compromise as a result of chronic exposure to trace concentrations of the inhalation anesthetics present in the operating room air. This occupational exposure may be reduced via waste anesthetic gas control measures including scavenging, low leakage preventive maintenance procedures for anaesthetic equipment, and low leakage work practices by the anaesthetist. The effectiveness of these measures is verified by air monitoring. The anaesthetist employing these techniques can maintain a gaseous environment containing less than 0.005 percent of the concentrations of the inhalation anaesthetics administered to the patient; for example, less than 30 ppm N_2O, 0.5 ppm halothane.[1]

National concern about occupational exposure to N_2O affects not only the personnel in the operating room but also the personnel in the dental suite. The unique problems of waste gas control in this setting are presently under investigation. The preliminary impression is that occupational exposure to N_2O in the dentist's treatment room need be no greater than in the operating room in the hospital.

THE HEALTH HAZARD OF THE OPERATING ROOM

The health hazard of the operating room was first recognized in Vaisman's study of the health of 303 Russian anesthesiologists (2). In this group an unusually high incidence of headache, fatigue and irritability was noted. Of the 110 women, an increased incidence of spontaneous abortion and a high incidence of abnormal pregnancies also were reported. Nitrous oxide and ether were the principle agents employed and in the absence of air conditioning and anaesthetic gas scavenging, the operating room probably contained high concentrations of these agents.

Subsequent epidemiological surveys of the health of operating room personnel have confirmed and extended these findings. The most compre-hensive study was initiated in 1972 under the combined auspices of an ad hoc committee on the Effects of Trace Anesthetic Agents on the Health of Operating Room Personnel of the American Society of Anesthesiologists (ASA) and the National Institute for Occupational Safety and Health (NIOSH). (3)

The data obtained from 40,044 respondents exposed to the operating room were compared to data obtained from control groups. Participants included the entire memberships of the ASA and the American Association of Nurse Anesthetists (AANA). The American Academy of Pediatrics (AAP), Association of Operating Room Nurses, The American Nursing Association (ANA), and the Association of Operating Room Technicians also partici-pated in this study.

The health hazards are indicated in figures 1 through 6. Figure 1 compares

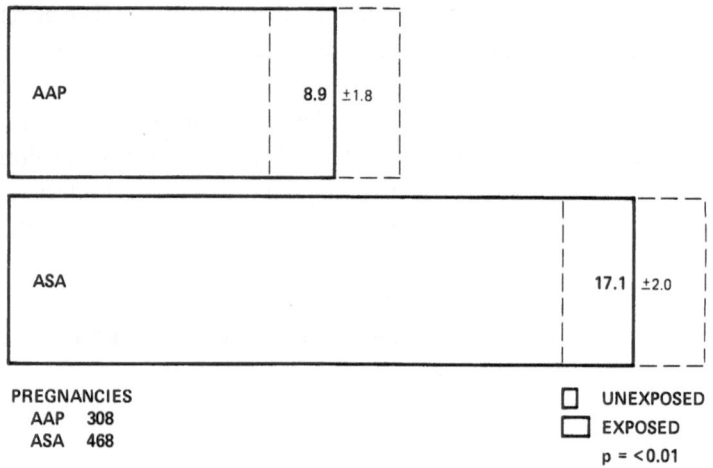

Fig. 1. Spontaneous abortion rates/100 pregnancies, female respondents. (Standardized for age and smoking habit).

the spontaneous abortion rate for occupationally exposed* members of the ASA with the AAP, and an approximately twofold difference is apparent. Figure 2 shows birth defects (skin excluded) in the same groups and they appear to be different by a factor of 2, but statistical significance is not achieved, probably due to the small number of births. Figure 3 shows birth

* Exposed personnel are defined as those who regularly administer anaesthetics or work in the operating room.

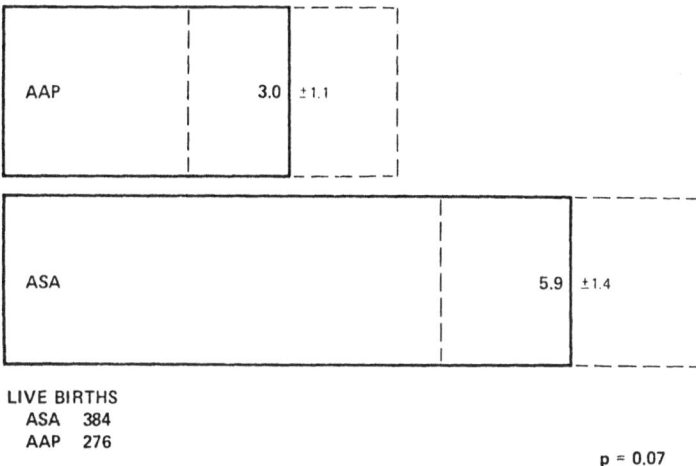

Fig. 2. Standardized congenital abnormality rates/100 live births female respondents (skin excluded).

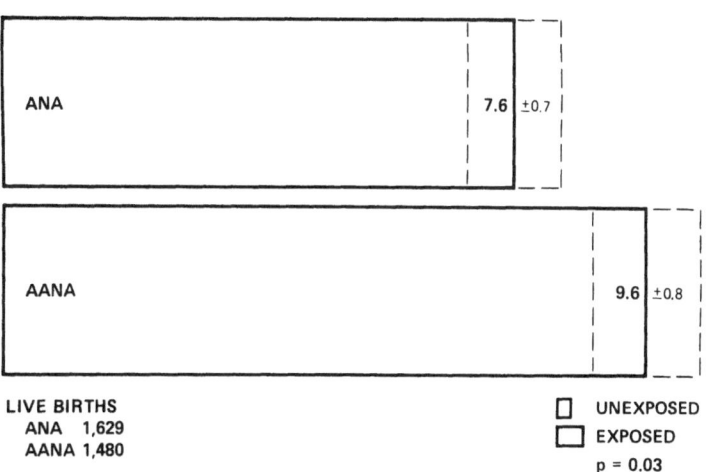

Fig. 3. Standardized congenital abnormality rates for female respondents/100 live births (skin excluded).

defects in a similar comparison of the membership of the ANA and the AANA where the number of births is larger, and significance is achieved. Figure 4 compares the birth defect rate of the membership of the AAP to the non-occupationally exposed wives of male members of the ASA working in the operating room. In this group, approximately 25 percent greater incidence of birth defects is reported. Figure 5 shows cancer data, comparing

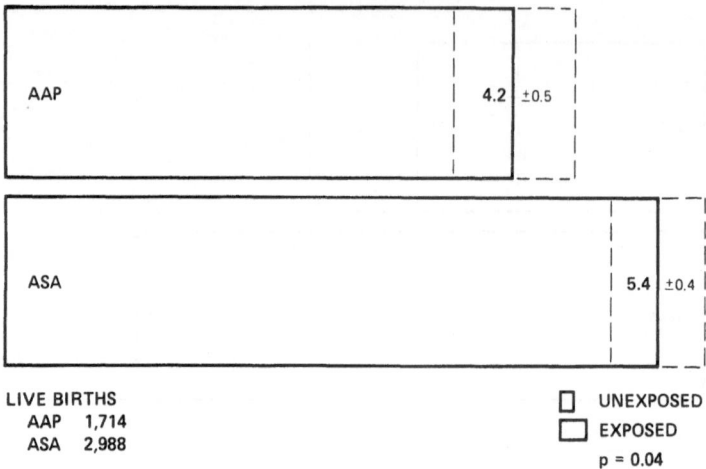

Fig. 4. Standardized congenital abnormality rates/100 live births, wives of exposed males (skin excluded).

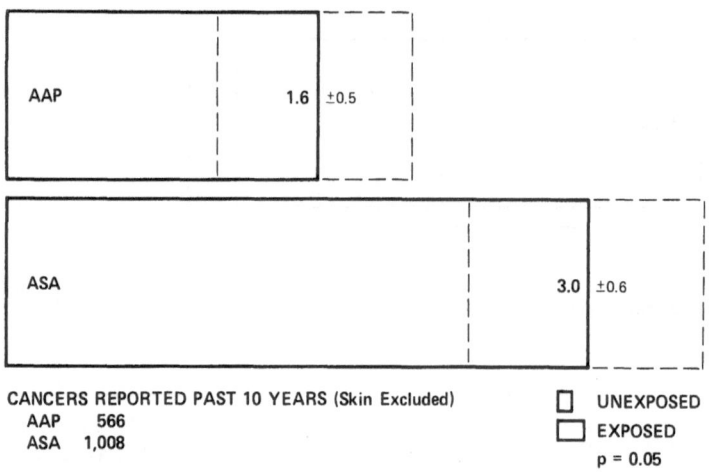

Fig. 5. Age standardized cancer rates/100 female respondents.

the female membership of the ASA and AAP groups. Nearly a twofold difference is apparent. Significance in this group is achieved at the 5 percent level and a similar comparison between the larger memberships of the AANA and ANA groups shows significance at less than the 1 percent level. Figure 6 shows the incidence of liver disease, serum hepatitis excluded. The rate for the pediatricians is 2.9, and for the anesthesiologists is 4.9.

The Ad Hoc Committee also compared the health of 2415 general dentists

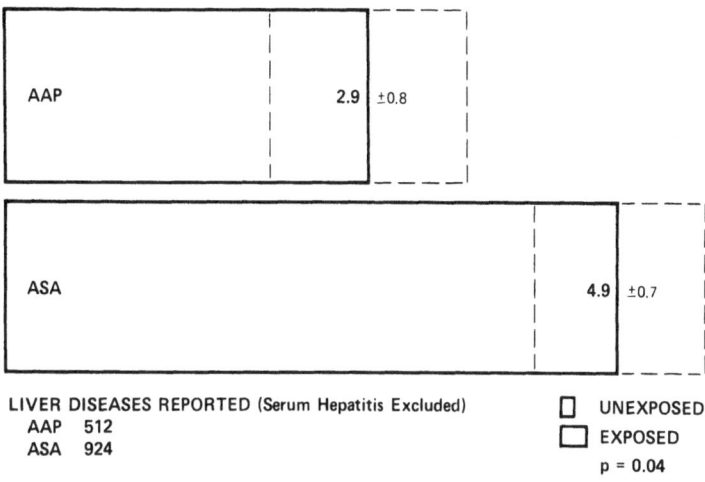

Fig. 6. Liver disease rates/100 female respondents (serum hepatitis excluded).

Table 1. Spontaneous abortion rates per 100 pregnancies (spouses) liver disease rate per 100 respondents.

	Exposed dentists		Unexposed dentists		
	Sample size	Standardized rate $\pm$ S.E.	Sample size	Standardized rate $\pm$ S.E.	p
Spontaneous abortion	887	16.0 $\pm$ 1.8	1541	9.0 $\pm$ 1.0	< 0.01
Liver disease	1528	5.9 $\pm$ 0.4	1249	2.3 $\pm$ 0.4	< 0.01

From Cohen *et al.*, JADA 90: 1291-1296 (June) 1975.

and oral surgeons who administer inhalation anesthesia more than 3 hours per week with 1790 dentists employing such anesthesia less than 3 hours per week. (4) The positive results (table 1) indicate that the spouses of the exposed dentists report spontaneous abortion 1.8 above controls and liver disease, serum hepatitis excluded, 2.6 over controls. This study is of special interest because of the presumed similarity of the experimental versus control groups.

The survey studies indicate an increased incidence of spontaneous abortion, birth defects, cancer, and liver disease in association with employment in the operating room; with the exception of liver disease, only females are affected. The relationship to chronic exposure to trace gases is not proven. Survey studies, no matter how carefully performed, are subject to errors in identifying comparable control groups and in differences of reporting. If a causal relationship actually exists, confirmation may be obtained in the next few years when the survey is scheduled to be repeated. This would occur after waste gas scavenging has been widely adopted and reduction in the incidence of the presumed toxic effects should be detectable.

A cause-effect relationship between the health hazard of the operating room and chronic exposure to the trace gases is strongly suggested by animal experiments. Various species, chronically exposed to any of the inhalation anesthetics tested (ether, cyclopropane, halothane, nitrous oxide, etc.) are subject to adverse effects, such as congenital malformations manifested by skeletal defects, interference with growth, anemia, and malignancy. (5) Corbett (6) has reported fetal lethality (human abortion equivalent) in rats exposed to N_2O at a concentration of 1000 ppm during critical stages of gestation, and Stevens (7) has shown decreased survival rate in various animal species chronically exposed to halothane 0.03 percent and Chang (8) has reported changes in the ultrastructure of the central nervous system and other organs in rats chronically exposed to halothane, and in their offspring.

An entirely different aspect of toxicity is the effect of trace concentrations of anaesthetics on efficiency in performing complex tasks. Quimby (9) has shown such effects in animals, and in man, Bruce has demonstrated decrements in response time to auditory and visual stimuli, impaired learning of memory passages and other adverse effects in response to 15 ppm of halothane (10) or enflurane (11) with 500 ppm N_2O. These concentrations are frequently reported in the unscavenged operating room.

It is notable that no distinction can be made in the relative toxicity of specific anesthetic agents, such as N_2O or halothane. Anaesthetics are frequently employed in combinations and relative toxicity cannot be defined. Moreover, laboratory experiments, both in man and animals, show similarities in the toxic effects of all inhalation agents evaluated.

The weight of the evidence of causal relationship between the health hazards of the operating room and chronic exposure to trace concentrations of inhalation anaesthetics is sufficiently strong that the ad hoc committee of the ASA has recommended that exposure be kept to a minimum.

All inhalation anesthetics are suspect, N_2O as well as potent agents. Because no 'safe' concentration can be defined at this time, it is desirable to maintain an environment containing the lowest concentrations reasonably attainable.

The principle sources of anaesthetic gases in the operating room air include the normal overflow from the unscavenged popoff valve of the CO_2 absorber, site of gas overflow from other breathing systems, leakage in the anaesthetic equipment, and leakage associated with the work practices of the anaesthetist. Relatively insignificant sources include diffusion through the rubber and plastic goods associated with the anesthetic equipment and the patient's skin. Excretion from the patient's lungs upon disconnection from the anaesthetic breathing system is a noticeable but transient source.

Leakage from the anesthetic equipment frequently occurs in worn out plastic and rubber goods, loose, defective, mis-seated or absent gaskets and seals, loose or deformed pipe fittings and slip joints, and cracks in plastic absorber cannisters. Inadequately designed scavenging equipment is a frequent source of leakage. Such equipment leakage is variable and highly influenced by the effectiveness of the equipment maintenance program.

In the absence of scavenging reported concentrations range from 9700 ppm N_2O, 10-85 ppm halothane (12). With scavenging these concentrations may be reduced to 1 ppm N_2O, 0.02 ppm halothane (1).

CALCULATION OF LEAK RATE OF ANAESTHETIC GAS FROM THE ROOM CONCENTRATION

For any known leak rate of an anaesthetic gas from a leak source, such as an anaesthesia machine, a correlation exists between the average mixed concentrations of such a gas present in the operating room air, whether measured by gas analysis or by calculation. This may be determined by measuring the concentrations of N_2O or halothane at the air-conditioning exhaust grille where an average mixed air sample may be obtainable. Assuming perfect mixing and the absence of gas leakage out of the room except via the air-conditioning system, a leak rate of 3 L/min N_2O escaping into the air in an average operating room (volume 4000 ft³), with a nonrecirculating air-conditioning flow rate of 667 ft³/min, the average concentration of N_2O is 159 ppm. Such a room has been considered as a 'standard operating room.' The calculation is shown by:

$$C = \frac{L \times 60 \times 10^6}{N\,V}$$

where

C = concentration of gas in room (ppm)
V = volume of room in liters (L)
N = nonrecirculated room air changes per hour
L = leak rate of gas (L/min)
Example:
Operating room = 20 × 20 × 10 ft = 4000 ft³

therefore

V = 4000 × 28.3 = 113000
N = 10 changes (667 ft³/min, 4000 ft³ room)
L = 3 L

$$C = \frac{3 \times 60 \times 10^6}{10 \times 113000} = 159 \text{ ppm}$$

A simplified expression applicable to a 'standard operating room' is:

leak rate N_2O 100 cc/min = 5.3 ppm room concentration

Similar principles are applicable to the calculation of the leak rate of halothane. This agent is likely to be administered in 1/60th the concentration of N_2O. At a leak rate of 1.7 cc/min of vapor the concentration in the standard room would be 0.9 ppm.

LEAKAGE FROM THE ANAESTHETIC EQUIPMENT

Leakage in the anesthesia machine is an important source of gas contamination in the operating room. A distinction is made between leakage in the high-pressure system (from the central gas source in the operating room to the flowmeter valves) and in the low-pressure system (from the flowmeter valves to the patient). This distinction is of importance because the causes of leakage and methods of detection are different in these major components.
   Leakage of N_2O was measured in a series of anaesthesia machines. These

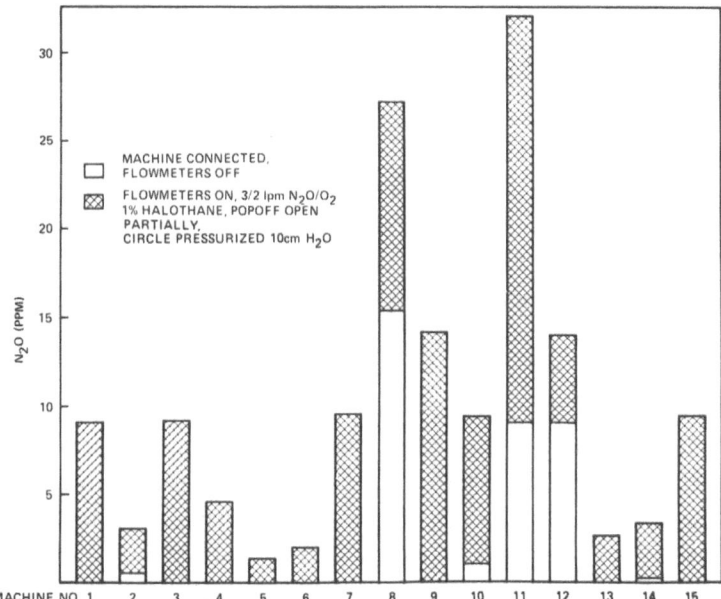

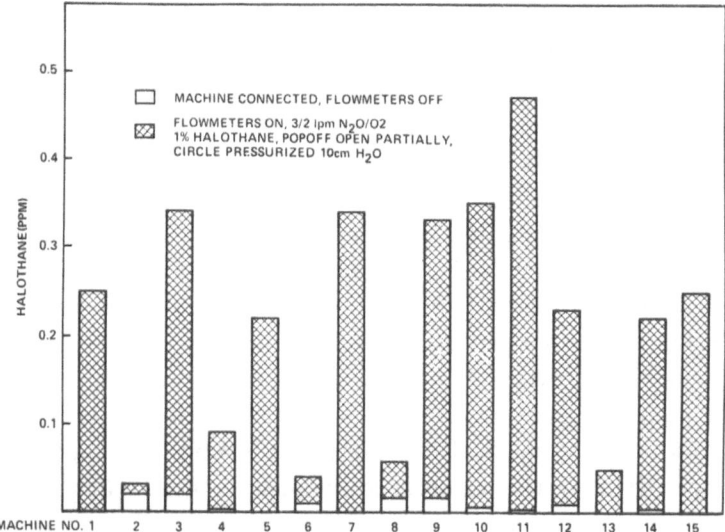

Fig. 7. Average room concentrations of N₂O and halothane from anesthesia machines.

machines had been kept in good repair through regular preventive maintenance at four-month intervals, provided by the manufacturers' service representatives. The tests were conducted in an operating room measuring
$10 \times 20 \times 20$ ft (4000 ft^3) provided with ten non-recirculating air changes
per hour. The doors were sealed; air samples for analyses were obtained at
the air-conditioning exhaust grille where an average mixed sample was
available. To determine the leakage in the high-pressure system, the high-
pressure hoses and scavenging lines were attached and the flowmeters were
turned off. Figure 7 shows the results. In the upper panel each bar represents
leakage in the 15 machines tested, expressed in terms of room concentrations
of N_2O. High pressure leakage of N_2O was detected in widely varying concentrations, represented by the clear areas of the bars. The high was 15 ppm
N_2O for Machine No. 8; the low was 0.5 ppm for Machine No. 14. High
pressure leakage was evaluated only in machines showing such leakage.

Following this test, the total leak was determined. The flowmeters were
turned on at $\frac{3}{2}$ L/min N_2O and O_2 and the absorber system was pressurized to
10 cm H_2O by closing the popoff valve sufficiently. Greater leakage is
apparent, ranging from a high of 32 ppm for Machine 11 to a low of 2 ppm
for Machine 5.

Similar measurements were made of halothane leakage (fig. 7, lower panel).
Again, the clear areas represent the room concentrations of halothane
measured with the machine in the room, attached to the highpressure hoses
with the flowmeters off. A range of concentrations is observed, 0.005 to 0.02
ppm. Following pressurization of the absorber system to 10 cm H_2O, the
total leakage ranged from approximately 4.6 to 0.03 ppm.

A dissociation of leak rates in comparing N_2O and halothane leakage is
evident; that is, a machine showing a high leak rate for one gas did not
necessarily show a high leak rate for another gas. For example, Machine 5
indicates a high leak rate for halothane but not for N_2O, and Machine 8 is
a case in reverse. As a result the fixed ratio 60:1 of N_2O to halothane delivered
by the gas machine is not necessarily present in the air.

Opportunities for such a dissociation of leak rates are evident in considering the design of the anesthetic machine. Relatively high halothane concentrations would be anticipated as a result of leakage from vaporizers of
the Copper Kettle type and associated components because this vaporizer
is located apart from the stream of N_2O. Relatively high N_2O concentrations
will result from any leakage upstream from the Copper Kettle vaporizer.
This dissociation suggests the advisability of measuring both gases in an
air monitoring program.

Following these studies it was found that the high pressure leakage was most easily measured from the room concentration of N_2O, as discussed in the sections on calculation of leak rate and air monitoring, with 1 to 2 ppm usually being found in an average operating room.

Low pressure leakage is classically determined by rapidly filling the absorber system with O_2 while occluding the Y piece and observing for the momentary retention of pressure in the breathing system. This test is inadequate in minimizing personnel exposure to the inhalation anaesthetics. Therefore, a quantitative leak test was developed.

Preparations for the quantitative test shown in figure 8 include removing

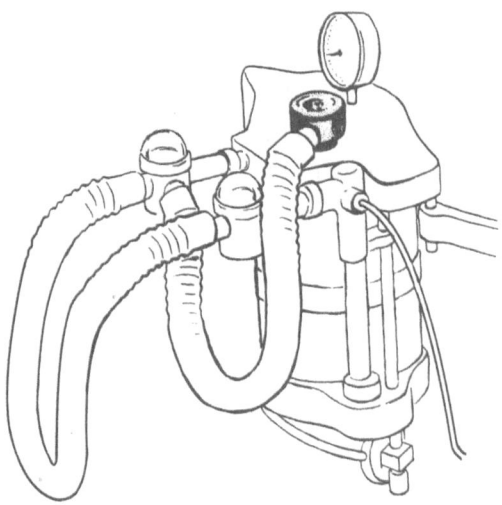

Fig. 8. Quantitative test for low-pressure leakage. 1. Arrange tubing as shown. 2. Open Popoff valve. 3. Adjust fresh gas flow to maintain 30 cm H_2O at absorber pressure gauge.

the breathing bag, attaching the high pressure hoses and connecting the inhalation and exhalation breathing valves with one length of breathing tubing. The other length of breathing tubing is employed in connecting the bag outlet with the scavenging popoff valve. This valve is fully open and the vaporizer switch is turned on in order to include these components. With these preparations, a low range O_2 flowmeter calibrated to 20 cc/min or less is turned on at a rate sufficient to maintain a constant static pressure of 30 cm H_2O measured on the absorber pressure gauge. Once equilibration has been achieved, the flow rate in cc per minute is taken as the leak rate of the low-pressure system. Caution is necessary in performing this test to avoid damaging the gauge by overpressurization. The gauge rather than the flowmeter is carefully observed during adjustment of O_2 flow. Following preventive maintenance by the manufacturer's service personnel, the low pressure leak rate should be less than 20 cc/min; following changes of soda-lime by in-house personnel a more rapid leak rate may be acceptable, up to 100 cc/min. This test can be completed in less than 1 min and is submitted as suitable for routine use.

For this test the use of an O_2 flowmeter is suggested in the interest of minimizing occupational gas exposure. However, a flowmeter for N_2O or O_2 via vaporizer could be employed.

The breathing bag must be removed from the gas machine for the quantitative test because its compliance excessively retards pressure equilibration. The bag may be quickly tested after replacement on the absorber by inflating it with oxygen to a pressure of at least 50 cm H_2O and then palpating the surface for any cooling sensation indicative of leakage.

The quantitative leak testing procedure serves to identify significant leakage in most anesthesia machines. The important exception is machines equipped with check valves located between the absorber pressure gauge and the flowmeter control valves. Such machines could appear to be gas tight despite gross leakage from the vaporizer or any flowmeter not actually turned on in performing the quantitative test. Indeed, a large leak in the oxygen system could result in severe hypoxia. To exclude possible accidents as well as leakage with these machines it is necessary to determine which circuits include check valves in the low pressure system. A knowledgeable service representative could provide this information. Each circuit with a check valve should be clearly marked on the machine. In the event that only circuits provided with low range flowmeters include check valves, each circuit so equipped is individually leak tested with the quantitative test as described above.

If high range flowmeters are protected with check valves, located downstream from the flowmeter control valve, the testing procedure is more complicated. These circuits may be tested via the following supplemental procedures:

Preparations include attaching a durable manometer, such as an aneroid blood pressure gauge, to the fresh gas outlet of the machine. The gas delivery tubing downstream from the gauge is occluded by kinking or clamping. In turn, each high range flowmeter protected by a check valve is momentarily turned on, barely long enough to observe a pressure increase of approximately 100 torr. Interpretation of this test is subjective, with a large momentary flow past the control valve suggesting a significant leak downstream. As with the quantitative test, possible damage to the gauge, due to overpressurization, is minimized by observing the pressure gauge rather than the flowmeter. The inconvenience of the test is reduced by permanently mounting and plumbing the gauge on the machine.

In conclusion, it is apparent that leak testing procedures enhance the safety of the patient while reducing personnel exposure to the trace anesthetics. A few conscientious anesthetists will carefully leak test their machines before each use or arrange for technicians to do so. Even the crude leak testing procedures offer a degree of protection both to the patient and to personnel; the more refined procedures offer a higher degree of protection. The safety of the patient is further enhanced by providing a carefully maintained O_2 analyzer in the breathing circuit. Personnel exposure, regardless of the leak testing procedures, requires periodic evaluation in the air monitoring program.

Gas leakage from the other scavenged breathing systems (nonrebreathing and T-tube) was insignificant because the design of these systems is inherently leakproof. Leakage could be determined by pressurization and immersion in water.

Despite scavenging attachments, the ventilator was identified as a significant source of gas leakage. This leak source was evaluated in nine ventilators, removed from routine clinical service and attached to a low leak anaesthesia machine in an operating room (surgery not in progress). Methods of air sampling and analysis were similar to those used in measuring leakage in the anesthesia machines. These ventilators were leak tested by measuring their contribution to N_2O in the room air during simulated clinical use inflating the test lung attached to an anesthesia machine. The contribution of the anaesthesia machine under static conditions without the ventilator was first determined. This was accomplished with the test lung in place and flowrates of N_2O and O_2, 3 to 2 L/min each, established on the machine. The popoff valve was then closed sufficiently to maintain a fixed pressure of 15 cm H_2O in the low pressure system measured on the absorber pressure gauge. Following equilibration the N_2O concentration present in the room air was recorded as the leak rate of the machine. Then the popoff valve was closed, and the ventilator was attached and adjusted to cycle at a rate of 20/min, at peak pressure of 30 cm H_2O. This value was chosen to approximate the 15 cm H_2O static pressure test of the anaesthesia machine alone. The room air was allowed to equilibrate to the leak rate of the ventilator

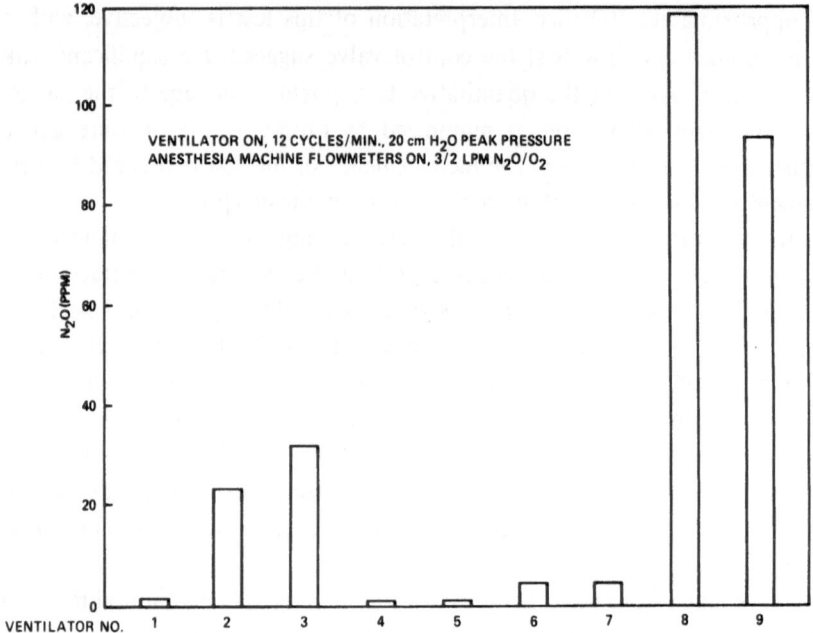

Fig. 9. Room concentrations of N_2O from scavenged ventilators.

plus gas machine. By subtracting the leak rate of the anaesthesia machine the leak rate of the ventilator was determined. Results shown in figure 9 indicate ventilator leakage ranging from 0.5 to nearly 120 ppm N_2O. A gas-tight ventilator should contribute no more than 1 to 2 ppm of N_2O in the 'standard operating room.'

This test should be performed at least when any ventilator is first placed in service following purchase or repair. It is a time-consuming test which most suites are likely to employ mainly with a special effort to identify an obscure source of leakage.

Other tests for leakage were conducted in other pieces of anaesthetic equipment. It was found that a few widely sold scavenging components were so designed that considerable leakage occurred under conditions of normal clinical use. It was apparent that devices marketed for waste gas control are not necessarily efficient. An example shown in figure 22 is a device designed for equalizing pressure differences when waste gases are removed by suction (tube-within-a-tube interfacing system). Unless a high suction flow rate was available, gross leakage could occur from the room air inlet every time the anesthetist squeezed the breathing bag. This underscores the observation that equipment sold for scavenging varies greatly in efficiency, not necessarily doing what is reasonably expected of it.

Assuming well designed and well maintained equipment, one important leak source remains. This is related to the work practices of the anesthetist. Leakage under the face mask may be insignificant, given an average face and a skilled anaesthetist fully informed on waste gas control measures. However, at least until an anaesthetist has administered anaesthesia during use of a trace gas analyzer, leakage under the face mask commonly occurs without his knowledge. A more obvious cause of leakage is failure to employ the available equipment; for example, the disposal hose may not be connected.

The contribution of the anaesthetist's techniques is highly variable. Under rigidly controlled conditions during clinical anaesthesia, anaesthetists have been observed to maintain room concentrations of N_2O below 1 ppm even with face mask technique. Other anaesthetists are frequently found to regularly maintain 50 to 100 ppm N_2O. It is reasonable to maintain less than 10 ppm. Such concentrations may be facilitated through the following procedures:

1. Equipment is purchased and maintained with low leakage in mind.
2. The anaesthetist is instructed in the use of low leakage techniques. These are:
   a. Confirm that the waste gas disposal lines are properly connected.
   b. Select a face mask that will ensure a tight fit with minimal pressure.
   c. When filling the vaporizer, use the funnel or keyed filler system to avoid spillage.
   d. Switch the vaporizer off when not in use.
   e. If it is your practice to turn on the N_2O before the induction of ana-esthesia, make use of a Y-piece provided with a shut- off valve; otherwise, cap the end of the Y-piece before the mask is attached and open the popoff valve. The gases will then escape via the scavenging system. Crutch tips may be used as caps.
   f. After anaesthesia has started, avoid disconnecting the patient from the breathing circuit unless flowmeters are turned off or the Y-piece is sealed.
   g. If it is necessary to empty the breathing bag, empty it into the scavenging system without disconnecting it from the absorber or patient.
   h. When terminating the case, try to wash the anaesthetic agents out of the patient with oxygen, leaving him attached to the breathing system as long as convenient. It is good patient care to give extra oxygen at this time.

The pump oxygenator employed in cardiopulmonary bypass procedures must be considered a potential leak source. Inhalation anaesthetics administered to the patient up to the time bypass is instituted are washed out of the blood as it passes through the oxygenator. If inhalation anaesthesia is continued via the oxygenator the gases flowing through will enter the operating room air. To prevent occupational exposure from this source the oxygenator must be attached to a waste gas disposal system.

The last source of anaesthetic gas contamination to be considered is the patient himself with his 30 liters of dissolved N_2O and other gases. Upon disconnection of the breathing system this N_2O is rapidly exhaled. As a result increased concentrations are regularly observed both in the operating room and in the recovery area. In the Stanford recovery room with its nonrecirculating air conditioning, personnel rarely inhale average concentrations greater than 5 to 10 ppm N_2O. However, when the patient first arrives much higher concentrations (hundreds to thousands of ppm) may exist in the expired air. The elimination of the more soluble agents would be sustained over a longer period of time. Occupational exposure could be minimized by avoiding the patient's expired air.

DISTRIBUTION OF GASES IN THE OPERATING ROOM

Any gases introduced into the air in the operating room are distributed by the air-conditioning system. This system is of prime importance because of its effect on the distribution of gases. It also provides a disposal pathway for the collected gases.

Significant factors in the distribution of gases include the dilution rate (fresh air exchange) and the method of dispersing the air as in enters the room. The higher the air exchange rate the lower the trace gas concentrations; however, high flow rates are costly and may cause drafts, and many people are uncomfortable at air exchange rates above 15/hour. Drafts are reduced by the careful choice and location of the supply grille. Efficient diffusers, including the aspirating and entrainment types, tend to mix the room air at uniform velocity, thereby reducing drafts and localized high concentrations of anesthetics ('hot spots'). Air-conditioning systems induce a slightly positive pressure in the operating room with respect to the adjacent hallway, and a slight outward movement of air is maintained.

Air-conditioning systems are either recirculating or nonrecirculating (fig. 10). The nonrecirculating system takes in exterior air and processes it

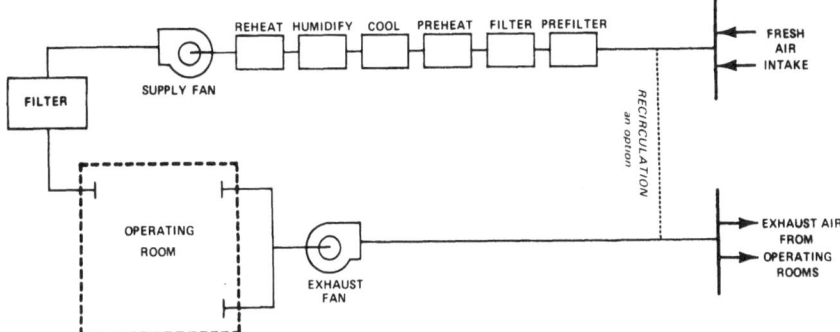

Fig. 10. Air-conditioning systems.

by filtering, heating, cooling, and adjusting humidity. This processed air is circulated through the operating room and then exhausted 100 percent to the atmosphere. The air exchange rate available in different suites may vary between 6 and 25 changes per hour although the latter is a minimum requirement.* With such air-conditioning, waste gases collected from the anaesthetic breathing system could be disposed of directly into the exhaust duct system.

In contrast, with recirculating air conditioning, a small amount of exterior air is taken in from the atmosphere, a minimum of five air changes per hour, and a similar small amount of air is exhausted. Most of the exhaust air (20 air exchanges per hour) is shunted back into the intake and recirculated into the operating room. In a recirculating system, waste gases may be disposed of at a carefully chosen site in the exhaust system, downstream from the shunt, thereby ensuring that the waste anaesthetics will not be circulated anywhere within the building.

In the past, recirculating systems were not used because of the danger of recirculating bacteria-contaminated air. With the high efficiency particulate air (HEPA) filters, recirculation is now possible; however, these filters do not remove anaesthetic gases.

Even if the waste gases are emptied into the exhaust duct beyond the bypass, the recirculating system is less effective in the removal of waste gases than the nonrecirculating system. Scavenging does not pick up 100 percent of leakage gases and the residual is always present in the operating room. This is removed in proportion to the fresh air exchange rate, which is low in most recirculating systems.

* Recommended *minimum* air exchange rate widely quoted[13] is 25/hr which is greater than actually found in many operating rooms.

Another consideration relating to the use of air-conditioning systems for waste gas disposal is the pressure drop downstream in the exhaust duct. If waste anaesthetic gases are introduced at the exhaust grille, negative pressure is low and does not interfere with the breathing systems. If such waste gases, however, are introduced at a distance downstream in the duct where the negative pressure is greater, interference with the breathing system may result. Pressure equalization then becomes necessary, as discussed in the section on scavenging.

Laminar-flow air conditioning must be considered in relation to anaesthetic gas scavenging. These systems usually recirculate. The air enters at a velocity typically 90 ft/min, spread over a large surface area approximately 90 percent or more of a wall or ceiling. A 'standard operating room' (10 × 20 × 20 ft with an end-wall area of 200 ft²) would be provided with a flow rate of at least 9000 ft³/min, and the amount of fresh air is approximately 5 percent of the recirculated air, or 450 ft³/min. Under these circumstances, the calculated trace gas concentrations are 32 percent higher than in a standard room provided with 667 ft³/min of nonrecirculated air.

A phenomenon conceivably occurring with laminar-flow systems is that, because of the lack of turbulence, any anaesthetic gases leaking into the air could be carried without much dilution toward personnel and could cause heavy exposure. This emphasizes the desirability of the working-room survey study of the distribution of gases during clinical anaesthesia, as described in the section on air monitoring.

In disposing of waste anaesthetic gases via the air-conditioning system, these gases must go directly out, without contaminating the air in other hospital areas. It may be difficult to ascertain that all such gases are actually exhausted. Errors in construction or an unfortunate choice of disposal site upwind from an air intake could result in the contamination of intake air and permit an insidious recirculation of anaesthetic gases. A gas analysis at the air conditioning inlet in the room could provide assurance that no internal contamination exists.

The rapid air exchange rates in operating rooms may result in prompt and thorough mixing of anaesthetic gases. Although the anaesthetic agents are heavier than air, specific gravity effects may be noticeable only at reduced air exchange rates, below 10/hr. A few areas of poor mixing are found where concentrations are lower or higher than the room average; these are referred to as 'hot spots.' Neglecting these, the predominating phenomenon can be rapid and complete mixing. In such operating suites, when scavenging is practices, it makes little difference where one samples in the room;

Table 2. Halothane (ppm) at Sampling Sites.

| Floor | Ceiling | Exhaust grille | 3 Ft level Ft from Popoff valve | |
			3	1
0.47	.40	0.44	.62	2.22
± 0.09	± 0.09	± 0.11	± 0.13	± 0.37

Conditions: Scavenging employed. Nonrecirculating air conditioning. Halothane delivery to patient ~ 1%, in 4 to 5 L/min diluent gas n = 11 measurements, each sampling site. ± S.E.
Adapted from Whitcher et al., Anesthesiology 35: 348 (1971).

all concentrations are similar, except in locations close to the anaesthesia machine (table 2). This has also been demonstrated for N_2O (section on air monitoring).

Discharging the waste gas at floor level in the mistaken belief that most of it will be swept out by the air-conditioning system without mixing has been recommended as a method of reducing personnel exposure. The ineffectiveness of this method is obvious.

WASTE GAS SCAVENGING IN THE HOSPITAL

One of the most important factors in waste gas control programs is scavenging. This is defined as collecting waste gases at the breathing system and eliminating them from the operating room. The purpose is to protect personnel from unnecessary exposure.

A scavenging system consists of two major components: a collecting device (or scavenging adapter) to collect waste gases, and a disposal system to carry the gases out of the room. The collecting device should trap the waste gases at the site of release from the breathing system in order to avoid spillage into the room air. The disposal system should exhaust the waste gases to the atmosphere without contaminating any air intakes in compliance with local state air pollution, building, and fire codes.

COLLECTION OF WASTE GASES FROM THE BREATHING SYSTEMS

Circle absorber

Figure 11 is a typical collection system for the circle absorber, consisting of an air-tight enclosure surrounding the popoff valve.

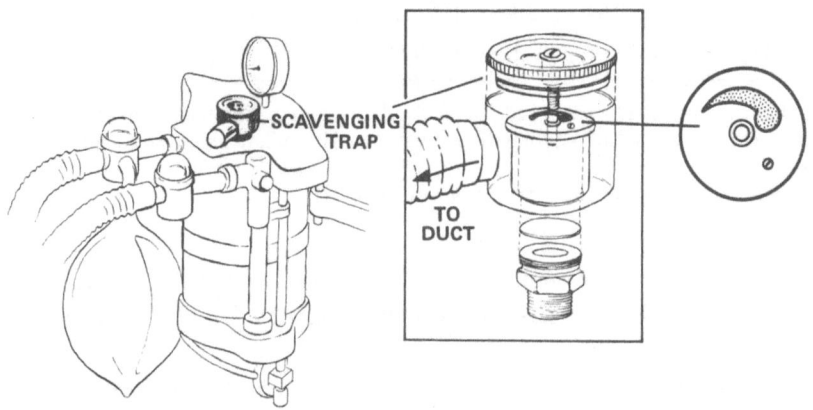

Fig. 11. Dupaco scavenging popoff valve for circle absorber.

Ventilator

The ventilators for anaesthesia use may be equipped with waste gas collecting devices; some are built into the ventilator, and others are attached accessories.

When the ventilators are used during anaesthetic administration, the scavenging collector device from the ventilator can be connected to a Y-piece (fig. 12) through which the effluent gases from the scavenging popoff valve and the ventilator are carried to the disposal system. The Y-piece eliminates the need to reattach the disposal tubing when alternating between ventilator and manual breathing.

The ventilators should be equipped with a one-way check valve located in the waste gas disposal line adjacent to the ventilator. This valve prevents waste gases from leaking from the anaesthesia machine through the ventilator and into the room when the ventilator is attached to the disposal system while detached from the patient.

It proved difficult to find a check valve that will not leak under any circumstance. The pressure present in many disposal systems approaches atmospheric and tends to discourage the firm seating of many of the available

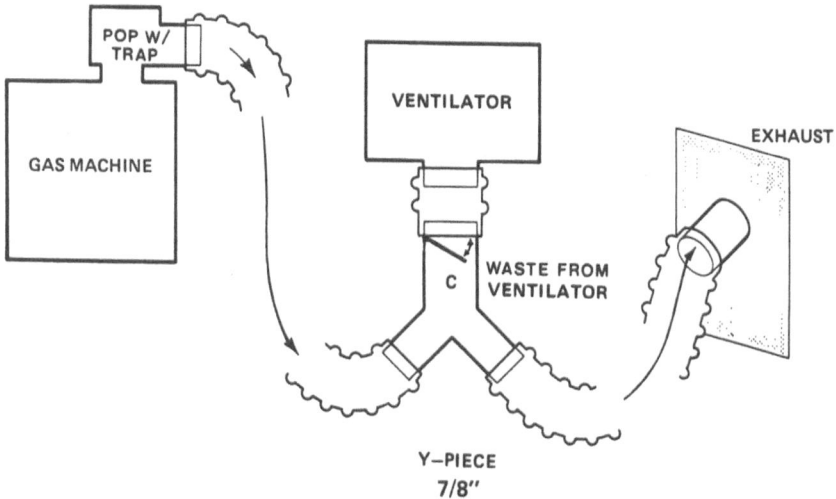

Fig. 12. Use of a Y-piece to collect waste gas from absorber and ventilator. Check valve (C) prevents leakage when ventilator is detached from breathing system.

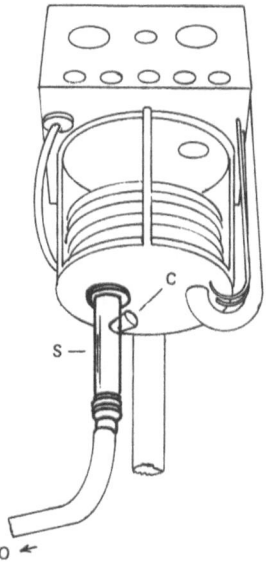

Fig. 13. Modification of gas collector device for Bennett Ventilator. Collector is indicated at S. Stopper at C occludes suction outlet. Waste gasses pass at O.

valves. This is not easy to recognize. Even the suggested Divilbiss valve was modified by sealing two small holes adjacent to the valve seat.

The Bennett scavenging trap (fig. 13) is intended exclusively for waste gas disposal into the suction system. This is an undesirable constraint and, in addition, there is no provision for receiving the effluent from the gas machine. As a result, this device was modified by sealing the suction outlet and attaching a Y-piece at the outlet.

The scavenging adapter, manufactured by Monaghan for the Ohio and Monaghan units, was found to be gas tight. The Ohio adapter, however, tended to leak.

The Air-Shields Ventimeter ventilator when provided with a specially lapped relief valve (an internal component of the ventilator) proved to be relatively gas tight. Current production units include this improvement. The manufacturer has indicated that field conversion kits for older units will be available. It was noted that this ventilator added 10 to 15 L/min of driving gas (the gas employed to operate the ventilator) to the disposal line. If the operating room suction system is used for waste gas disposal, this extra capacity must be available.

Nonrebreathing system

In the nonrebreathing system evaluated in this study, with a scavenging adapter (fig. 14), fresh anaesthetic gases enter at the breathing bag and all excess gases leave through the adapter. This valve is especially sensitive to negative pressure; the bag tended to empty unless the system was vented into a disposal pathway presenting a slight positive pressure.

T-tube, modified (Jackson-Reece; Summers)

With this T-tube (fig. 15), fresh anesthetic gases enter the system at the side arm. All exhaust leaves the tail of the bag and, employing the collection system developed in the present study, this exhaust passes through an adapter attached to the disposal line. Accidental occlusion of the tail of the bag, by twisting on itself, is prevented by inserting a length of plastic tubing or a plastic wafer through the tail into the lumen. When the plastic tubing method is employed, accidental disassembly is prevented by tightly fitting the tubing into the tail (an assembly operation facilitated by the use of a stylet). The tubing, being resilient, allows the pinch clamp to compress the tail of the bag together with the contained plastic tubing, thereby achieving the desired degree of occlusion required for intermittent positive pressure breathing. With the plastic wafer method, the outflow may be

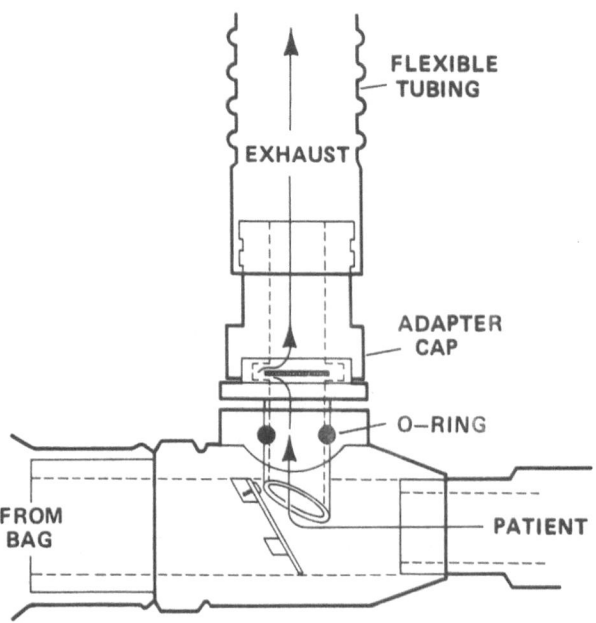

Fig. 14. Waste gas collector for Dupaco nonrebreathing valve. Effluent gases captured by adapter cap.

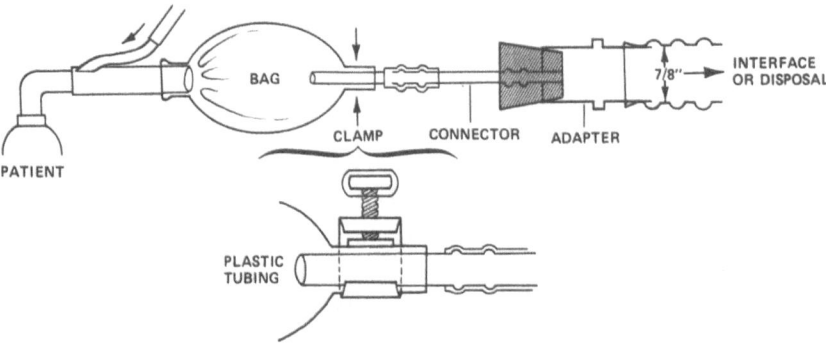

Fig. 15. Waste gas collector for T-tube. Effluent gases are captured at tail of bag. Occlusion of outflow at tail of bag due to twisting is prevented by plastic tubing.
System begins with plastic tubing tightly fitted into tail of bag and projecting into lumen. This prevents accidental occlusion due to twisting of tail. Adjustment of screw clamp permits deliberate partial occlusion of tail, necessary for IPPB. Connector, cork and adapter provide a disposal route not subject to accidental disconnection.

occluded either with the fingers or the clamp. A tight connection between the cork and the disposal system is facilitated by inserting a plastic adapter. It is emphasized that the convenience of this method is enhanced by the use of a short length of highly flexible lightweight disposal tubing, with a loop fixed to the operating table to prevent traction on the breathing bag.

Disposal of waste anaesthetic gases
Waste anaesthetic gases once collected at the anesthetic breathing system must be disposed of, usually into the atmosphere. Any applicable codes related to building, fire, and air pollution must be considered. A functionally gas-tight connection between the breathing system and the disposal system is required because the air-conditioning system does not efficiently remove waste gases escaping into the air in the operating room. With the low pressure disposal techniques (air-conditioning exhaust and special low velocity duct), the collector device may be directly connected to the disposal system. In contrast, disposal into the central vacuum system requires special components for equalizing the pressure, and a flowmeter is desirable for monitoring the suction flow.

It is emphasized that waste gas disposal must be engineered to avoid contamination of intake air or of areas where personnel are working.

Air-conditioning exhaust
The simplest disposal system routes the anaesthetic waste gases from the scavenging trap directly to the room's air-conditioning exhaust grille (fig. 16) where the sweeping effect of the air flowing into the grille carries all waste gases outside. A minor hazard to the patient may result from an accidental occlusion of the tubing that connects the scavenging collector to the grille, which may cause a temporarily overfilled breathing bag; this problem can be prevented by providing a positive pressure relief valve. No such valve was employed in the present studies and this type of disposal system has been used at Stanford University Hospital since 1969 and in another large operating suite without significant complications. In the present experimental studies, the negative pressure measured at the junction of the anaesthetic breathing and disposal systems was in the range of 0 to -4.4 mm H_2O.

One device intended for waste gas disposal into the air conditioning system (Ohio) discharges the waste gases at right angles to the flow of the air-conditioning exhaust; however, leakage into the operating room may occur in the presence of low air-conditioning flow rates. It is safer to di-

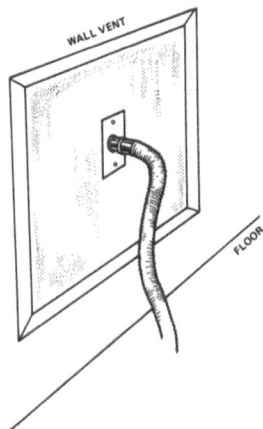

Fig. 16. Waste gas disposal to grille of non-recirculating air conditioning system located in operating room.

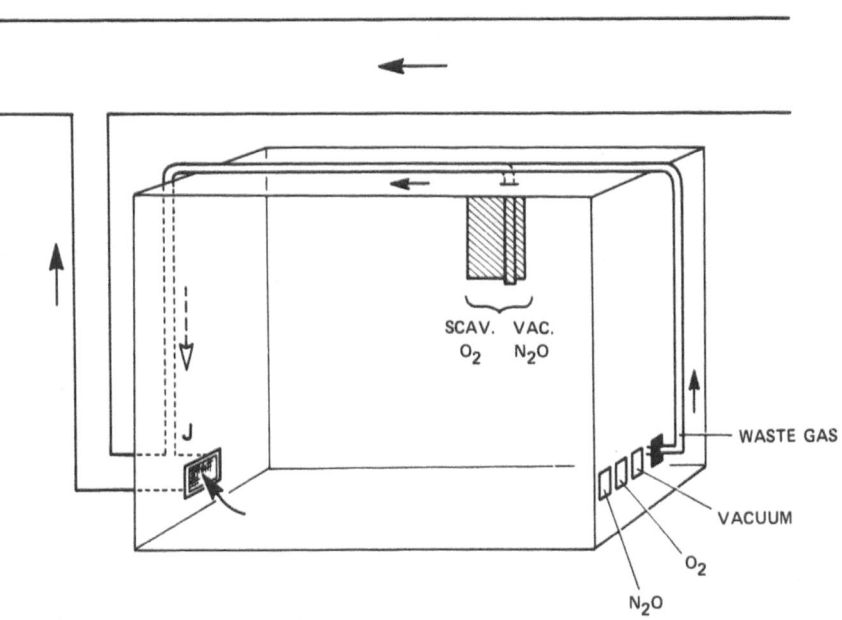

Fig. 17. Concealed access to air-conditioning exhaust.

scharge the waste gases in line with the exhaust stream. The simple method illustrated in figure 16 uses a metal plate drilled to accept a 1 inch length of $\frac{7}{8}$ inch copper tubing for receiving the disposal line.

In recirculating air-conditioning systems, the exhaust can be employed if the waste gases are introduced into the exhaust duct by entering downstream from the point of recirculation (fig. 10). Negative pressure increases downstream in the exhaust system and may be sufficient to empty the breathing bag. If so, interfacing equipment is required.

In some operating rooms, the air-conditioning exhaust vent is separated from the anesthesia machine, thereby requiring a long length of disposal tubing. This objectionable feature is eliminated by arranging the tube to follow the same path as the anaesthetic gas supply hoses. A wall or ceiling service panel may be connected to a permanently concealed waste gas line joined to the air-conditioning exhaust duct in the crawl space. The location of this junction can be critical. Because negative pressure increases with the proximity to the exhaust fan, a large enough pressure imbalance may exist to empty the breathing bag. In such rooms, the negative pressure is balanced by locating the junction in a concealed site close to the exhaust grille (J, fig. 17). Other pressure balancing methods also are applicable. If electrical outlets are close to the service area and flammable agents are used, this disposal route could be hazardous.

Low velocity specialized duct system
Another disposal route for the waste anaesthetic gases is a separate low velocity duct system leading to the atmosphere (fig. 18). As with all waste gas disposal, any applicable codes related to building, fire, and air pollution must be considered.

In this study, and by this technique, waste gases from two operating rooms were collected into a common duct that led to a duct main and were discharged at the roof. A fan provided sufficient negative pressure and air flow to ensure that cross contamination in the operating room did not occur.

With the special duct system it was found that negative pressure was sufficient to open certain popoff valves (Ohio and Dupaco) and to empty the breathing bag. It was noted that, under the clinical conditions of this study, all the anaesthetists, without special instructions, compensated for this condition by partially closing the popoff valves. Excessive negative pressures also may be compensated for, using pressure balancing devices.

In planning the installation of a special duct system, all factors that could

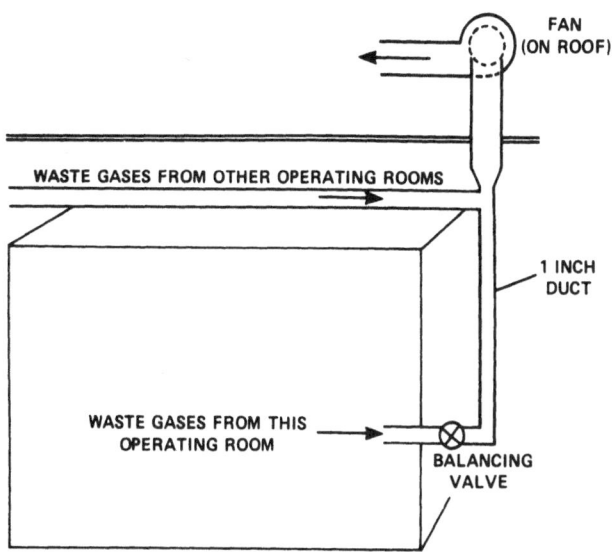

Fig. 18. Low-velocity duct system for waste gas disposal.

possibly influence its performance must be considered. For example, markedly varying positive pressures among certain operating rooms could cause reduced flow in one of the room disposal ducts and result in leakage. Leakage also could occur if the reservoir volume in the short lengths of disposal tubing is very small. The volume between gas machines must be sufficient to accept the short rapid pulses that occur when the anaesthetist compresses the breathing bag. Any possibility of leakage could be reduced by inserting a scavenging reservoir bag near the breathing system.

Suitable materials for the duct must be selected. Special duct systems installed during the present study employed polyvinyl chloride or stainless steel piping. Nylobraide* could have been used.

A separate duct for venting waste gases directly outside without the use of a fan may be an acceptable alternative, but several limitations are apparent. A separate line would be required for each operating room to prevent the cross contamination with waste gases among the operating rooms. A safe disposal site would be necessary. The possible effects of variations in wind velocities and direction suggests the necessity of a means for preventing a reverse flow in the disposal system. A standard gravity ventilator diverter

* A flexible plastic tubing armored with molded-in plastic mesh; available from dealers in plastic tubing

should be considered (available through heating and air-conditioning dealers).

Despite these limitations, the separate duct without the use of a fan may be ideal in older hospitals constructed with windows that are not opened and in the absence of nonrecirculating air conditioning.

In the present studies, the special duct system was designed to function at approximately atmospheric pressure. However, a continuum of designs is conceivable, beginning with systems operating at atmospheric pressure and extending up to standard line vacuum.

Fire, building, and air pollution codes do not specifically provide for low velocity anesthetic waste gas disposal systems. Exhaust fans in areas intended for the storage of flammable agents, however, must be installed near the disposal site and have nonsparking wheels (14).

Central vacuum system

The central vacuum system available in operating rooms can be used for waste gas disposal. A prime consideration is to ensure that the lines and vacuum pump have the capacity required for the extra burden of scavenging. Even more important is a vacuum break (an interface or pressure balancing system, described later this section) located between the suction outlet in the operating room and the anaesthetic breathing system. This interface must not leak anesthetic gases and must provide absolute assurance that the unrestricted negative pressure cannot enter the anaesthetic breathing system and possibly cause atelectasis (collapse of the patient's lungs).

One method of waste gas disposal by suction is to install three separate outlets that enter the same suction line, one for the surgeon, one for the anaesthetist for removal of secretions, and one reserved exclusively for waste gas disposal. A completely separate suction system with its own lines and vacuum pump may be ideal and has been employed in new construction.

In the absence of the three suction outlets, a single outlet can be branched to provide separate lines, one each for patient secretions and for waste gas disposal. In figure 19 the branch is indicated by the letter T. This system includes a suction flowmeter and control valve, plus a shut-off valve for the line intended for secretions. This equipment is mounted on the anaesthesia machine within easy reach of the anaesthetist. With an efficient interfacing system requiring a relatively small amount of suction, sufficient suction was available for scavenging and secretion. In an emergency, the convenience of the controls permitted dedication of all suction to the removal of secretions. Although the diagram (fig. 19) is quite complicated, the anesthesia machine with this equipment properly attached appears reasonably tidy.

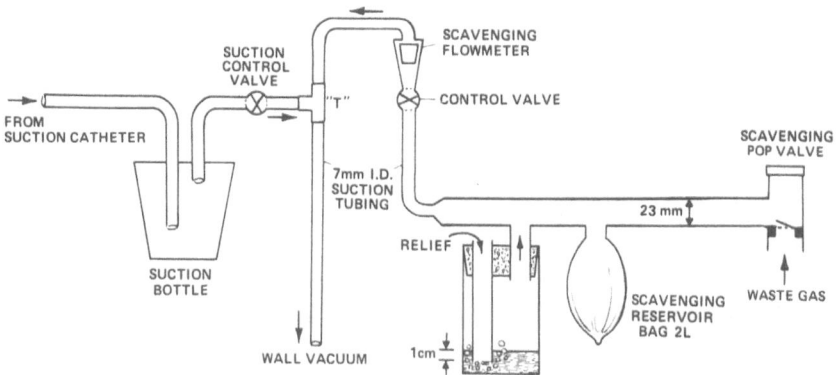

Fig. 19. Disposal into wall suction – one outlet.

A questionable objection to the use of suction for waste gas disposal relates to possible corrosive effects of the anaesthetic gases on the vacuum pump. The exclusive use of suction for scavenging would maximize the possibility of corrosion, but the shared use for surgical purposes would result in a massive dilution of the anaesthetic mixture. The average flow rate of anaesthetic gases rarely exceeds 5 L/min, and the surgical suction alone flowing at 30 L/min or more would result in a maximum increase in the concentration of oxidants (N_2O and O_2) of 11 percent above room air values which would be unlikely to damage the pump.

One difficulty with the normal wall suction system is that its use in the disposal of flammable agents is prohibited. (14) Nevertheless, there appears to be no conflict with the requirements of this code if the usual oil lubricated suction pump is replaced by a water-sealed unit.

The disposal of halogenated anesthetics into a canister containing activated charcoal has been recommended. The concentration of halothane is reduced, but N_2O is not significantly absorbed by this method.

One ineffective disposal method vents the waste gases from the popoff valve to the floor in the mistaken belief that anaesthetic gases, being heavier than air, will settle to the floor away from personnel. Clinical and laboratory tests indicate that the distribution of N_2O and halothane may be essentially uniform throughout the operating room and the gases are thoroughly mixed by the movement of the personnel and by the air-conditioning system (table 2). These factors discount this 'floor venting' method.

Pressure balancing or interfacing

Any marked pressure differential between the anaesthetic breathing system and the disposal piping or duct must be equalized to prevent interference with the breathing system, such as a collapse of the breathing bag or a collapse of the patient's lungs.

If the disposal system presents a slight negative pressure, up to 5 torr, pressure balancing can be achieved by adjusting the scavenging popoff valve. The spring loaded Ohio valve, for example, can be regulated by turning the adjustment screw; the disk-type Dupaco valve can be adjusted by substituting a metal disk for the lightweight plastic disk usually provided. Appropriately weighted disks are available from the manufacturer, and installation requires disassembly of the valve.

It has been noted that the nonrebreathing system is particularly sensitive to slightly negative pressures. Such pressures can be controlled by the popoff valve on the absorber (fig. 20). The bag outlet and the inhalation valve are

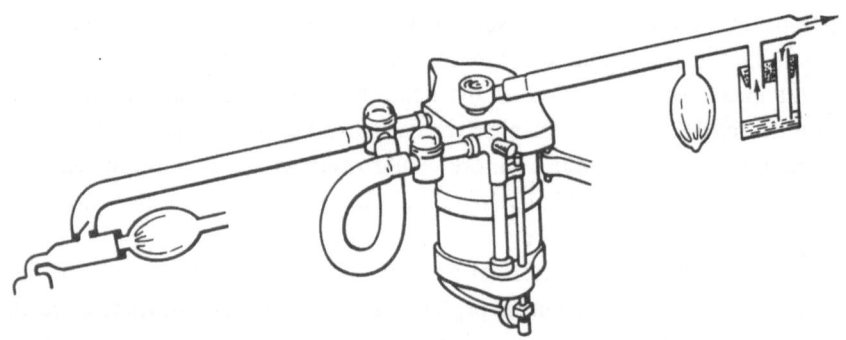

Fig. 20. Use of Absorber circuit for waste gas disposal.

connected, and the fresh gas inlet is closed. The effluent from the nonrebreathing valve is then introduced into the exhalation valve and passed through the popoff valve to the disposal system. This method is particularly satisfactory with the Ohio popoff valve because it is easily adjusted.

Negative pressure greater than 5 torr requires special interfacing equipment for additional pressure equalization. In the present studies the equipment requiring the least suction flow was the liquid-sealed interface shown in figure 19. The liquid employed was a nonflammable, nonvolatile silicone liquid (Dow Corning 550 or 200). During use, the waste gases leave the anesthetic breathing system, and the scavenging reservoir bag temporarily stores high peak flow rates, thereby contributing to pressure relief and the prevention of leakage.

This method developed by Summitt Services is simple in principle with its similarity to the underwater seal for chest drainage. It presents a combination of advantages not realized by any other method, such as low leakage at minimum suction flow, universal applicability to all scavenging traps and disposal systems, and a visible indication when its functioning is efficient or not. But it may prove to be uneconomical for routine use because of its complexity and the availability of improved interfacing devices from other manufacturers.

Another commercially available interfacing system, designed exclusively for use with the wall suction, was evaluated (Dupaco, fig. 21). A valve is

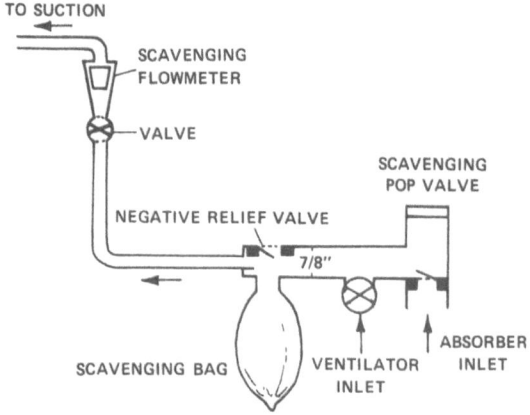

Fig. 21. Dupaco interface.

installed for negative pressure relief, and a degree of protection against excessive positive pressure is supplied by the scavenging reservoir bag. Inputs to receive waste gases from the ventilator and absorber are provided. Considerable difficulty was encountered in adjusting the suction because resistance to flow through the relief valve can cause inappropriate emptying of the breathing bag. This problem was reduced by improving the control of suction through the addition of a flowmeter and adjusting the scavenging popoff valve.

Other interfaces designed for use with the wall suction have recently appeared on the market. Foregger has an interface with relief valves for both positive and negative pressures. Boehringer has a largevolume, tube-within-a-tube interface. These devices appear to be less likely to leak at lower suction flow rates than some of the equipment offered earlier.

Several interfacing systems were considered unsuitable because of difficulty in monitoring the scavenging efficiency or because of leaky operation. The older Ohio and Foregger tube-within-a-tube interfaces (fig. 22) present both deficiencies unless rapid suction flow rates are provided.

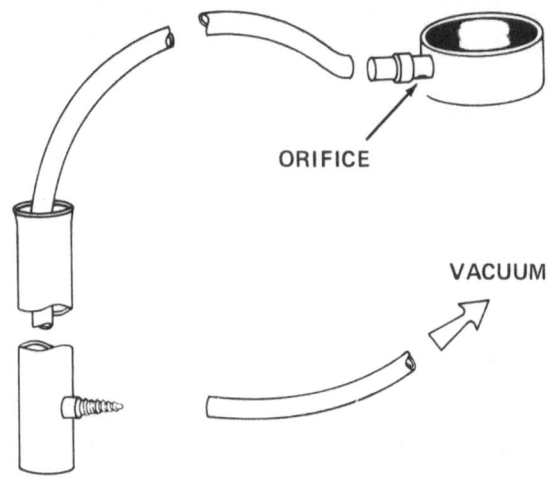

Fig. 22. Foregger tube-within-a-tube.

Tubing for the intraoperating room portion of waste gas disposal systems
The requirements for the tubing that connects the anesthetic breathing system to the disposal system vary according to the breathing system employed and to the scavenging components. The ideal tubing should be kinkproof, free of leaks, and capable of forming a gas-tight seal at any connection. In addition, it must be easy to assemble and disassemble without accidental disconnections. When long lengths are required, those portions exposed to occlusion should be nonresilient; however, the use of long lengths is considered an expediency until appropriate permanent connections are provided. The location of the high pressure gas supply hoses and the location of the disposal line are carefully planned. The first or primary length of tubing is attached to the anesthetic breathing system. For the T-tube and nonrebreathing systems, this primary length must be lightweight and flexible. Away from these breathing systems, a less resilient material is suitable. Industrial grade garden hose is essentially collapse-proof.

The bore of the tubing should be sufficient to avoid undue back pressure in the breathing system. A $\frac{7}{8}$ in. bore was chosen in these studies because of its availability and low resistance to breathing; however, $\frac{1}{2}$ in. bore is acceptable. The bore of the tubing that eventually will be employed in waste gas disposal systems should be noninterchangeable with any breathing system components. Further protection against misconnections is provided by color coding.

Flammable anesthetics
Flammable anesthetic agents, such as ether and cyclopropane, must be considered in waste gas disposal systems because the use of such agents continues in certain hospitals. When flammable mixtures are present in the breathing system they are also present in the disposal system in locations close to the site of gas overflow. Downstream, past the interfacing device, or at the air-conditioning exhaust, dilution occurs and flammability is reduced. The special duct system employed in the present studies carries the undiluted anesthetic gases outside, but other duct systems have been designed to entrain room air, thus diluting the mixture. Tubing containing high concentrations of flammable agents should be kept away from electrical connections and electronic monitoring equipment and be made of nonsparking materials. Diffusion of diluted flammable agents through plastic tubing is probably insignificant.

CONCLUSIONS

In disposing of waste gases it is reasonable to employ the simplest and least expensive methods of proven effectiveness which are compatible with all regulations, building, fire, and air pollution. With nonrecirculating air conditioning this is usually the air-conditioning exhaust. Otherwise the low velocity duct system could be considered, with the central vacuum system probably the most expensive and complex method.

ALTERNATIVES TO THE PROPOSED SCAVENGING TECHNIQUES

Thus far, the assumption has been made that inhalation anesthetics are to be used only with adequate scavenging.

In the absence of scavenging, totally closed system inhalation anesthesia reduces exposure, but most anesthetists prefer not to use this technique. In addition, few 'closed system' anesthetics are actually closed 100 percent of the time, and the semiclosed technique is employed, particularly at induction and recovery. Nevertheless, the use of the closed system could be encouraged for other reasons – economy and reduced pollution of the air outside the hospital. An additional factor is the availability of analyzers for O_2 and anaesthetic agents, resulting in increased safety of the patient. Regional anaesthesia theoretically obviates the need for waste gas control measures, but many patients prefer to be asleep.

It would be ideal if the waste gases could be absorbed at the breathing system, eliminating the need for complicated scavenging hoses and plumbing. Activated charcoal filters absorb halogenated anesthetics but not N_2O.

INITIATING A SCAVENGING PROGRAM

The following set of instructions should be of value to those who are interested in setting up a scavenging program.

1. Examine all anesthetizing locations such as operating rooms, delivery suites, X-ray, outpatient clinic, emergency room, psychiatry to determine local in-house differences in options available for scavenging. For example, in the operating room, the air-conditioning exhaust may be suitable for waste gas disposal because it is nonrecirculating; however, it may be unsuitable in X-ray because there it recirculates.

2. Consider disposal system alternatives and arrange for parts and installation:

    Air-conditioning exhaust: Assemble and install grille adapter; install duct work if gases are to be introduced downstream.

    Special duct system: duct work and fan (if required).

    Central vacuum system: Purchase and install interfacing device, flowmeter, and control valves.

3. Order scavenging popoff valve for circle breathing system. The gas-tight valves used in the present studies were:

    Ohio: Simple to adjust
    Dupaco: Impedance adjustable by adding weights
    Berner: Requires no critical adjustment of leak rate during assisted
                or controlled breathing
    Boehringer: Will be preferred by certain users
    Dameca: Inexpensive

4. Order scavenging nonrebreathing valve (if nonrebreathing is used).
5. Assemble scavenging collector device for T-tube (if T-tube used).
6. Select interfacing equipment if central vacuum system is used – Boehringer, Dupaco, Foregger – depending on preference.
7. Decide whether to convert existing ventilators for scavenging or to purchase new units. The least leaky ventilators in the present studies were:

Bennett:	Scavenging adapter is modified (fig. 13).
Ohio DO 300 and Monaghan:	Easily converted, using factory equipment made by Monaghan
Ohio Fluidic:	Provided with built-in scavenging equipment.

Ventimeter (Air Shields) – latest model only.
8. Plan for air monitoring, considered either purchasing or leasing the equipment or contracting with an extramural company or laboratory (see section on air monitoring).

EQUIPMENT MAINTENANCE

Equipment maintenance is a key factor in the prevention of anesthetic gas leaks and in the prompt correction of leaks that do occur. The objective is to secure low leak performance (defined as a maximum leak rate of 100 cc/min at a presure of 30 cm H_2O) for all anaesthesia machines. It must be emphasized that such performance requires rigid standards of preventive maintenance and servicing beyond that necessary for the administration of clinical anaesthesia.

The maintenance procedures presented are based on the findings of the studies on equipment leakage discussed in a previous section.

MAINTENANCE SCHEDULES AND LEAK TOLERANCES FOR ANAESTHESIA MACHINES & RELATED EQUIPMENT

1. Anaesthesia machines receive preventive maintenance at fourmonth (minimum) intervals by manufacturer's service representatives or by other qualified personnel. Following such maintenance, high pressure leakage should be the equivalent of less than 2 ppm N_2O in room air. The low pressure leak rate should be less than 50 cc/min at 30 cm H_2O.

2. The low pressure systems of the anaesthesia machines (from the flow-meters to the breathing tubes) are leak tested daily, preferably before each case. Leakage should be less than 100 cc/min at 30 cm H_2O.
3. Ventilators receive preventive maintenance at four-month (minimum) intervals by service representatives or other qualified personnel.
4. Breathing hoses attached to the anaesthesia machines are leak tested as part of the low pressure test. Breathing hoses associated with the T-tube, nonrebreathing system, and ventilators are tested at four-month intervals. All leaky hoses are replaced.
5. Breathing bags attached to the anaesthesia machines are leak tested when changed. Other breathing bags associated with the T-tube, non-breathing system, and ventilators are tested at four-month intervals.
6. Waste gas disposal tubing, if fragile, is leak tested at fourmonth intervals. Leaky tubing is replaced.
7. New equipment should be leak tested by the manufacturer before being placed in service. Minimum standards should be met.

AIR MONITORING IN THE OPERATING ROOM

Proof of the success of such waste gas control measures as scavenging, the cooperation of the anaesthetist, and equipment maintenance is based in the air-monitoring program.

In the present study, the gas of primary interest was the widely employed inhalation anaesthetic, N_2O. The technique for measuring trace concentrations of N_2O by infrared spectroscopy proved technically simple and reliable. In contrast, the halogenated anesthetics were less frequently used and, because the concentrations are relatively lower, a highly sensitive analyzer is required. Such infrared analyzers working at high gain are subject to electronic noise and drift. An additional difficult problem was interference from alcohols, employed in cleaning the operating room and in sterilizing the patient's skin for surgery. Other analytical methods were considered too expensive or cumbersome for routine use.

Samples for the monitoring studies were collected at the air-conditioning exhaust grille where the trace gas concentrations representative of personnel exposure were obtainable.

A gas is required for zero adjustment on the infrared analyzer. With non-recirculating air conditioning, room air obtained at a fresh air inlet of the air-conditioning system provides a suitable source. Clean air is ensured by inserting the sampling tubing well into the inlet duct. With recirculating air conditioning and with certain heat exchangers, the 'fresh' air entering the room may contain N_2O; if so, a convenient gas source is the central oxygen system. (Oxygen should not be taken from the anaesthesia machine because of possible contamination with N_2O.) A difference in the zero baseline due to contaminants was regularly observed between inlet air and pure O_2. If uncorrected, this would introduce an error in the N_2O concentrations equivalent to 1-2 ppm depending on the analyzer employed.

The frequency of air sampling is intended to reflect minute-to-minute changes in the average trace concentrations of inhalation anaesthetics, plus long-term exposure averages. Short-term changes were observed by continuously sampling and analyzing and were found to be closely related to the anaesthetist's activities. A small battery-powered analyzer detected abnormally high levels and immediately displayed the results of any corrective measures that were applied.

A monitoring technique, employing samples collected in syringes, was developed for evaluating long-term changes. Such changes were also determined by collecting samples in gas-tight bags, filled over a period of hours.

SAMPLES OBTAINED IN SYRINGES

The feasibility of analyzing room air samples obtained in syringes depended on the availability of a trace gas analyzer capable of responding to the relatively small samples (100 cc).

Two 50 cc glass syringes were rapidly filled with air obtained at the air-conditioning exhaust grille located in each operating room. Prior to analysis, these syringes were capped and then stored until all rooms had been sampled. Their contents were then injected into the infrared gas analyzer. The entire procedure for the 14-room suite was completed within 30 min.

The first group of samples was obtained before the arrival of the anaesthetists so as to determine the high pressure leakage of the gas machines. Subsequent samples were obtained to determine the concentrations of N_2O relating to the exposure of personnel during the workday and to search for low pressure leaks. To secure randomization, samples were collected at a different hour each day.

The results of early morning sampling are shown in figure 23. In 73 out of 137 samples, N_2O concentrations were 1.0 ppm or less. In five instances, the values were 25 ppm or above; one measurement (110 ppm) resulted when

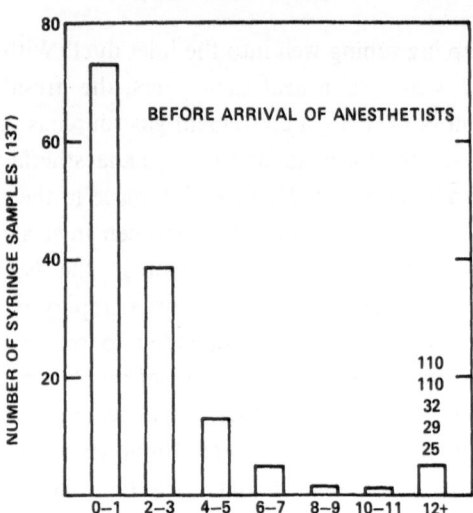

Fig. 23. Ranges of room air concentrations (ppm).

the N_2O flowmeter on the anaesthesia machine was accidently left on. Another elevated value was caused by a high pressure leak in a N_2O hose connection. The mean concentration was 4.1 ± 1.2 ppm ($\pm$ S.E.). All results were obtained using the fresh air zero reference.

The results obtained from 461 N_2O analyses of samples collected in syringes during a workday are presented in figure 24. 344 samples (74

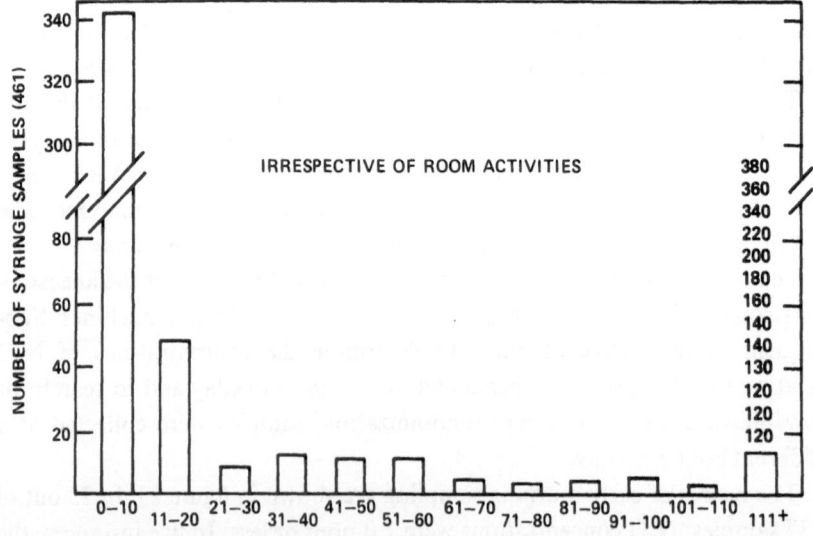

Fig. 24. Ranges of room air concentrations (ppm).

percent) contained N_2O in the range from 0 to 10 ppm, and 13 samples (2.7 percent) contained N_2O above 111 ppm. The mean concentration was 16 $\pm$ 1.9 ppm. This study included samples obtained during the intervals between cases plus those taken during the induction, maintenance, and recovery phases of anesthesia. Scavenging procedures were in effect, and the anaesthesia equipment, with the exception of a few ventilators, was relatively gas tight.

These results, during the administration of anaesthesia, were separated into groups, with a breakdown according to choice of the face mask, endotracheal tube, or ventilator technique (table 3). Separation of these groups is not statistically achieved although the average concentration of N_2O in the syringe samples appears to be minimum (15 ppm) when the endotracheal tube was used. When the face mask and endotracheal tube with ventilator were applied, the mean concentrations were approximately twice as high (36 and 34 ppm, respectively).

Figure 25 shows the distribution of room concentrations found in the

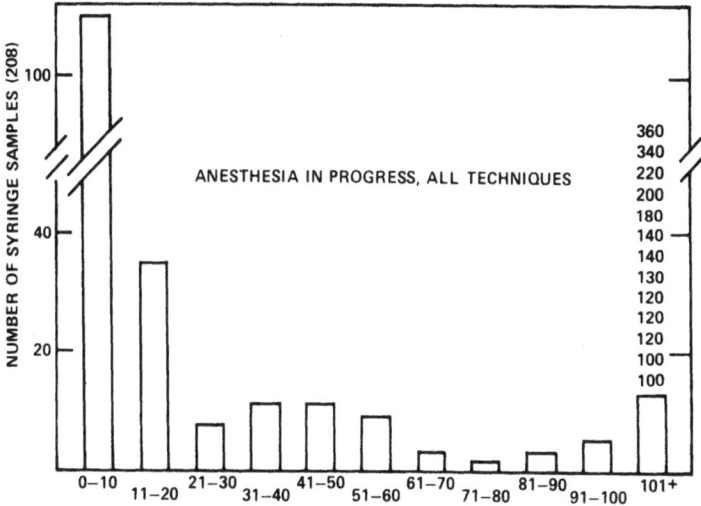

Fig. 25. Ranges of room air concentrations (ppm).

208 samples taken during the administration of N_2O. The anaesthetic technique is not considered. It can be seen that waste gases in the 0 to 10 ppm concentration range predominate, being observed in 110 of the 208 samples.

Figure 26 represents specific anaesthetic techniques including face mask, endotracheal tube, and endotracheal tube with ventilator. All demonstrate

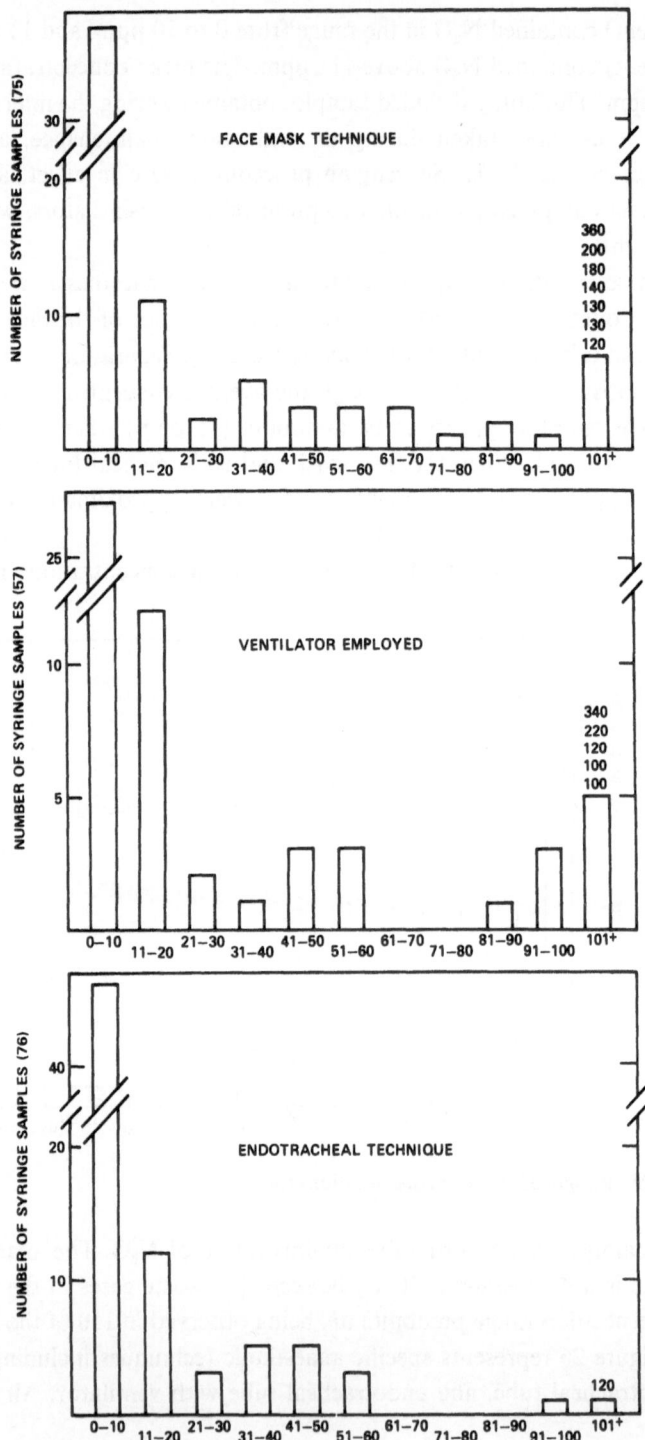

Fig. 26. Ranges of room air concentrations (ppm).

Table 3. Concentrations of N_2O in room air during anesthesia.

Anesthetic Technique	No. of Syringe Samples	Average Concentration of N_2O (ppm)
Mask	75	36 ± 6.7*
Endotracheal tube	76	15 ± 2.4
Endotracheal tube with ventilator	57	34 ± 7.8
All samples	208	28 ± 3.4

* ± S.E.

similar distribution patterns, and the 0 to 10 ppm range again predominates. A few samples containing 100 ppm N_2O and more are noteworthy. In samples obtained when the face mask was used (upper panel), six contained over 100 ppm because of leakage under the mask. When the ventilator was employed (center panel), values in five samples were 100 ppm or greater. These were probably the result of leaky ventilators. These data are inter-

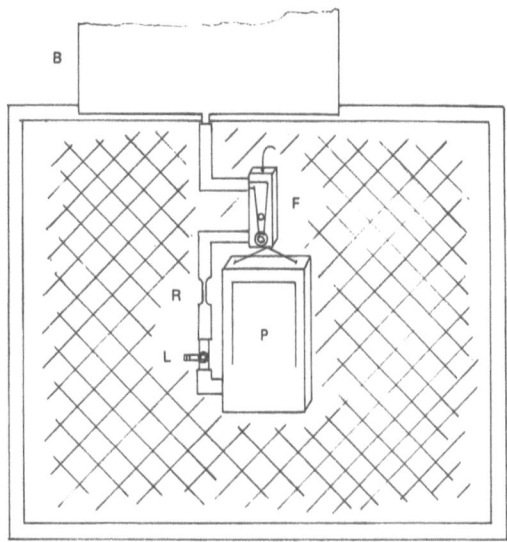

Fig. 27. Bag sampling equipment at exhaust grille.
Ba= gas-tight bag (44 L). F = flowmeter (20 to 200 cc/min).
R = resistance (27 gauge needle hub tightly fitted in tubbing).
L = aquarium bleed valve. Pr= aquarium pump.

preted to indicate the need for greater care in the use of the face mask and for nonleaking ventilators, rather than for increased use of the endotracheal tube.

SAMPLING IN BAGS

Gas-tight bags were filled at a constant rate over a period of several hours to obtain average data on long-term exposure to the inhalation anaesthetics. The collection system (fig. 27) consists of a modified hometype aquarium pump for filling the bags and a flowmeter for monitoring the filling rate. The aquarium pump was located at the exhaust grille of the air-conditioning system and at several other locations. The bag samples were analyzed for N_2O by infrared methods; halogenated anaesthetics were determined by gas chromatography. The operating rooms chosen for these studies were heavily scheduled for inhalation anaesthesia.

Analysis of the samples obtained included normalization to predict the concentrations of gases that would have been present in the bag had the anaesthetic agents been administered over the entire collection period. Nitrous oxide calculations rarely required such correction because it was usually administered throughout the case. The exception occurred during local anaesthesia. In contrast, halothane was less frequently used. As an example of the normalization procedure, when halothane was detected in a bag, the duration of administration was first determined by inspection of the anaesthesia record. If halothane had been administered during 50 percent of the total sampling period, the normalized value would be twice the value actually measured. Such normalization indicated the room concentration, if halothane had been administered throughout the sampling period, and corrected the bias related to the lower incidence of halothane anaesthesia.

The following results were obtained from the samples collected.

	No of bag samples	Measured concentration (ppm)	Normalized concentration (ppm)
Nitrous oxide	48	19 ± 3.0	28 ± 4.5
Halothane	27	0.24 ± 0.05	0.45 ± 0.11

The concentrations of N_2O measured in the bags represent actual exposure levels and are comparable to the 467 syringe samples. The average for these syringes samples was 16 ppm which is lower than the 19 ppm determined for the bag samples. The reason for this difference may be the limited number of samples; however, the bags were placed deliberately in heavily scheduled rooms, whereas the syringes were filled in succession without regard for the activities within the rooms.

The distributions of these bag samples are illustrated in fig. 28 for N_2O (top panel) and for halothane (lower panel). Similar to the samples in

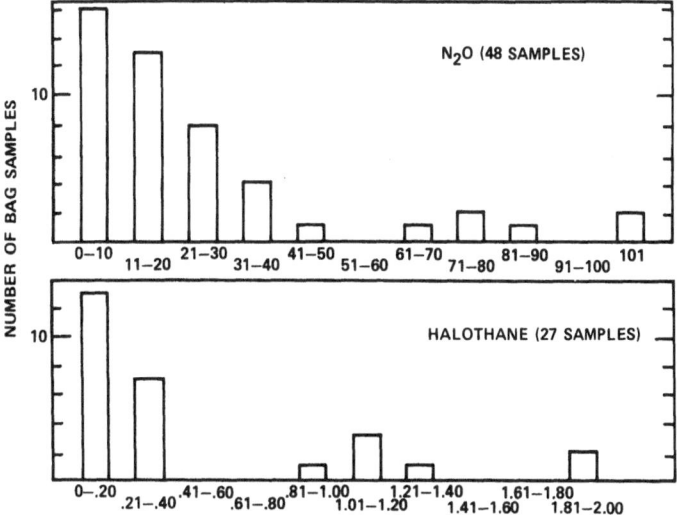

Fig. 28. Ranges of Room air concentrations (ppm).

syringes, predominating concentrations are found at the lower ranges, 0 to 20 ppm for N_2O any 0 to 0.40 ppm for halothane.

The normalization procedure allows the bag samples to be compared to the syringe samples collected during the administration of anaesthesia. Correlations in the average values of N_2O obtained by the two methods were 28 ± 4.5 and 28 ± 3.4 ppm for the bag and syringe samples, respectively.

These values for N_2O (28 ppm) determined from the samples collected both in syringes and in bags (normalized) and for halothane collected in bags (normalized to 0.45 ppm) lead to the suggested maximum concentrations, 30 ppm for N_2O and 0.5 ppm for halothane. These equal 0.005 percent of the administered concentrations of 60 percent N_2O and 1.0 percent halothane and provide a 'rule of thumb' for estimating reasonable concentrations of other inhalation agents.

It is reiterated that, during the present studies, not all reasonable precautions were taken to minimize trace gas concentrations. Leaky ventilators had not been replaced, equipment maintenance procedures were not fully refined, and personnel did not always connect the scavenging equipment or secure the best possible mask fit. With the support of the anesthetists, lower concentrations in the range of 5 to 10 ppm N_2O and 0.1 to 0.2 ppm halothane were and can be regularly achieved.

SAMPLES OBTAINED IN PROXIMITY TO PERSONNEL

Up to this point, the air monitoring methods presented in this report have been based on the average room concentration of N_2O sampled at the air-conditioning exhaust grille. This procedure was considered to represent personnel exposure because of the essentially uniform distribution of the leakage gases in the particular rooms studied. Nevertheless, the question remained whether, because of his proximity to the leak source, the anaesthetist might inhale higher concentrations of N_2O than the room air average. As a result, the present study was designed to compare various sampling sites including operating room personnel during the performance of their normal duties.

The sampling sites included the air-conditioning exhaust grille at its center; an area near the center hinge of the door of the operating room, and selected personnel (the anaesthetist, surgeon, and the circulating and scrub nurses). The sampling site for these personnel was an area immediately posterior to the back of the neck, a location chosen for its accessibility during surgery and its proximity to the air actually inhaled while avoiding the exhaled CO_2 which interferes with the IR analysis. The analytical instrument was a small battery-powered continuously sampling infrared trace gas analyzer with interferance filtering at a wavelength of 4.48 μ and a calibrated range of 1 to 200 ppm N_2O. This instrument was hand-carried into the operating rooms, and the sampling probe was first held at the air-conditioning exhaust grille. After equilibration (10 to 30 sec), the personnel were sampled, then the door, and finally a repeated measurement was taken at the grille. Following these measurements, the instrument was carried to the next room. In this manner, all available rooms were sampled in sequence with more than one set of samples obtained in each room.

A total of 334 samples resulted, comprised of 54 sets of 7 samples each, except that in 44 instances a sampling site was omitted because of inaccessibility. These data were obtained by a single technician in 2.5 working days at approximately 4 hours per day. In reducing these data, four sets were discarded because the analyzer was overloaded by concentrations exceeding 100 ppm N_2O. The instrument range was then extended to 200 ppm to include the succeeding higher concentrations. Nineteen additional data sets were deleted because of a difference between grille measurements indicating nonsteady state conditions ($> \pm 20$ percent at concentrations greater than 10 ppm and $> \pm 2$ ppm at concentrations below 10 ppm).* The results below comprise the 202 remaining samples including 60 at the grille sites, and 142 near the personnel.

Sampling Site	Grille	Anes-thetist	Surgeon	Nurses Scrub	Nurses Circu-lating	Door	Grille
N_2O (ppm) $\pm$ S.E.)	15 ± 2.7	18 ± 2.9	17 ± 5.0	13 ± 3.2	14 ± 2.8	14 ± 2.8	14 ± 2.8

These results reveal little or no significant differences among the various sampling sites employed. Area monitoring at the grille or at the door appears to be representative of personnel exposure under the conditions prevailing in the present operating suite. In fact, sampling could be accomplished through a small hole in the door, thus avoiding the inconveniences of entering the room. Other operating suites interested in establishing representative sampling sites could easily complete the necessary studies, given the speed and the convenience of the portable trace gas analyzer. The lower mean N_2O values reported above as compared to the concentrations reported in the gas-tight bag and syringe samples, 15 ppm versus 28 ppm, are explained by the recent results of the present study and the anticipated effect of an increased experience with the waste gas control measures.

CONTINUOUS MONITORING

Specific operating rooms were selected for continuous monitoring of N_2O. The instrumentation was the portable infrared monitoring unit.

Initial experience indicated that the members of the operating room team were very interested in the ambient trace gas concentrations and in the rapid changes noted during anaesthesia. This was particularly true of

* These criteria seemed reasonable upon inspecting the data.

the anaesthetist who could immediately observe the effects of his clinical techniques on trace gas concentrations and could modify them to achieve a further reduction in gas leakage.

Inspection of the continuous recordings indicated that N_2O in the air could be maintained below 5 ppm throughout the period of anaesthesia, both with mask and endotracheal tube; however, any momentary disconnection of the breathing system produced transient elevations. A chronic leak was reflected promptly in sustained elevated concentrations. Many of the observed elevations could not be explained by the anaesthetist's techniques. Disconnections in the disposal system or leaks in the high pressure hose connections occasionally were responsible. Following correction of the problem, a reduction in the air concentrations of N_2O rapidly (within 30 min) become apparent. If such reduction did not occur, the leaks were located through more careful search.

When moving the monitoring station about the surgical suite, many unexpected events were encountered. The following are examples of such occurrences.

1. A hot spot, with N_2O at 100 ppm, was found in a hallway, leading to the discovery of a leaky connection in the room control valve system that probably was present since its original installation.
2. On entering the operating room during the early morning rounds, high concentrations were discovered because flowmeters were left on overnight.
3. A cylinder with a leaky valve was found to be flooding the storeroom with N_2O.
4. A machine developed a high pressure leak during an operation, and the roomair concentration of N_2O increased to above 120 ppm.
5. An accidental dislodgement of an endotracheal tube during a cleft palate repair was suspected as the cause of a sudden increase in N_2O concentration.

The mobile N_2O monitoring unit is considered a valuable tool. It not only identifies leaks in the equipment, but it can inform the anaesthesia staff on the impact of their techniques and provide a method for immediately observing the results of their improved or modified work practices.

DISCUSSION

The air monitoring program should be executed by an interested and qualified person, preferably an anaesthetist, nurse, technician, or environmental engineer. A major factor in determining the type of personnel is whether the hospital chooses to operate its own monitoring program or to depend on an outside contractor.

Ideally, the gases to be monitored include all inhalation agents employed in an operating suite. Meeting such a standard may be difficult, and a decision to monitor only selected agents could depend on the frequency of their use, availability of an appropriate analytical method, and cost of instrumentation.

Nitrous oxide is the most important anaesthetic in a monitoring program because it is the most widely administered. It is easily monitored and is found in many components of the anaesthesia equipment. Because, in the anaesthesia machine, many parts are subject only to leakage of N_2O and because more suitable analyzers are available for monitoring N_2O than for halothane, assessment of N_2O leakage alone is often sufficient. The components subject solely to leakage of halothane are few and largely confined to the 'copper kettle' type of vaporizers and associated plumbing. Because these vaporization parts are localized to a small area and can be leak tested and serviced easily, the need for their monitoring is reduced.

Despite the above considerations, a case can be made for monitoring halothane and other agents such as enflurane, ether, and cyclopropane in operating suites frequently using these agents. During the present studies, it was found that solo leakage of halothane regularly occurs when the vaporizers are filled; furthermore, leakage of halothane did not always occur in the same proportions as delivered with N_2O, indicating independent leakage rates of the two agents. At present, the only generally available proven program for monitoring gases other than N_2O is the collection of samples for analysis in an outside laboratory.

Air samples for the monitoring program may be obtained from a location close to the inspired air of one or more persons in the operating room (personnel sampling) or from other sites in the general area occupied by personnel (area samp.ing). Personnel sampling is usually considered the preferable method (15) but experience with monitoring in the operating room during the present studies indicates that scrubbed personnel may be disturbed by the risk of accidental contact with the sampling equipment. For this reason it is best if possible to rely on area sampling. This requires the establishment of a reasonable correlation between area and personnel samples, a test which is easily accomplished with the portable, battery powered N_2O analyzer. If such tests are not feasible it may be reasonable to sample in close proximity to a single person, such as the anaesthetist, or a single area in the exhaust stream of the air-conditioning system such as the grille.

Area sampling is convenient, inexpensive, and easily accomplished. The methods include 1. measurement of multiple samples or 2. continuous monitoring by means of the infrared analyzers or sampling pumps and gas-tight bags. Either method can yield time-weighted exposure patterns. Battery-powered pumps are the most suitable for personnel monitoring because the movements of the staff in the operating room are not restricted. The cost is high, however, in comparison to aquarium pumps.

Aquarium pumps are suitable for area monitoring when equipped with a bleed valve, resistance, and a flowmeter. Their usefulness can be extended by the addition of a sampling probe. This modification can be made simply by sealing the case from room air except for a length of sampling tubing which opens into the case. Some models are so small, lightweight, and quiet that they can be easily carried by personnel.

Regardless of the type of pump employed, means must be provided for the temporary storage of samples. The minute capillary tubes filled with activated charcoal are convenient for the storage of halogenated anaesthetics; unfortunately, however, they cannot store N_2O, and bags must be employed. The size of the bag is determined by the requirements of the analyzer; certain IR units with a cell volume of 5 L require a sample larger than 15 L. A careful technique and a tactful approach are important factors in attaching the larger bags in such a way that movements will not be restricted, thereby minimizing objections of personnel to such paraphernalia.

The significance of the time period over which an air sample is obtained should be emphasized. Unless the air is thoroughly mixed, an air sample from a single rapidly filled syringe may be unrepresentative. Uneven data can be smoothed out if a number of samples are averaged. Gas-tight bags filled at a constant rate over a period of hours could produce the most representative averages.

Analyzers suitable for N_2O monitoring are available (table 4) as well as instruments capable of measuring trace concentrations of the halogenated anaesthetics, ether and cyclopropane. Halothane analysis is less satisfactory than N_2O analysis in the operating room because of interfering substances such as alcohols, freons, and halogenated cleaning solutions. Solid-state ionizing halogen leak detectors adapted for continuous monitoring are under development, and a preliminary evaluation of a prototype model is promising in that it revealed minimal sensitivity to interfering substances. Other problems, particularly zero drift, are being investigated by the manufacturer.

Table 4. Methods and equipment for trace N_2O analysis in the operating room.

	Special advantages	Disadvantages
A. Samples mailed to an outside laboratory:		
1. Boehringer Laboratories $ 28.50 to $ 36.50 per analysis depending on number.*	Complete equipment is available for all types of air sampling. All gases and vapors are reported.	Delay in reporting of results reduces chances of correlating reported N_2O to circumstances at time of sampling. Duration and site of sampling must be carefully planned to relate to personnel exposure.
2. Summit Services. $ 20 to $ 22.50 per analysis depending on the number.*	Includes all equipment for time-weighted N_2O measurements.	Delay in reporting of results is as above.
B. Samples analyzed on the premises:		
1. Foregger Model 410 N_2O Monitor. Ranges 0-100 & 0-1000 ppm $ 2.500.*	Low cell volume (58 cc) requires small samples (200 cc). Fast response in leak detection mode, a superior leak detector. Linear output facilitates time weighted sampling (accessory equipment needed).	Optical filters for agents other than N_2O are not presently available. A relatively expwnsive inverter is required for mobile operation.
2. Ohio Trace Gas Analyzer for N_2O. Ranges 0-25 and 0-.250 ppm $ 2.900.*	Filters and path length can be changed (difficult), providing the capability of measuring various gases and concentration ranges. Operates mobile via inexpensive battery/inverter.	Cell volume (2.25 L) requires large (7 L) sample and slows response for leak detection.
3. Wilks Miran 101 Gas Analyser for N_2O. Ranges as for Ohio $ 2200*.	Self contained and battery powered. Otherwise similar to the Ohio.	Similar to the Ohio
4. Wilks Miran IA Gas Analyzer with variable 20 m sampling cell and variable filters. $ 5.000.*	Designed for rapid conversion to measure a wide variety of gases and concentrations. Available accessories extend versatility. Will operate on battery/inverter.	Bulky in comparison to the above analyzers which were designed for operating room use.

* Prices quoted October 15, 1975.

The advantages of a monitoring program that makes use of a continuously measuring gas analyzer should be considered. The program in operation at Stanford University Hospital includes area monitoring during anaesthesia at one-week intervals and the measurement of early morning samples (before the arrival of the anaesthetists) at one-week intervals. The advantages of this method include the development of the desired record of trace gas concentrations and the resultant incidental but ongoing public-relations program to encourage cleaner techniques. In rooms selected for continuous monitoring, the anaesthetist can appreciate the responsiveness of the room air concentrations of N_2O to the usual changes in leakage rates resulting from his techniques. An additional use of the continuous monitor is the analysis of bag samples obtained from peripheral anaesthetizing locations.

WASTE ANAESTHETIC GAS MANAGEMENT IN THE DENTIST'S TREATMENT ROOM

This chapter although primarily concerned with waste gas management in the hospital would be remiss in not mentioning the extensive and severe occupational exposure to N_2O which occurs in the dentist's treatment room. Concentrations are frequently observed in the thousands of ppm and the dentist is not only the original user of N_2O but also is said to be the largest consumer of this gas at the present time.

Waste gas scavenging in the dentist's treatment room presents a unique set of problems. The nasal mask is frequently fitted very loosely to the face; the patient's mouth must be open; air conditioning if present at all is usually recirculating at low flow rates. These factors tend toward high levels of occupational exposure which may exceed 10,000 ppm N_2O. Preliminary studies indicate that a specially designed double nasal mask (fig. 29) developed by Summit Services) with suction between the two major componnnts can reduce inhaled N_2O concentrations to levels comparable to those considered reasonably achievable in the operating room. The use of this mask preserves the dentist's customary practices. Gas disposal must be via the central vacuum system which is vented to the outside. A complete report on waste gas control in the dentist's operatory is presently being drafted, as the Final Report for Research Contract No. CDC 210-75-0007, National Institute for Occupational Safety and Health.

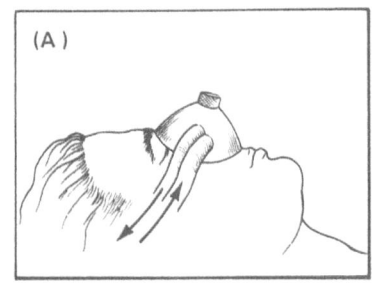

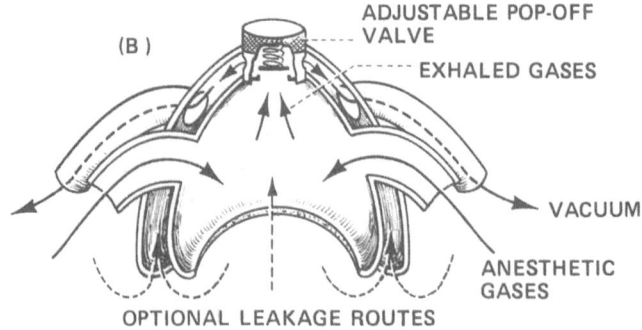

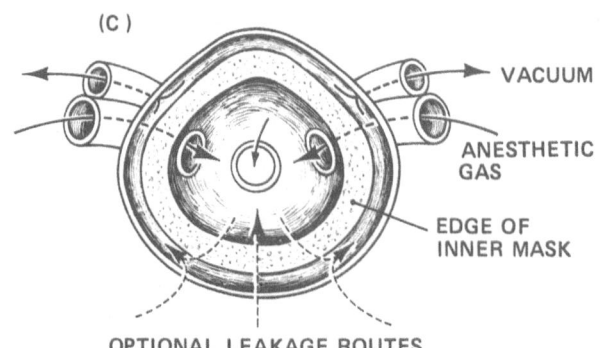

Fig. 29. Double suction nasal mask.

ACKNOWLEDGEMENTS

Equipment for leak detection and measurements of trace concentrations of inhalation anaesthetics present in the operating room air was loaned by the General Electric Company; Inficon, Incorporated; Sensors, Incorporated; and Wilks Scientific Corporation.

The engineering expertise of Mr. A. Reid Chappell and Mr. Charles Drace of the Stanford University Hospital Department of Engineering and Mr. Glenn Brown of Summit Services, Los Gatos, California, is acknowledged as is the consultation on gas analysis provided by Dr. James Trudell of Stanford University. The participation of graduate students at Stanford University is appreciated, including Mr. James Eastwood, Mr. Donald Harter, and Mr. Thomas Yackle. The technical assistance of Mrs. Jeanne Daney and Mr. Daniel Chin is acknowledged.

Funding for the work leading to this chapter was provided by the National Institute for Occupational Safety and Health, U.S. Department of Health, Education, and Welfare, pursuant to Contract Numbers HSM 99-73-73 and CDC 210-75-0007.

Mechanical engineers from Stanford University sharing in the receipt of these research contracts and actively collaborating in all phases of the development of measures for reducing occupational exposure to inhalation anaesthetics include: Robert L. Piziali, Ph. D., Assistant Professor, Robert J. Moffat, Ph.D., Professor, Rudolph Sher, Ph.D., Professor.

REFERENCES

1. Whitcher, C., R. Piziali, R. Sher, R. Moffat, *Development and Evaluation of Methods for the Elimination of Waste Anesthetic Gases and Vapors in Hospitals.* National Institute for Occupational Safety and Health, May 1975. HEW Publication No. (NIOSH) 75-137, Superintendent of Documents, U.S. Government Printing Office, Washington, D. C., 20402.
2. Vaisman, A. I., Working Conditions in Surgery and Their Effect on the Health of Anesthesiologists: *Eksp Khir Anesteziol* 3: 44-49 (1967).
3. Cohen, E. N., B. W. Brown, D. L. Bruce, H. F. Cascorbi, T. H. Corbett, T. W. Jones and C. Whitcher, Occupational Disease Among Operating Room Personnel: A National Study. Report of an Ad Hoc Committee on the Effects of Trace Anesthetic Agents on the Health of Operating Room Personnel, American Society of Anesthesiologists. *Anesthesiology* 41: 321-340 (1974).
4. Cohen, E. N., B. W. Brown, D. L. Bruce, H. F. Cascorbi, T. H. Corbett, T. W. Jones and C. Whitcher, A Survey of Anesthetic Health Hazards Among Dentists: Report of an Ad Hoc Committee on the Effects of Trace Anesthetic Agents on the Health of Operating Room Personnel, American Society of Anesthesiologists. *J. Am. Dental Assoc.* 90: 1291-1296 (1975).

5. Fink, B. R., Editor. *Toxicity of Anesthetics*. Baltimore, The Williams and Wilkins Company, 1968. Part Four, Teratogenic Effects. pp. 259-323.

6. Corbett, T. H., R. G. Cornell, J. L. Endres, R. I. Millard, Effects of low concentrations of nitrous oxide on rat pregnancy. *Anesthesiology* 39: 299-301 (1973).

7. Stevens, W. C., E. I. Eger, II, A. White, M. J. Halsey, W. Munger, R. D. Gibbons, W. Dolan and R. Shargel, Comparative Toxicities of Halothane, Isoflurane, and Diethyl Ether at Subanesthetic Concentrations in Laboratory Animals. *Anesthesiology* 42: 408-419 (1975).

8. Chang, L. W., A. W. Dudley Jr., J. Katz and A. H. Martin, Nervous System Development Following In Utero Exposure to Trace Amounts of Halothane. *Teratology* 9: 15 (1974).

9. Quimby, K. L., J. Katz, L. J. Aschkenase and R. E. Bowman, Behavioral Consequences in Rats from Chronic Exposure to 10 ppm Halothane During Early Development. *Anesthesia and Analgesia* 54: 628-633 (1975).

10. Bruce, D. L., M. J. Bach and J. Arbit, Trace Anesthetic Effects on Perceptual, Cognitive, and Motor Skills. *Anesthesiology* 40: 453-458 (1974).

11. Bruce, D. L. and M. J. Bach, Laboratory report: Psychological Studies of Human Performance as Effected by Traces of Enflurane and Nitrous Oxide. *Anesthesiology* 42: 194-196 (1975).

12. Corbett, T. H., Anesthetics as a Cause of Abortion. *Fertility and Sterility* 23: 866-869 (1972).

13. ASHRAE Handbook and Product Directory. Published by the American Society of Heating, Refrigerating and Air-Conditioning Engineers, Inc., 345 East 47th Street, New York, N.Y. 10017. p. 7.8, Chapter 7, 1974 Applications Handbook.

14. National Fire Codes, Volume 2. Gases. 1973-74. National Fire Protection Association, 470 Atlantic Avenue, Boston, Massachusetts 02210. p. 65A-47 (fans); p. 56A-73 (suction) and other sections.

15. *Evaluation of Ambient Air Quality by Personnel Monitoring*. A. L. Lynch. CRC Press, Cleveland, Ohio (1974).

29. CONCLUSION AND RECOMMENDATIONS

JOH. SPIERDIJK

Finally we want to go back to the questions that we have mentioned in the introduction.

1. Are there good scavenging systems available which satisfy two requirements:
a. No danger to the patient,
b. Simple to regulate?
Safe methods for scavenging anaesthetic gases are available. Although the influence of chronic exposure to anaesthetic gases has not yet been sufficiently investigated, we think that scavenging should be recommended.

Before installing a system the effect on the patient as well as on the concentration of the gases should be considered.

2. What steps should personnel be advised to take in the absence of scavenging systems, particularly women who are or wish to become pregnant.
This question is still difficult to answer. The effects of exposure to anaesthetic gases on the incidence of abortion and congenital malformation is still unclear and has to be further investigated. As mentioned before, we believe that as long as certain working rules are adhered to, such as a 5 day working week, coffee, tea and lunch breaks, a pregnant employee need not fear working in these operating theatres.

We would advise against permitting pregnant personnel to assist in dental anaesthesia and in tonsillectomies.

We further wish to point out that in most instances total removal of anaesthetic gases is impossible.

Should there be a nurse or a female anaesthetist who wishes to have children and with a history of one or more abortions during the period in which she has worked in an operating theatre, or with a child who already has a congenital malformation, our advise would be for her to change her environment.

If a pregnant woman is worried about working in a poorly air conditioned

operating room we should consider employing her in a different department where no anaesthetic gases and less stress are present.

3. Is it necessary to perform further studies on the chronic toxicity of
anaesthetic gases?

Until now little is known about chronic toxicity. What is known is mostly
derived from retrospective studies. Future prospective studies and animal
experiments are necessary to point out whether chronic toxicity exists and
to what extent. The influence of other factors like stress and workload should
also be investigated.

4. Is further analysis of the work and performance of the anaesthetist
necessary?

The answer to this question is very similar to the answer to the previous
question. The effect of low doses of anaesthetics on work performance has
not been investigated extensively. Further studies in this field are necessary.

5. Should there be international approved standards?
     Is it therefore necessary to issue recommandations for
a. health authorities
b. hospital designers.

In several countries the health authorities have given instructions or re-
commendations on operating room environment. In Holland as yet there
are no rules on this subject. We think it is important that good cooperation
should exist between the people directly involved (people working in
operating rooms), the health authorities, hospital management and hospital
designers, because this will be the only way to achieve a common agreement
and direction in dealing with the problem. The introduction of international
approved standards is necessary.

INDEX